Pathophysiology of Kidney Disease and Hypertension

A. Vishnu Moorthy, MD
Professor
Department of Medicine
University of Wisconsin School of Medicine
and Public Health
Madison, Wisconsin

Associate Editors:

Bryan N. Becker, MD
Professor
Department of Medicine
University of Wisconsin School of Medicine
and Public Health
Madison, Wisconsin

Frederick J. Boehm III, MD
Postdoctoral Senior Fellow
Department of Biostatistics
University of Washington
Seattle, Washington

Arjang Djamali, MD, MS, FASN
Assistant Professor
Department of Medicine
University of Wisconsin School of Medicine
and Public Health
Madison, Wisconsin

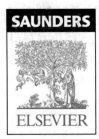

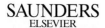
SAUNDERS
ELSEVIER

1600 John F. Kennedy Blvd.
Ste 1800
Philadelphia, PA 19103-2899

PATHOPHYSIOLOGY OF KIDNEY DISEASE AND HYPERTENSION   ISBN: 978-1-4160-4391-1

Notice

Knowledge and best practice in this field are constantly changing. As new research and experience broaden our knowledge, changes in practice, treatment, and drug therapy may become necessary or appropriate. Readers are advised to check the most current information provided (i) on procedures featured or (ii) by the manufacturer of each product to be administered, to verify the recommended dose or formula, the method and duration of administration, and contraindications. It is the responsibility of the practitioner, relying on their own experience and knowledge of the patient, to make diagnoses, to determine dosages and the best treatment for each individual patient, and to take all appropriate safety precautions. To the fullest extent of the law, neither the Publisher nor the Editors assume any liability for any injury and/or damage to persons or property arising out of or related to any use of the material contained in this book.

The Publisher

Library of Congress Cataloging-in-Publication Data
Pathophysiology of kidney disease and hypertension / [edited by] A. Vishnu Moorthy ; associate editors, Bryan N. Becker, Frederick J. Boehm III, Arjang Djamali.—1st ed.
  p. ; cm.
  Includes bibliographical references.
ISBN 978-1-4160-4391-1
1. Kidneys—Pathophysiology. 2. Renal hypertension. I. Moorthy, A. Vishnu.
  [DNLM: 1. Kidney Diseases—physiopathology. 2. Kidney Diseases—therapy. 3. Acid-Base Imbalance. 4. Hypertension, Renal. 5. Renal Replacement Therapy. 6. Water-Electrolyte Imbalance. WJ 300 P2977 2009]
  RC903.9.P366 2009
  616.6′107—dc22

                                                                    2008021065

Acquisitions Editor: William Schmitt
Developmental Editor: Andrea Vosburgh
Project Manager: David Saltzberg
Design Direction: Louis Forgione

Printed in China
Last digit is the print number: 9   8   7   6   5   4   3   2   1

DEDICATION

"I want to beg you, as much as I can, dear sir, to be patient toward all that is unsolved in your heart and to try to love the questions themselves."
Rainer Maria Rilke, Letters to a Young Poet.

This work is dedicated to all students and teachers of the health sciences—past, present, and future. May you continue to enjoy the questions.

Contributors

Bryan N. Becker, MD
Professor
Department of Medicine
University of Wisconsin School of Medicine and
Public Health
Madison, Wisconsin

Yolanda T. Becker, MD
Associate Professor
Department of Surgery
University of Wisconsin School of Medicine
and Public Health
Madison, Wisconsin

Tracy C. Blichfeldt, MD
Resident
Department of Medicine
Gundersen Lutheran Medical Foundation
La Crosse, Wisconsin

Frederick J. Boehm III, MD
Postdoctoral Senior Fellow
Department of Biostatistics
University of Washington
Seattle, Washington

Peter C. Brazy, MD
Emeritus Professor of Medicine
Department of Medicine
University of Wisconsin School of Medicine
and Public Health
Madison, Wisconsin

Arjang Djamali, MD, MS, FASN
Assistant Professor
Department of Medicine
University of Wisconsin School of Medicine
and Public Health
Madison, Wisconsin

Theodore L. Goodfriend, MD
Emeritus Professor
Departments of Medicine and Pharmacology
University of Wisconsin School of Medicine
and Public Health;
Associate Chief of Staff for Research
William S. Middleton Memorial Veterans Hospital
Madison, Wisconsin

Claire Elliott Herrick, MD
Resident
Department of Obstetrics, Gynecology,
and Reproductive Sciences
University of California, San Francisco
San Francisco, California

Jonathan B. Jaffery, MD
Assistant Professor
Department of Medicine
University of Wisconsin School of Medicine
and Public Health
Madison, Wisconsin

Paul S. Kellerman, MD, FACP
Associate Professor
Department of Medicine
University of Wisconsin School of Medicine
and Public Health
Madison, Wisconsin;
Medical Director
Wisconsin Dialysis, Inc.
Fitchburg, Wisconsin

Ryan Kipp, MD
Resident
Department of Medicine
University of Wisconsin School of Medicine
and Public Health
Madison, Wisconsin

Joshua David Lindsey, MD
Resident
Department of Orthopaedics
University of Washington Affiliated Hospitals
Seattle, Washington

Kristin M. Lyerly, MD
Master of Public Health Student
Department of Population Health Sciences
University of Wisconsin School of Medicine
and Public Health
Madison, Wisconsin

A. Vishnu Moorthy, MD
Professor
Department of Medicine
University of Wisconsin School of Medicine
and Public Health
Madison, Wisconsin

Terry D. Oberley, MD, PhD
Professor and Vice Chairman
Department of Pathology and Laboratory Medicine
University of Wisconsin School of Medicine
and Public Health;
Chief, Electron Microscopy
Pathology and Laboratory Medicine Service
William S. Middleton Veterans Administration
Hospital
Madison, Wisconsin

Byram H. Ozer, BA
MD/PhD Candidate
Department of Biomolecular Chemistry
Medical Scientist Training Program
University of Wisconsin School of Medicine
and Public Health
Madison, Wisconsin

Milagros D. Samaniego, MD
Associate Professor
Department of Medicine
University of Wisconsin School of Medicine
and Public Health
Madison, Wisconsin

Kelly Ann Traeger, MD
Resident
Department of Anesthesiology
Froedtert Hospital
Milwaukee, Wisconsin

Sung-Feng Wen, MD
Emeritus Professor
Department of Medicine
University of Wisconsin School of Medicine
and Public Health
Madison, Wisconsin

Weixiong Zhong, MD, PhD
Assistant Professor
Department of Pathology and Laboratory Medicine
University of Wisconsin School of Medicine
and Public Health;
Staff Pathologist
Pathology and Laboratory Medicine Service
William S. Middleton Memorial Veterans Hospital
Madison, Wisconsin

Preface

The goal of this project was to produce a text appropriate for an introductory study of the pathophysiology of kidney diseases and hypertension for health professional students and medical students in particular. In many medical schools, including the University of Wisconsin School of Medicine and Public Health, students study kidney pathophysiology during their pre-clinical years. When the University of Wisconsin student authors, many of whom are now resident physicians, began working on the text, they had recently completed the kidney disease and hypertension pathophysiology course offered during their second year of medical school. They knew the course's strengths and weaknesses and believed that they could make a difference in improving its impact and ability to deliver comprehensive, understandable information about kidney and hypertensive diseases to students who were not yet overly familiar with the clinical environment. The University of Wisconsin students had studied other texts that had resulted from student–faculty collaborations, and they believed that their final, much-needed product would fill a vacancy in the medical school curriculum. Their interest, perseverance, and determination resulted in

a unique experience for the student and faculty authors in learning how to work together across knowledge and experiential gaps and still produce a product worthy of use in any basic student course addressing pathophysiology of kidney disorders and hypertension.

The need for the text was apparent to all the contributors. Although the practicing nephrologist could find comprehensive and recently published books, review articles, and even outstanding online resources, an up-to-date and accessible text targeted at health professional students was unavailable. We hope that this text fulfills its purpose of introducing the pathophysiology of kidney diseases and hypertension to health professional students and piques their interest and curiosity. Finally, we hope that health professional students, regardless of their discipline, will find the text enlightening, enjoyable, and worthwhile.

A. Vishnu Moorthy, MD
Bryan N. Becker, MD
Frederick J. Boehm III, MD
Arjang Djamali, MD, MS, FASN

Acknowledgments

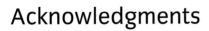

We would like to acknowledge the administrators and support staff in the Section of Nephrology, the Department of Medicine, and the school infrastructure at the University of Wisconsin School of Medicine and Public Health. We have been fortunate to have their support for this project from its infancy. Furthermore, we would like to thank our students and teachers, who continue to inspire us and to enrich our lives.

Special thanks go to Theodore L. Goodfriend, MD, and Sung-Feng Wen, MD, who spent numerous hours reading and commenting on many chapters in this text other than the ones they contributed to themselves.

We would also like to expressly thank Bill Schmitt and Andrea Vosburgh of Elsevier. They guided us through the production process and continuously offered advice, support, and encouragement. Their leadership in this project has been a key to its success.

Last, but certainly not least, we wish to thank our families for their support and patience while we wrote and edited this text.

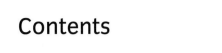

Contents

Preface   vii

Acknowledgments   ix

1. **Anatomy and Physiology of the Kidney**   1
   A. Vishnu Moorthy and Tracy C. Blichfeldt

2. **Body Fluid Compartments and Their Regulation**   17
   Byram H. Ozer and Peter C. Brazy

3. **Disorders of Water Metabolism**   29
   Ryan Kipp and Peter C. Brazy

4. **Disorders of Sodium Metabolism**   41
   Claire Elliott Herrick, Jonathan B. Jaffery, and Arjang Djamali

5. **Pathophysiology of Potassium Metabolism**   49
   Kelly Ann Traeger and Sung-Feng Wen

6. **Acid–Base Homeostasis and Metabolic Alkalosis**   63
   Kelly Ann Traeger, Frederick J. Boehm III, and Arjang Djamali

7. **Metabolic Acidosis and Approach to Acid–Base Disorders**   79
   Frederick J. Boehm III, Kelly Ann Traeger, and Arjang Djamali

8. **Glomerular Diseases**   89
   A. Vishnu Moorthy, Byram H. Ozer, Terry D. Oberley, and Weixiong Zhong

9. **Cystic Diseases of the Kidney**   109
   Kristin M. Lyerly and Arjang Djamali

10. **Urinalysis and an Approach to Kidney Diseases**   121
    A. Vishnu Moorthy and Frederick J. Boehm III

11. **Acute Kidney Injury**   131
    Paul S. Kellerman and Tracy C. Blichfeldt

12. **Chronic Kidney Disease**   145
    Ryan Kipp and Paul S. Kellerman

13. **Replacement Therapy for Kidney Failure: Dialysis**   159
    Joshua David Lindsey and Paul S. Kellerman

14. **Replacement Therapy for Kidney Failure: Transplantation**   169
    Milagros D. Samaniego, Yolanda T. Becker, and Joshua David Lindsey

15. **Essential Hypertension**   179
    Theodore L. Goodfriend and Kristin M. Lyerly

16. **Secondary Hypertension**   197
    Kristin M. Lyerly and Theodore L. Goodfriend

Answers to Practice Questions   212
Appendix: Some Common Laboratory Tests and Their Normal Values as Reported by the Clinical Laboratory at the University of Wisconsin Hospital and Clinics   219
Index   221

Anatomy and Physiology of the Kidney

A. Vishnu Moorthy
Tracy C. Blichfeldt

OUTLINE

I. Introduction
II. Anatomy of the Kidney
  A. The Nephron
  B. The Vascular System
  C. The Glomerulus
  D. The Kidney Tubule
III. Glomerular Filtration
IV. Autoregulation and Tubuloglomerular Feedback
V. Tubular Transport Processes
  A. Proximal Tubule
  B. Loop of Henle

  C. Distal Convoluted Tubule
  D. Collecting Duct
VI. Endocrine Functions of the Kidney
  A. Renin–Angiotensin–Aldosterone System
  B. Erythropoietin
  C. 1,25-Dihydroxyvitamin D_3 (Calcitriol)
VII. Measurement of Kidney Function: The Glomerular Filtration Rate
  A. Measurement of Creatinine Clearance
  B. Estimation of Creatinine Clearance and the Glomerular Filtration Rate

Objectives

- Know the anatomy of the kidney and its vasculature.
- Know the structure of the glomerulus and the various segments of the nephron.
- Understand the juxtaglomerular apparatus and tubuloglomerular feedback.
- Appreciate the factors that regulate glomerular filtration.
- Review the major transport functions of the different segments of the nephron.
- Know the kidney as an endocrine organ, particularly with regard to the production of renin, 1,25-dihydroxy vitamin D_3, and erythropoietin.
- Know how to assess kidney function with the measurement of creatinine clearance, the Cockcroft–Gault equation to estimate creatinine clearance, and the Modification of Diet in Renal Disease (MDRD) formula to estimate the glomerular filtration rate.

Clinical Case

A 62-year-old Caucasian man with a 10-year history of diabetes mellitus type 2 visits the primary care clinic where you, a second-year medical student, are working with your preceptor. The patient tells you that he has no new symptoms and that he is visiting the doctor for a routine health assessment and diabetes check. While reviewing the patient's chart, you see that his most recent visit to your preceptor was approximately 1 year ago. His weight has been stable at 62 kg, and his blood pressure is 130/80 mm Hg. His only prescription medication is glipizide to lower his blood sugar, and his serum creatinine level is 1.6 mg/dl.

The patient is concerned that his kidney function might be impaired. How will you address his concerns?

I. INTRODUCTION

The kidneys regulate the excretion of excess ingested water, electrolytes, and products of metabolism as well as foreign substances, including drugs and toxins. The kidneys maintain the volume of body fluid as well as its electrolyte composition, pH, and osmolality. The stability of this milieu is necessary for the proper functioning of cells and organs. Various sensing mechanisms that determine the extracellular fluid volume and the osmolality of the body fluids help the kidneys with this vital work. Hormones such as antidiuretic hormone (ADH), aldosterone, angiotensin II, and atrial natriuretic peptide (ANP) have important roles in the functions of the kidneys. The kidneys are also important endocrine organs that produce a variety of hormones, including erythropoietin, renin, and 1,25-dihydroxyvitamin D_3 (calcitriol), that are necessary to sustain health.

II. ANATOMY OF THE KIDNEY

The kidneys are located behind the peritoneal cavity (retroperitoneal) in the abdomen on either side of the midline. Each kidney weighs approximately 150 g and

measures 10 to 12 cm in length. The kidneys are highly vascular organs, receiving 20% of the cardiac output (the greatest amount of blood per 100 g of tissue in the body) via the renal arteries that originate from the abdominal aorta. Each kidney contains 400,000 to 1,200,000 functional units called *nephrons*. The arterial blood perfusing the kidney is later drained by the renal veins into the inferior vena cava (Fig. 1-1).

A. The Nephron

The nephron is the functional unit of the kidney, and it consists of a glomerulus and a tubule. Glomeruli are clusters of specialized capillaries contained within the Bowman's capsule in the cortex of the kidney. Blood enters glomeruli through the afferent arterioles and leaves through the efferent arterioles. The urine begins as a glomerular ultrafiltrate (blood minus plasma proteins) that drains from the glomerulus to the tubule. The kidney tubule has distinct segments, namely the proximal tubule, the hairpin-shaped loop of Henle, and the distal tubule, all of which connect the glomerulus to the collecting duct, which ultimately drains into the renal pelvis. As the glomerular ultrafiltrate traverses the tubules, its volume decreases, and its composition changes by the processes of tubular reabsorption and secretion. Finally, the urine drains into the renal pelvis and down the ureter into the urinary bladder, where it is stored before elimination.

B. The Vascular System

Each kidney is usually supplied by a single (at times double) renal artery, which arises from the aorta. The glomerular capillaries are unique in that they are situated between two arterioles: the afferent arteriole, which arises from branches of the renal artery and brings blood to the glomerular capillaries, and the efferent arteriole, which drains the glomerular capillaries. After the glomerulus, the efferent arteriole branches into a cluster of peritubular capillaries that intimately surrounds the tubules. Thus, there are two capillary beds in series in the kidney parenchyma. This arrangement is vital for glomerular filtration and for tubular reabsorption and secretion (Fig. 1-2).

The segments of postglomerular capillaries, which are known as the *vasa recta*, supply the medullary portion of the kidney. The vasa recta are hairpin-shaped blood vessels that arise in the cortex and descend into the medulla before turning back into the cortex and leading to the venous system. The medullary circulation removes solutes and fluid reabsorbed by the tubules. In the descending loops of the vasa recta, water moves out of the vessels and solutes move in. In the ascending loops of the vasa recta, this process is reversed: water moves into the vessel, and solutes move out into the interstitium. By this process of counter-current exchange, the vasa recta minimize the removal of excessive medullary interstitial solutes and maintain a high medullary tonicity. This high medullary interstitial tonicity is essential for the production of concentrated urine.

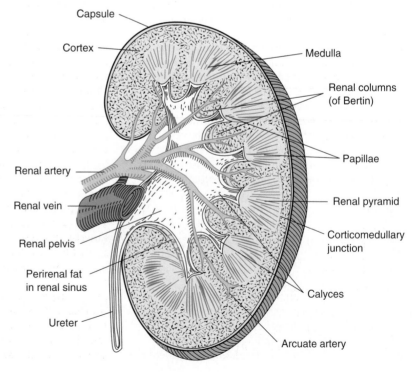

Figure 1-1. Anatomy of the kidney. A coronal section through the kidney showing the renal cortex and medulla. The capsule surrounds the kidney. The cortex contains the glomeruli and the medulla, which are mostly tubules that drain into the renal calyces and then into the pelvis and connect to the ureter. The renal blood vessels (the artery and the vein) are shown in the hilum of the kidney. *(Modified from Brenner B: Brenner and Rector's The Kidney, 7th ed. Philadelphia, Saunders, 2004.)*

Capsule

Cortex

Medulla

Renal columns (of Bertin)

Papillae

Renal artery

Renal vein

Renal pyramid

Corticomedullary junction

Renal pelvis

Perirenal fat in renal sinus

Calyces

Ureter

Arcuate artery

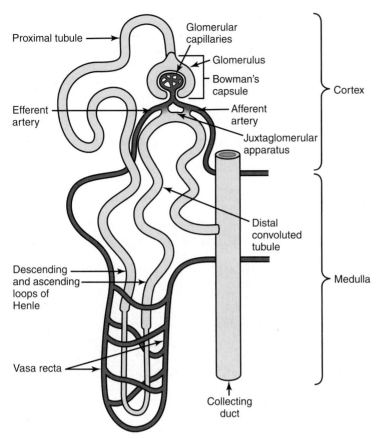

Proximal tubule

Glomerular
capillaries

Glomerulus

Bowman's
capsule

Afferent
artery

Juxtaglomerular
apparatus

Efferent
artery

Distal
convoluted
tubule

Descending
and ascending
loops of
Henle

Vasa recta

Collecting
duct

Cortex

Medulla

Figure 1-2. The structure of the kidney showing the nephron and its vascular supply. The nephron with its various components: the glomerulus and the proximal tubule in the cortex, the descending and ascending loops of Henle in the medulla, and the distal tubule that returns to the glomerulus of its origin in the cortex and ultimately connects to the collecting duct. The afferent artery supplies the glomerulus. The efferent artery arises from the glomerular capillaries, branches one more time into the peritubular capillaries, and descends into the renal medulla as the vasa recta before connecting into the venous system. *(Modified from Andreoli T, Loscalzo J, Carpenter C, Griggs R: Cecil Essentials of Medicine, 6th ed. Philadelphia, Saunders, 2004.)*

C. The Glomerulus

Glomeruli are clusters of capillaries that are surrounded by Bowman's capsules and lined with a single layer of epithelial cells called the *parietal epithelium*. The *afferent arteriole* supplies the glomerulus, and the *efferent arteriole* drains it; the proximal tubule drains filtrate from the Bowman's space. Glomerular capillaries are unique in that they are placed between two arterioles (Box 1-1 and Fig. 1-3).

Glomerular capillaries, like capillaries elsewhere in the body, have a basement membrane with an endothelial cell lining. The glomerular endothelium is fenestrated with the individual fenestra, and it measures 70 to 100 nm in length. The glomerular basement membrane (GBM) is an acellular matrix about 300-nm thick, with a central lamina densa and with the lamina rara interna and externa on either side. It is composed of extracellular matrix proteins, including type IV collagen and laminin. It also contains negatively charged glycoproteins, such as heparan and chondroitin sulfates. The triple helical collagen type IV molecule in the GBM of adults contains α-3, α-4, and α-5 chains of collagen (Box 1-2). The collagen chains in the GBM are cross-linked, and they provide tensile strength to the GBM.

The glomerular capillaries also have a unique cell called the *glomerular epithelial cell* that is located external to the GBM; this cell is also called the *podocyte*. In the past, podocytes were known more commonly as *visceral epithelial cells*. Podocytes are large cells that give rise to several interdigitating foot processes anchored to the GBM. The adjacent foot processes, which arise from different podocytes, are attached to one another through cytoplasmic connections called *slit diaphragms*. The slit diaphragm forms a zipper-like structure between adjacent podocytes. It has pores that are about 40 nm across, and it serves as a size-selective barrier to prevent molecules from entering Bowman's urinary space (Figs. 1-4 and 1-5).

Box 1-1. The Glomerulus

The glomerulus is a cluster of capillaries that is surrounded by Bowman's capsule. The capillary wall has a central basement membrane with endothelial and epithelial cells (the podocyte) on either side. Mesangial cells with matrix surround the capillaries. The podocyte is anchored to the basement membrane with fingerlike foot processes. Slit diaphragms connect adjacent foot processes. The glomerular capillary wall and the podocyte serve as barriers to exclude cells and protein in the blood from entering the Bowman's space.

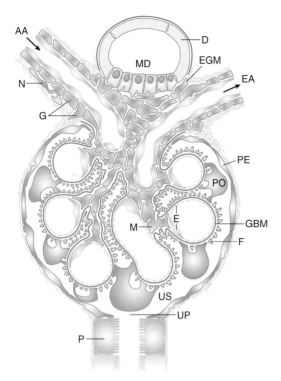

Figure 1-3. The glomerulus with the capillary wall, the cellular constituents, and the Bowman's capsule. The mesangium with the matrix and the mesangial cell is noted. Also illustrated is the juxtaglomerular apparatus, which is comprised of the macula densa and the renin-producing cells. *AA*, Afferent arteriole; *D*, distal tubule; *E*, endothelial cell; *EA*, efferent arteriole; *EGM*, extraglomerular mesangial cell; *F*, foot process; *G*, granules (renin); *GBM*, glomerular basement membrane; *M*, mesangial cell; *MD*, macula densa; *N*, nerve endings (sympathetic); *P*, proximal tubule; *PE*, parietal epithelial cell lining the Bowman's capsule; *PO*, podocyte; *UP*, urinary pole; *US*, urinary space. *(Modified from Greenberg A: Primer on Kidney Diseases, 4th ed. Philadelphia, Saunders, 2005.)*

Box 1-2. Inherited Disorders of the Glomerulus

Alport syndrome is a kidney disease that is usually the result of an X-linked inherited defect in the composition of type IV collagen in the glomerular basement membrane. This leads to hematuria and kidney failure.

Congenital nephrotic syndrome of the Finnish type is caused by an inherited defect in nephrin, which is a protein in the slit diaphragm of the podocytes. This causes excessive protein leakage into the urine during the first year of life and progressive kidney failure.

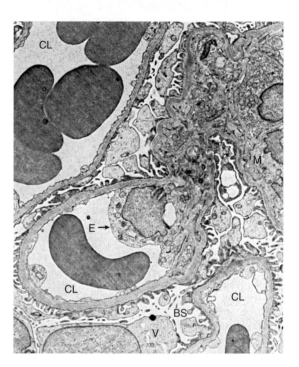

Figure 1-4. Electron micrograph of a normal glomerulus showing the capillary loops (CL) with red blood cells. Bowman's urinary space (BS), endothelial cell (E), mesangial cell (M), and visceral epithelial cell (V) are also seen. *(Modified from Brenner B: Brenner and Rector's The Kidney, 7th ed. Philadelphia, Saunders, 2004.)*

Proteins such as nephrin, podocin, and α-actinin 4 have been identified in the podocyte and in the slit diaphragm. These proteins are essential for the integrity of the glomerular capillary barrier. Inherited defects in genes that encode these proteins can lead to the leakage of plasma proteins into the urine and the eventual loss of kidney function.

The glomerular capillary wall includes the GBM and the filtration slits that are formed by the podocytes. It serves as a barrier that separates the blood in the glomerular capillaries from the ultrafiltrate in the Bowman's space, and it prevents cellular elements and protein from entering the urine. This is known as the *filtration barrier* (Box 1-3). The negatively charged proteins of the GBM exclude negatively charged molecules (e.g., albumin) from entering the ultrafiltrate from the glomerular capillaries. Studies using differently charged (i.e., anionic,

neutral, or cationic) dextran molecules have shown that glomerular capillaries are both size- and charge-selective barriers. Smaller or cationic molecules are easily filtered in the glomerulus, whereas larger and anionic molecules are retained in the glomerular capillaries.

In addition to endothelial cells and podocytes, the glomerulus also contains mesangial cells, which are surrounded by the mesangial matrix. Some of the mesangial cells possess contractile properties like smooth muscle cells, and they are anchored to glomerular capillaries. Other mesangial cells belong to the reticuloendothelial system. They have phagocytic activity, and they secrete a variety of cytokines. The

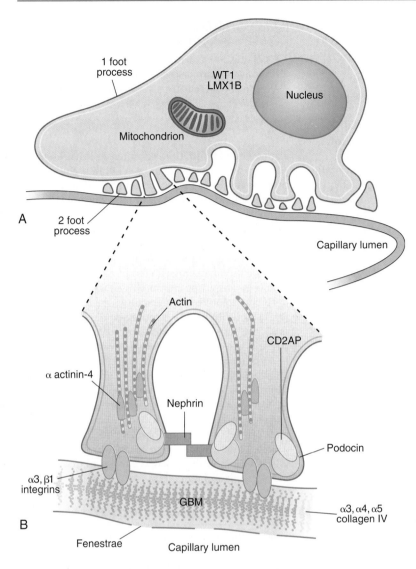

A

- 1 foot process
- WT1 LMX1B
- Nucleus
- Mitochondrion
- 2 foot process
- Capillary lumen

B

- Actin
- CD2AP
- α actinin-4
- Nephrin
- Podocin
- α3, β1 integrins
- GBM
- α3, α4, α5 collagen IV
- Fenestrae
- Capillary lumen

Figure 1-5. A schematic view of the podocyte resting on a capillary loop. *A,* Primary foot processes give rise to secondary foot processes that are anchored to the basement membrane with integrins. *B,* Nephrin proteins extend from adjacent foot processes and interdigitate to form the zipper-like slit diaphragm. Nephrin is anchored onto the cell membrane by podocin and CD2AP. α-Actinin-4 connects actin filaments to cellular structures. Inherited defects in proteins such as nephrin, podocin, CD2AP, and the transcription factors (WT1, LMX1B) have been found to cause focal glomerulosclerosis. Inherited defects in the α-3, α-4, and α-5 collagen type IV chains in the glomerular basement membrane (GBM) are seen in patients with Alport syndrome. *(Modified from Greenberg A:* Primer on Kidney Diseases, *4th ed. Philadelphia, Saunders, 2005.)*

Box 1-3. Filtration Barrier

The components of the glomerular filtration barrier are as follows:
1. The endothelial cell, with its fenestrae
2. The glomerular basement membrane
3. The podocyte, with the slit diaphragm

mesangial matrix is less dense than the GBM, and it extends outside of the hilum of the glomerulus into the juxtaglomerular apparatus.

D. The Kidney Tubule

The tubule of the nephron is divided into several segments. The different segments of the tubules have different structures and play different roles in modifying the content and amount of the final urine that is excreted. The proximal tubule arises from the glomerulus in the cortex. After a convoluted course, the proximal tubule descends into the medulla and becomes the loop of Henle. The nephrons in the outer zone of the renal cortex have short loops of Henle, whereas the deeper (juxtamedullary) nephrons have longer loops of Henle that descend almost to the tip of the papillae. The loops of Henle make an acute turn and return to the cortex to become the distal convoluted tubules in close proximity to the glomerulus from which they originated. A segment of the distal convoluted tubule is in contact with both the afferent and the efferent arterioles at the hilum of the glomerulus. At this site, the cells of the distal tubule are called the *macula densa,* and they are able to sense sodium and chloride concentrations in the tubular urine. Renin-containing granular cells are found in the wall of the afferent arterioles; this area also has rich sympathetic nerve endings. The macula densa and the renin-containing cells of the afferent

arterioles constitute *the juxtaglomerular apparatus*. The distal tubule then becomes the collecting duct, which returns again to the medulla and then leads into the renal pelvis.

III. GLOMERULAR FILTRATION

Hydrostatic pressure in glomerular capillaries drives glomerular filtration, and it is regulated by the tone of the afferent and efferent arterioles. Vasoconstriction of the efferent arteriole and vasodilatation of the afferent arteriole increases glomerular hydrostatic pressure and consequently glomerular filtration. Also contributing to glomerular filtration is the hydrostatic pressure in Bowman's space, the permeability of the glomerular capillary, and the oncotic pressure caused by plasma proteins. The oncotic pressure in the glomerular capillaries will decrease glomerular filtration, whereas that of the ultrafiltrate in the Bowman's space will oppose it. All of these forces are known as *Starling forces,* and they can be used to study the glomerular filtration using the following equation:

$$\text{Glomerular filtration} = K_f[(P_{GC} - P_{BS}) - (\pi_{GC} - \pi_{BS})]$$

K_f is the ultrafiltration coefficient (combining glomerular capillary permeability and surface area), P_{GC} and P_{BS} are the hydrostatic pressures in the glomerular capillary and Bowman's space, respectively, and π_{GC} and π_{BS} are the oncotic pressures in the glomerular capillary and Bowman's space, respectively.

Glomerular filtration can be decreased by reducing capillary hydrostatic pressure with one of the following: (1) a decrease in glomerular blood flow as a result of low blood pressure or low cardiac output; (2) the constriction of the afferent arteriole as a result of increased sympathetic activity or drugs (e.g., norepinephrine) that cause vasoconstriction; (3) the dilatation of the efferent arteriole by angiotensin blockade; (4) a loss of capillary wall surface area and permeability as occurs in glomerular diseases; and (5) an increase in hydrostatic pressure in the Bowman's space as a result of renal tubular obstruction or urinary tract obstruction downstream.

IV. AUTOREGULATION AND TUBULOGLOMERULAR FEEDBACK

Normally, kidney blood flow and glomerular filtration remain fairly constant over a wide range of mean arterial blood pressures. This phenomenon, called *autoregulation,* is the result of an intrinsic pressure-sensitive myogenic mechanism of the afferent arterioles (Box 1-4). As kidney perfusion pressure rises, an increase in afferent arteriole resistance occurs, thereby preventing the transmission of the increased pressure to the glomerulus. When the kidney perfusion pressure falls, the relaxation of the afferent arterioles maintains the glomerular hydrostatic pressure and

Box 1-4. Components of Autoregulation

1. Intrinsic pressure-sensitive myogenic mechanism of the afferent arteriole
2. Renin release from the juxtaglomerular apparatus and angiotensin-mediated efferent arteriolar vasoconstriction

also glomerular filtration. Angiotensin II has an important role in autoregulation. A fall in perfusion pressure results in increased renin release by the kidney and increased angiotensin II production. The angiotensin-II–mediated constriction of efferent arterioles leads to an increase in glomerular hydrostatic pressure that maintains glomerular filtration. Autoregulation is impaired by renin–angiotensin blockade, with the use of angiotensin receptor blockers or angiotensin-converting enzyme (ACE) inhibitors.

The juxtaglomerular apparatus is sensitive to sodium (Na^+) and chloride (Cl^-) concentrations in the tubular fluid, and it regulates glomerular blood flow. An increase in the delivery of Cl^- to the macula densa results in afferent arteriolar constriction and a decrease in the glomerular filtration; this is called the *tubuloglomerular feedback.* The exact mechanisms of tubuloglomerular feedback are unknown, but adenosine influenced by angiotensin and nitric oxide likely contribute. The major functions of autoregulation and tubuloglomerular feedback are to maintain the glomerular filtration rate (GFR) within relatively narrow limits and to prevent excessive salt and water losses.

V. TUBULAR TRANSPORT PROCESSES

Several different mechanisms are used to transport different substances across the tubules. A general model for the transport of solutes is shown in Figure 1-6. The tubular epithelial cells have polarity with apical (luminal) and basal (basolateral) surfaces. The tubular epithelial cells are attached to one another at tight junctions. There are generally two types of tubular transport mechanisms: transcellular and paracellular. Solutes and water can move across the cell (transcellular transport) or tight junctions (paracellular transport) by different active and passive processes. Luminal sodium ions can move across the cell membrane and be reabsorbed via the cotransport of glucose, amino acids, and phosphate. In some segments of the kidney tubule, sodium absorption is in exchange for other substances, such as hydrogen ions (H^+), as is seen in the proximal tubule. The Na^+/K^+-ATPase pump located on the basolateral side of the tubular cell extrudes sodium out of cells and into the peritubular fluid. Adenosine triphosphate hydrolysis provides the energy that is required for this active transport process. Some solutes, such as calcium and magnesium, are transported across the ascending limb

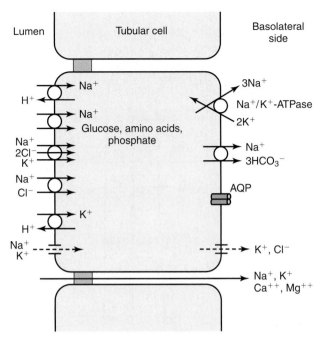

Figure 1-6. A general model for tubular cell transport processes in the kidney (e.g., those at the proximal tubule). The movement of solutes from the lumen into the tubular cell is mediated by several different types of transport mechanisms, including exchanger or antiporter (Na^+ for H^+) or cotransporter or symporter (Na^+ with Cl^-, Na^+ with glucose, or Na^+ with amino acids). Ion channels allow for the movement of Na^+, K^+, and Cl^- across membranes. The sodium pump on the basolateral membrane of the cell derives energy from adenosine triphosphate and hence is called *Na⁺/K⁺-ATPase*. It is the key mechanism for maintaining a low intracellular Na^+ and a high K^+ concentration relative to the extracellular concentrations. This facilitates the entry of Na^+ into the cell. *AQP,* Aquaporin.

of the loop of Henle in a paracellular route through the tight junction.

Water transport across the cell into the peritubular space is the result of the osmotic gradient that is created by the movement of these solutes. Water transport across tubular cells occurs through transmembrane water channels (aquaporins) or through paracellular routes across the tight junctions. In the proximal tubule, the tight junctions are leaky and permit the movement of water. Several segments of the tubule, such as the ascending limb of the loop of Henle, are impermeable to the passage of water. In the medullary collecting duct, the passage of water is controlled by ADH, which inserts aquaporins in the luminal membrane. Several hormones, such as angiotensin II, aldosterone, and ADH, influence tubular functions (Fig. 1-7).

A. Proximal Tubule +See Errata

The proximal tubule has convoluted and straight segments. It is lined with columnar epithelial cells that are rich in mitochondria. The proximal tubular cells have a brush border on their luminal surface. The proximal tubule actively reabsorbs the bulk of the small solutes, including 66% of the glomerular-filtered Na^+, Cl^-, K^+, calcium, and water; 90% of the filtered bicarbonate; and all of the filtered glucose and amino acids. It reabsorbs phosphate under the regulation of parathyroid hormone. It also secretes organic anions and cations into the urine, and it is able to eliminate drugs and toxins. Sodium reabsorption via the proximal tubule is an active process by the Na^+-dependent cotransporter (symporter) with glucose, phosphate, or amino acids and by the Na^+/H^+

exchanger (antiporter). Angiotensin II produced in response to renin release increases Na^+ reabsorption in the proximal tubule by the stimulation of the Na^+/H^+ exchanger. Proximal tubular cells reabsorb Cl^- passively across the tight junctions between the cells in the proximal tubule. Water reabsorption in the proximal tubule is passive and follows the concentration gradient that develops in response to solute reabsorption (Fig. 1-8).

The proximal tubule reabsorbs the bulk of the filtered bicarbonate. It secretes hydrogen (H^+), produces ammonia (NH_3), and has a very important role in eliminating the H^+ produced by cellular metabolism throughout the body. Weak acids (e.g., phosphate) in the tubular filtrate buffer the H^+ that is secreted by the tubule cells; this is called *titratable acidity.* Of greater importance for H^+ excretion is its combination with ammonia (NH_3) in the tubular urine and the formation of ammonium (NH_4^+). Ammonia (NH_3), which is produced in the proximal tubular cells, can diffuse freely through both sides of the cell membrane. In the distal tubular lumen, where the pH is low, ammonia (NH_3) combines with the H^+ that is secreted by the tubule cell and is converted into ammonium (NH_4^+). As a result of its charge, ammonium (NH_4^+) is much less diffusible than ammonia (NH_3); therefore, it is trapped in the lumen and excreted in the urine. Ammonia synthesis in the proximal tubule and subsequent ammonium excretion gives the healthy kidney the ability to excrete a significant amount of acid produced in the body during chronic metabolic acidosis.

An important function of the proximal tubule is the reabsorption of the glucose and amino acids filtered by the glomerulus. Both Na^+ and glucose bind

SEGMENTAL NEPHRON FUNCTION

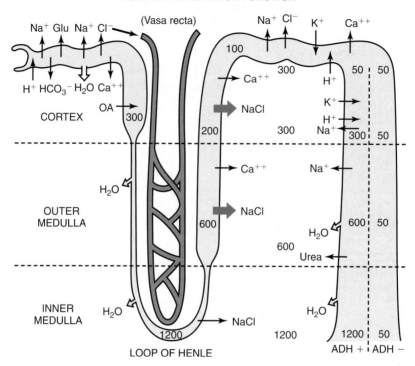

Figure 1-7. The transport processes of various substances in the different segments of the renal tubule. In the proximal tubule, Na^+ and glucose are absorbed by an active process. H^+ is secreted in exchange for Na^+. Water and K^+ absorption into the cell and NH_3 ammonia entry into the lumen are passive processes. The descending limb of the loop of Henle is impermeable to solutes. Water leaves the cell and goes into the hyperosmotic interstitium. The urine thereby becomes more concentrated as it passes down to the bend in the loop of Henle. The ascending limb of the loop of Henle absorbs Na^+ and Cl^- by an active process, but it is impermeable to water; this is the diluting segment of the nephron. The distal tubule reabsorbs Na^+ along with Cl^-. The late distal tubule and the cortical collecting duct absorb Na^+ in exchange for K^+, and they secrete H^+. The medullary collecting duct is the site of absorption of water and urea in the presence of ADH (ADH+), thereby producing a concentrated urine. In the absence of ADH (ADH−), hypotonic urine is excreted. The numbers in the tubule refer to tubular fluid osmolality. *OA*, Organic acid. *(Modified from Andreoli TE, Carpenter CCJ, Plum F, et al [eds]: Cecil Essentials of Medicine. Philadelphia, WB Saunders, 1986.)*

to the transporter. The transporter then changes conformation to enable both Na^+ and glucose release into the cytoplasm. This process is very efficient under normal conditions. In patients with diabetes mellitus, excessive blood sugar levels lead to excessive amounts of glucose entering the tubular lumen. This overwhelms the capacity of the proximal tubule to absorb filtered glucose, and glucose appears in the urine (this condition is known as *glycosuria*). Amino acids that may be filtered by the glomerulus are also completely reabsorbed by the proximal tubules by specific transport proteins. In patients with inherited disorders of proximal tubular function (e.g., Fanconi syndrome), substances that are normally completely absorbed by the proximal tubule (e.g., glucose, amino acids) may be present in the urine. In patients with Fanconi syndrome, which represents a generalized reabsorptive defect of the proximal tubule, other unreabsorbed solutes (e.g., bicarbonate, phosphate, uric acid) may also be added to the urine.

B. Loop of Henle

The loop of Henle plays an important role in the concentration of urine by the countercurrent mechanism. The tubular fluid at the end of the proximal tubule, although decreased in volume, is isotonic to the ultrafiltrate in Bowman's space. The descending limb of the loop of Henle allows for the selective passage of water into the medulla, thereby increasing the osmolality of the tubular fluid in the lumen. The osmolality of the tubular fluid is greatest at the tip of the loop of Henle. The ascending limb of the loop of Henle is different from the descending limb in that the ascending limb is impermeable to water but permits the reabsorption of Na^+ and Cl^-. This segment is also called the *diluting segment of the nephron*. As the tubular fluid returns to the cortex in the distal tubule, it becomes increasingly hypotonic.

Up to 25% of filtered Na^+ is reabsorbed by the ascending limb of the loop of Henle. The cells that line

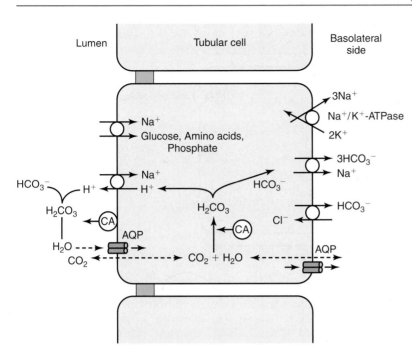

Lumen   Tubular cell   Basolateral side

Figure 1-8. The important transport processes in the proximal tubule cell include the following: Na^+/H^+ exchange, aquaporin (AQP)-facilitated water transport, basolateral Na^+/K^+-ATPase activity, and basolateral HCO_3^- transport coupled with Na^+ transport. Carbonic anhydrase (CA) present in the brush border breaks down H_2CO_3 (formed by the filtered HCO_3^- and secreted H^+) into CO_2 and water, both of which are passively absorbed into the cell. The CA in the cell facilitates HCO_3^- formation, which then exits the cell across the basolateral membrane coupled with Na^+ or in exchange for Cl^-.

the thick ascending limb contain the $Na^+/K^+/2Cl^-$ transporter on their luminal surface. This transporter actively reabsorbs Na^+ into the tubular cell. Sodium then leaves the tubular cell and enters the peritubular space by the Na^+/K^+-ATPase pump. Chloride leaves the tubular cell by the Cl^- channel located on the basal surface of the tubule cell. K^+ enters the cell by two processes: in exchange for Na^+ driven by the Na^+/K^+-ATPase at the basolateral surface and by cotransport with Na^+ and Cl^- across the luminal membrane ($Na^+/K^+/2Cl^-$ cotransporter). The ascending limb of the loop of Henle also reabsorbs magnesium and calcium via the paracellular pathway. The secretion of Na^+ into the interstitial space by ascending limb tubular cells sets up an osmotic gradient between the interstitial space and the descending limb, which leads to the passive movement of water from the descending limb into the interstitium (Fig. 1-9).

C. Distal Convoluted Tubule

The distal tubule reabsorbs Na^+ (7% of the filtered load) by the Na^+/Cl^- cotransporter that is present on its apical surface. Sodium reabsorption in the distal tubule is dependent on the tubular fluid flow rate. The distal tubule is also the site for calcium reabsorption through apical calcium channels and a vitamin-D–dependent calcium-binding protein (Fig. 1-10).

D. Collecting Duct

The collecting duct arises in the cortex from the distal tubule, returns to the medulla, and drains into the pelvis. The cortical and medullary portions of the collecting duct have different transport processes and functions.

The cortical collecting duct has two types of cells: the principal cells and the intercalated cells. The principal cells reabsorb Na^+ and secrete K^+. Sodium leaves the principal cell from the basal side into the peritubular space via the Na^+/K^+-ATPase pump, thus producing an Na^+ concentration gradient between the tubular space and the cell. Na^+ moves across the tubular lumen through the epithelial sodium channel down its concentration gradient. This results in electronegativity in the tubular lumen, which leads to potassium secretion from the cell through potassium channels. The cortical collecting duct is the final determinant of potassium excretion by the kidney. Aldosterone increases the number of open Na^+ channels on the luminal side of the principal cell as well as the activity of the Na^+/K^+-ATPase pump.

The collecting duct also has an important role in acid–base regulation by the kidney (for more information, see Chapter 6). Type A intercalated cells of the cortical collecting duct secrete H^+ by H^+/K^+-ATPase located on the luminal side of the cell. Type B intercalated cells in the cortical collecting duct secrete bicarbonate via a chloride–bicarbonate exchanger located in the luminal membrane. They reabsorb chloride and excrete bicarbonate when there is metabolic alkalosis (Fig. 1-11).

The medullary segment of the collecting duct is the final determinant of water excretion by the kidney. The proximal segments of the nephron passively reabsorb considerable amounts of the water and thereby reduce urine volume significantly. The osmolality of the urine as it enters the medullary collecting duct is hypotonic. If conditions warrant the loss of water from the body, the medullary collecting duct remains impermeable to

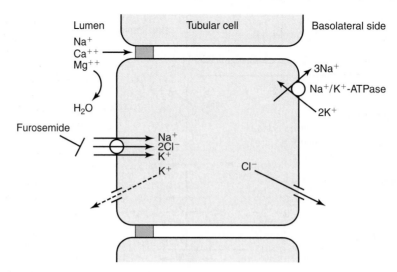

Figure 1-9. The transport mechanisms in the thick ascending limb of the loop of Henle. The entry of filtered NaCl into the cells is mediated by a neutral $Na^+/K^+/2Cl^-$ cotransporter in the apical (luminal) membrane; reabsorbed Na^+ is pumped out of the cell by the Na^+/K^+-ATPase pump in the basolateral (peritubular) membrane. K^+ must recycle back into the lumen through K^+ channels in the apical membrane to allow for continued NaCl reabsorption. Cl^- is reabsorbed out of the cell into the peritubular capillary via a Cl^- channel. Na^+ and, to a lesser degree, Ca^{++} and Mg^{++}, are absorbed via the paracellular pathway between the cells. The loop diuretics inhibit Na^+, K^+, and Cl^- (and Ca^{++} and Mg^{++}) reabsorption by competing for the Cl^- site on this transporter. *(Modified from Costanzo L: Physiology, 3rd ed. Philadelphia, Saunders, 2006.)*

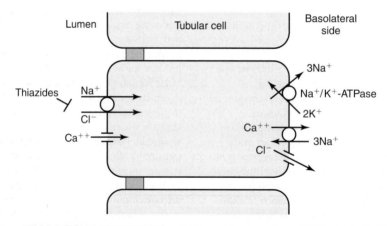

Figure 1-10. The transport processes in the distal convoluted tubular cell. The entry of filtered NaCl into the cell is mediated by a neutral Na^+/Cl^- cotransporter in the apical (luminal) membrane. At the basolateral (peritubular) membrane, reabsorbed Na^+ is pumped out of the cell by the Na^+/K^+-ATPase pump, whereas reabsorbed Cl^- exits via a chloride channel. Thiazides inhibit NaCl reabsorption by competing for the Cl^- site on the apical Na^+/Cl^- cotransporter. The distal tubule is also the major site of active Ca^{++} reabsorption. Ca^{++} enters the cell via a Ca^{++} transporter that is probably a Ca^{++} channel, and it is then extruded at the basolateral membrane by a $3Na^+:1Ca^{++}$ exchanger. *(Modified from Minneman K: Brody's Human Pharmacology, 4th ed. Philadelphia, Mosby, 2005.)*

water, and this hypotonic urine is excreted. However, when there is a need to conserve water, the medullary collecting duct absorbs considerable amounts of water from the urine, thereby progressively increasing urine osmolality. This "antidiuresis" is accomplished by ADH (vasopressin). ADH is secreted from the hypothalamus and released into the circulation from the posterior pituitary gland. ADH combines with V2 vasopressin receptors on the basal side of cells in the medullary collecting duct. This leads to the generation of cyclic adenosine monophosphate via adenyl cyclase and the activation of protein kinase A, which results in the insertion of aquaporin-2 (a water channel) into the luminal membrane from preformed cytoplasmic vesicles. This allows water to flow into cells. Water then moves into the hyperosmolar interstitium via aquaporins-3 and -4, which are located on the basal side of the cell. The medullary collecting duct can

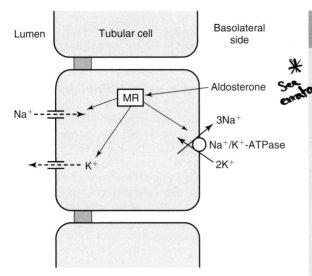

Lumen   Tubular cell   Basolateral side

Figure 1-11. The action of aldosterone on potassium secretion at the principal cell of the cortical collecting tubule. Aldosterone binds with mineralocorticoid receptors (MR) of the principal cell, where it sends signals to activate sodium channels at the luminal membrane. It also stimulates Na^+/K^+-ATPase at the basolateral membrane and increases the permeability of the luminal membrane to potassium by activating potassium channels. The net results are increased sodium reabsorption to generate lumen-negative electrical potential and the creation of a steep downward concentration gradient of potassium. Thus, a favorable electrochemical gradient is created by the action of aldosterone to enhance the passive secretion of potassium via the activated potassium channels and the intercellular space.

increase the osmolality of the final urine from 50 mOsm/kg in the absence of ADH to as high as 1000 mOsm/kg in the presence of ADH. The amount of water that can be reabsorbed is regulated by medullary tonicity. Urea, which is a waste product of protein catabolism, has an important role in providing nearly half of the medullary tonicity. A reduction in urea synthesis by a decrease in protein intake impairs the concentrating ability of the kidney. Drugs have been developed to block vasopressin receptors, and they can increase urinary water excretion in patients with conditions that involve the inappropriate excess production of ADH.

The medullary collecting duct also has a role in sodium excretion. ANP is stored in cardiac myocytes and released in patients with congestive cardiac failure when the atrium is stretched. ANP causes vasodilatation and lowers blood pressure. In the kidney, ANP increases sodium excretion by decreasing the number of epithelial sodium channels in the inner medullary collecting duct and decreasing sodium entry into cells. Not surprisingly, ANP is an excellent antagonist of the renin–angiotensin–aldosterone axis. However, the role of ANP in normal physiology is unclear.

Box 1-5. Major Functions of the Different Tubule Segments

Proximal tubule: This structure reabsorbs 66% of filtered sodium with chloride and bicarbonate, 90% of filtered phosphate, and all glucose and amino acids. Water is transported passively with the solutes.

Descending loop of Henle: This allows for the passive diffusion of water into the medulla. The tubular fluid becomes hypertonic. The tubular fluid is most hypertonic at the tip of the loop of Henle.

Ascending loop of Henle (the diluting segment): The active transport of chloride and sodium into the medulla without the passage of water makes the tubular fluid dilute.

Distal tubule: This provides for the further reabsorption of sodium and the dilution of the fluid.

Cortical collecting duct: This structure reabsorbs sodium in exchange for potassium and hydrogen.

Medullary collecting duct: The reabsorption of water in the presence of antidiuretic hormone makes the final urine concentrated. In the absence of antidiuretic hormone, this segment remains impermeable to water and allows for the passage of dilute urine.

VI. ENDOCRINE FUNCTIONS OF THE KIDNEY

The kidney has several important endocrine functions, including the production of hormones that regulate fluid status, the maintenance of blood pressure, red blood cell production, and the body's potassium and calcium balance.

A. Renin–Angiotensin–Aldosterone System

By producing renin, the kidney plays a vital role in maintaining volume and electrolyte balance in the body. Renin is a proteolytic enzyme that is released into the blood by a number of different cells but most importantly by granular cells in the juxtaglomerular apparatus in response to extracellular fluid volume depletion and sympathetic stimulation. Renin converts angiotensinogen (a globulin in the blood that is formed by the liver) into angiotensin I. Angiotensin I is then converted by ACE into angiotensin II. ACE is located on the capillary endothelium of blood vessels, especially in the lungs, the kidneys, and the brain. Acting through the AT-1 receptor, angiotensin II acts as a potent vasoconstrictor. Angiotensin II increases Na^+ retention by the kidney by direct and indirect mechanisms. In the proximal tubule, angiotensin II enhances Na^+ reabsorption by an increase in Na^+/H^+ exchanger activity. Angiotensin II also stimulates aldosterone production in the adrenal cortex. Aldosterone then acts on the cortical collecting duct to stimulate Na^+ reabsorption in exchange for K^+ secretion.

Renin, angiotensin, and (usually) aldosterone are increased in the blood in the following situations, all of
which are characterized by reduced perfusion of the
kidneys or reduced sodium and chloride concentrations
in the tubular fluid in the distal tubule, which bathes
the juxtaglomerular apparatus:

1. Hemorrhage
2. Diuresis
3. Salt depletion (low-sodium diet)
4. Extracellular volume depletion
5. Adrenal insufficiency (renin and angiotensin are increased but aldosterone is decreased because the
   adrenal gland is unable to make it)
6. Upright posture
7. Nephrotic syndrome
8. Heart failure
9. Cirrhosis with ascites

Note that, in the last three conditions, the total body
sodium and water content may be high, but the blood
flow to the kidney is decreased. This is because the extracellular fluid is largely sequestered in tissue spaces,
apart from the blood.

In the glomerulus, angiotensin II causes efferent
arteriolar constriction to a greater degree than that of
the afferent arteriole. Glomerular hydrostatic pressure rises, and glomerular filtration is maintained.
Other effects of angiotensin II include the stimulation of thirst, the release of ADH, the stimulation
of sympathetic nerve activity, and the release of
catecholamines.

Drugs such as lisinopril can block the effects of
the renin–angiotensin system by inhibiting ACE,
thus preventing the conversion of angiotensin I to
II. These drugs are referred to as *ACE inhibitors.* A
similar effect can be obtained by drugs (e.g., losar-
tan) that antagonize the angiotensin II (AT-1) receptor. Both of these agents are effective for lowering
blood pressure in patients with hypertension. These
drugs also lower glomerular hydrostatic pressure
and decrease glomerular filtration. In patients with
chronic kidney disease, the lowering of glomerular
hydrostatic pressure by these drugs decreases proteinuria and slows the progressive loss of kidney
function.

B. Erythropoietin

Erythropoietin is a glycosylated protein that is produced in the kidney by proximal tubular epithelial
cells and cortical interstitial cells. It stimulates the
maturation of erythrocytes in the bone marrow.
Erythropoietin deficiency or underproduction, as
has been demonstrated in patients with chronic

kidney disease, leads to anemia. Recombinant
erythropoietin preparations are very effective for
the treatment of anemia in patients with chronic
kidney disease.

C. 1,25-Dihydroxyvitamin D_3 (Calcitriol)

Calcitriol is the active form of vitamin D, and it is
essential for calcium absorption and bone mineralization. Vitamin D_3 is a steroid that is ingested in
the diet or synthesized in the skin in the presence
of ultraviolet light. It is converted in the liver into
25-hydroxyvitamin D_3 and then hydroxylated again
in the proximal tubular epithelial cells of the kidney by the enzyme 1-α hydroxylase into the active
metabolite 1,25-dihydroxyvitamin D_3 (calcitriol).
Parathyroid hormone stimulates calcitriol production in the kidney by increasing the synthesis of 1-α
hydroxylase.

Calcitriol has several important functions in the
body. It maintains serum calcium levels by increasing
calcium absorption in the gastrointestinal tract. It
promotes healthy bone formation by the calcification
of osteoid tissue. It also directly inhibits parathyroid
gland activity by decreasing parathyroid hormone
synthesis and release. In patients with chronic kidney
disease, a lack of calcitriol can result in metabolic
bone disease. Calcitriol and several synthetic vitamin
D analogs are now available for patients with kidney
disease.

VII. MEASUREMENT OF KIDNEY FUNCTION: THE GLOMERULAR FILTRATION RATE

As one can see from this discussion, the kidney has
several important metabolic, excretory, regulatory,
and endocrine functions. These functions can be
impaired, at different times, either separately or
globally. A customary method to assess global kidney function is the measurement of the glomerular
filtration rate (GFR). The GFR is the amount of
plasma that is filtered by all functioning nephrons
in a period of time. It can be measured by finding

1. **Renin production:** Renin is released in response to a
   decrease in extracellular fluid volume, and it stimulates
   the production of angiotensin II, which leads to the
   reabsorption of sodium and water.
2. **Erythropoietin production:** Erythropoietin stimulates
   the production of red blood cells in the bone marrow.
3. **1,25-dihydroxyvitamin D_3 production by the enzyme
   1-α hydroxylase:** 1,25-dihydroxyvitamin D_3 stimulates
   the absorption of calcium in the intestine, inhibits the
   parathyroid gland, and aids in bone calcification.

the clearance of a substance that is freely filtered by the glomerulus and neither secreted nor reabsorbed by the tubules. *Clearance* is defined as the volume of plasma of a given substance that is completely cleared during a given time period. The clearance of any substance may be measured using the following equation:

$$\text{Clearance} = (U \times V)/P$$
$$U = \text{Urinary concentration of the substance (mg/ml)}$$
$$V = \text{Urine flow rate (ml/min)}$$
$$P = \text{Plasma concentration of the substance (mg/ml)}$$

A. Measurement of Creatinine Clearance

The substance that was used initially for the measurement of GFR was inulin, which is a large carbohydrate-like molecule that is freely filtered by the glomerulus. Today, creatinine, which is an endogenous substance produced from creatine that originates in the muscles, is used to calculate the GFR. However, it is more appropriate to call this *creatinine clearance*, because the renal tubule does secrete a small amount of creatinine. Measuring creatinine clearance using creatinine concentrations in plasma and timed urine collections can create an error of 10% or more as a result of the tubular secretion of creatinine in the kidney. Because creatinine production is related to muscle mass, creatinine clearance can also be an inaccurate measure of GFR in individuals with decreased muscle mass (e.g., elderly patients), in those with severe malnutrition, and in patients who do not ingest meat in their diets. Radioisotopes (including ^{99m}Tc DTPA and ^{99m}Tc MAG3) have been used to measure GFR in patients. However, these are expensive for routine clinical use.

B. Estimation of Creatinine Clearance and the Glomerular Filtration Rate

Timed collections of urine over a 24-hour period can be cumbersome and difficult to obtain, and they are often inaccurate as a result of missed samples. Hence, several formulae have been developed to estimate kidney function from serum creatinine measurements alone. The oldest of these for the estimation of creatinine clearance is the Cockcroft–Gault formula:

$$\text{Men:} \frac{(140 - \text{age in years})(\text{Weight in kg})}{72 \times \text{Serum Cr(mg/dL)}}$$

$$\text{Women:} \frac{(140 - \text{age in years})(\text{Weight in kg})}{72 \times \text{Serum Cr(mg/dL)}} \times 0.85$$

The weight of the patient is used as a surrogate for muscle mass, and the age and gender of the patient are required because muscle mass is decreased in women and older adults. The Cockcroft–Gault formula is superior to serum creatinine measurements alone and also to the measured creatinine clearance with a 24-hour urine collection. However, newer formulae may be more accurate. The formula currently recommended by the National Kidney Foundation to estimate GFR is called the modification of diet in renal disease (MDRD) study formula. This formula is complex and requires a computer program for its calculation.

Several versions of the MDRD equation exist. An abbreviated version that estimates GFR (ml/min/ 1.73 m^2) is as follows:

$$\text{eGFR} = 186 \times (\text{serum creatinine})^{-1.154} \times (\text{age})^{-0.203} \times$$
$$(0.742 \text{ if female}) \times (1.210 \text{ if African American})$$

Several Web sites are available that can estimate the GFR using the MDRD formula, and programs in personal digital assistants are available for this purpose as well. Many clinical laboratories routinely provide the eGFR when a patient's serum creatinine is measured (Box 1-8).

The use of the MDRD formula and the measurement of eGFR has improved clinical care by diagnosing patients with chronic kidney disease earlier in the course of the illness, when the patient has no clinical symptoms. The MDRD formula for estimating the GFR is very useful for patients with chronic kidney disease who have a stable serum creatinine level. However, it is not accurate in the hospitalized patient whose serum creatinine level can fluctuate for a variety of reasons. The value of the MDRD formula is also less in adults with near-normal levels of kidney function. The underestimation of the GFR can be substantial in patients with values of more than 60 ml/min/1.73 m^2. Chronic kidney disease is defined as more than 3 months' duration of either kidney damage or an eGFR of less than 60 ml/min/1.73 m^2. Kidney damage is defined as pathologic abnormalities or markers of damage, including abnormalities in blood or urine or imaging studies of the kidney. In patients with chronic kidney disease, the eGFR estimated by the MDRD formula can be used to measure disease progression and response to therapy and as a general guide for patient management. Table 1-1 provides a

---

Box 1-8. Estimation of Kidney Function

Cockcroft-Gault equation:

$$\text{Men:} \frac{(140 - \text{age in years})(\text{Weight in kg})}{72 \times \text{Serum Cr(mg/dL)}}$$

$$\text{Women:} \frac{(140 - \text{age in years})(\text{Weight in kg})}{72 \times \text{Serum Cr(mg/dL)}} \times 0.85$$

Modification of Diet in Renal Disease study formula for estimated glomerular filtration rate:

$$\text{eGFR} = 186 \times (\text{serum creatinine})^{-1.154} \times (\text{age})^{-0.203} \times$$
$$(0.742 \text{ if female}) \times (1.210 \text{ if African American})$$

Table 1-1. Stages of Chronic Kidney Disease

Stage	Description	Estimated glomerular filtration rate (ml/min/1.73 m^2)
1	Kidney damage with normal glomerular filtration rate	>90
2	Kidney damage with mild decrease in glomerular filtration rate	60–89
3	Moderate decrease in glomerular filtration rate	30–59
4	Severe decrease in glomerular filtration rate	15–29
5	Kidney failure	<15

framework for classifying patients in the different stages of chronic kidney disease.

Urea is produced by protein catabolism in the liver, and it is excreted by glomerular filtration. The level of blood urea nitrogen (BUN) varies inversely with GFR, but it is not a reliable measure of kidney function. More than 50% of filtered urea is reabsorbed by the proximal tubule passively after the reabsorption of sodium and water. BUN levels are higher when this reabsorption is increased, as is the case in patients with decreased extracellular fluid volume, decreased urinary flow rate, or urinary obstruction. BUN levels are also higher for a given level of kidney function in patients with kidney failure if there is increased protein intake, gastrointestinal bleeding (because blood is a good source of protein), or increased tissue breakdown and protein catabolism.

Other markers are being developed to measure kidney function. Cystatin C is a cysteine protease inhibitor that is produced by nearly all human cells and excreted into the bloodstream. At a molecular weight of 13 kD, cystatin C is freely filtered by the renal glomerulus and then metabolized by the proximal tubule cells. Serum levels of cystatin C are a reliable measure of kidney function; they correlate well with the GFR and increase predictably in patients with kidney failure. Cystatin C may eventually be adopted as a measure of kidney function if the testing procedure becomes easier and less expensive.

Clinical Case

A 62-year-old Caucasian man with a 10-year history of diabetes mellitus type 2 visits the primary care clinic where you, a second-year medical student, are working with your preceptor. The patient tells you that he has no new symptoms and that he is visiting the doctor for a routine health assessment and diabetes check. While reviewing the patient's chart, you see that his most recent visit to your preceptor was approximately 1 year ago. His weight has been stable at 62 kg, and his blood pressure is 130/80 mm Hg. His only prescription medication is glipizide to lower his blood sugar, and his serum creatinine level is 1.6 mg/dl.

The patient is concerned about whether his kidney function is impaired. How will you address his concerns?

Patients with diabetes mellitus (both types 1 and 2) are at increased risk for developing kidney disease. Long duration of diabetes, poor control of blood sugar levels, and elevations in blood pressure will increase the likelihood of kidney damage in a patient with diabetes. The patient does not demonstrate any clinical symptoms until kidney damage is far advanced. Blood and urine tests are needed to determine whether the patient has kidney disease as a result of diabetes. The earliest manifestation of kidney damage in a patient with diabetes is the leakage of small amounts of albumin through the glomerular capillary wall into the urine; this is called *microalbuminuria* (see Chapter 10). As the kidney damage progresses, the amount of protein excreted in the urine increases, and kidney function declines. The decline in kidney function is diagnosed by estimating GFR using the MDRD formula from the serum creatinine level. In this particular patient, a serum creatinine level of 1.6 mg/dl results in an estimated GFR of 47 ml/min. He has stage III chronic kidney disease, and he has lost nearly half of his kidney function, most likely as a result of diabetic nephropathy.

Suggested Readings

Briggs JP, Kriz W, Schnermann J: Overview of kidney function and structure. In Greenberg A (ed): *Primer on Kidney Diseases,* 4th ed. National Kidney Foundation, Philadelphia, 2005, pp 2–19.

National Kidney Foundation: K/DOQI clinical practice guidelines for chronic kidney disease: Evaluation, classification and stratification. *Am J Kidney Dis* 39(Suppl 1): S1–S266, 2002.

Scheinman SJ, Guy-Woodford LM, Thakker RV, Warnock DG: Genetic disorders of renal electrolyte transport. *N Eng J Med* 340:1177–1187, 1999.

Stevens LA, Levey AS: Measurement of kidney function. *Med Clin North Am* 89(3):454–473, 2005.

PRACTICE QUESTIONS

1. A 50-year-old, 80-kg man had some routine laboratory work done. His laboratory values are a blood urea nitrogen level of 10 mg/dl and a creatinine level 0.9 mg/dl. Estimate this patient's creatinine clearance using the Cockcroft–Gault equation.

   A. 80 ml/min
   B. 90 ml/min
   C. 110 ml/min
   D. 130 ml/min

2. A 75-year-old woman who has had decreased kidney function for several years visits her doctor. She has been feeling more tired lately, and she becomes short of breath when walking up the stairs. On examination, she is a pale-appearing woman with tachycardia. The remainder of her examination is normal. Her laboratory values include a hemoglobin level of 8.9 g/dl and a creatinine level of 2.0 mg/dl. The lack of which hormone produced by the kidney is contributing to this patient's anemia?

   A. 1,25-dihydroxyvitamin D_3
   B. Angiotensin II
   C. Renin
   D. Erythropoietin

3. A medical student notices that, when she is taking an examination, her blood pressure is increased from normal. She is worried that this increase in blood pressure may damage her kidneys. What is she forgetting about?

   A. Autoregulation
   B. Renin–angiotensin
   C. Aldosterone
   D. That the glomerulus can handle high pressures

Body Fluid Compartments and Their Regulation

2

Byram H. Ozer
Peter C. Brazy

OUTLINE
I. Importance of Fluid Homeostasis
II. Body Fluid Compartments
III. Body Fluid Regulation
   A. Movement of Water between Intracellular Fluid and Extracellular Fluid Regulated by Osmotic Pressure
   B. Movement of Water from Intravascular to Interstitial Space: The Starling Relationship
IV. Pathophysiology of Fluid Compartment Changes
   A. Methods of Monitoring Body Fluid Status and Distribution
   B. Losing Fluid from the Body Compartments
   C. Additions to the Body Fluid Compartments
   D. Shifts in Fluid from One Compartment to Another
V. Summary

Objectives

- Know the distribution of water and electrolytes within the compartments of the body.
- Understand the factors that affect the distribution of fluid among these compartments.
- Learn to assess the volume in each of the body compartments.
- Understand the mechanisms that lead to an imbalance in distribution or in the amount of fluid in a compartment.

Clinical Case

A 55-year-old man has kidney failure and is receiving hemodialysis three times a week. He has negligible urine output, and he does not follow the prescribed dietary advice. He comes to the emergency department on the night before his next dialysis appointment with increased shortness of breath and the inability to lie flat. He has gained 6 kg since the last dialysis treatment. He has increased jugular venous pressure, rales in his lung bases, and pedal edema. His blood pressure is 160/90 mm Hg. His laboratory tests reveal a serum sodium level of 128 mmol/L, a blood urea nitrogen level of 80 mg/dl, and a blood glucose level of 98 mg/dl.

What do you think has happened to this patient's body fluid compartments since the last dialysis treatment to account for his symptoms and laboratory findings?

I. IMPORTANCE OF FLUID HOMEOSTASIS

A person may vary his or her amount of food and fluid intake from day to day over an extremely wide range of types and quantities, and the net effect on the composition and content of their body fluids is usually negligible. If this were not the case, significant changes in fluid composition would occur, and these changes would have dramatic effects on cell and tissue function. Cellular metabolism, cell-to-cell signaling, and other vital processes require a constant composition (homeostasis) of the intracellular and extracellular fluid compartments. In a hyperosmotic (high-solute) environment, water flows out of cells and they shrink. Alternatively, in a hypoosmotic (low solute) environment, water flows into cells, thereby causing them to swell and even burst. In either case, cell function is disrupted. Therefore, one of the key functions of the kidneys is to maintain the homeostasis (constant composition) of body fluids while the daily intake varies.

Part of maintaining proper osmotic homeostasis within the body is regulating the water content within the body fluid compartments. In this case, the principle is that "what goes in must come out," and intake through drinking, eating, or intravenous administration must be matched by excretion through urine, feces, sweat, or other forms of fluid loss. This chapter explores how water is distributed throughout the body, what forces determine its distribution, and how water homeostasis is achieved. The discussion concludes with an examination of how homeostasis is challenged and sometimes limited by certain disease states.

II. BODY FLUID COMPARTMENTS

Under normal conditions, total body water (TBW) makes up about 60% of the body's weight. However, this number depends on the percentage of body fat in

an individual; fat cells exclude water and, therefore, contain less water than other tissues, such as muscle and blood cells. It is this difference in body fat percentage that accounts for the discrepancies in TBW composition that occur as a result of age and sex. For example, water makes up about 75% of body weight in newborns, and it decreases to adult values by the age of 1 year. Furthermore, women generally have a higher percentage of body fat than men, and water makes up only about 50% of their total body weight.

The TBW is distributed into several body compartments. The first division is between intracellular fluid (ICF; water within the cells) and extracellular fluid (ECF). Extracellular fluid is further divided into interstitial fluid (the fluid that bathes the cells) and intravascular fluid (plasma; the fluid in the blood vessels). The volume of fluid in each compartment may be estimated by multiplying typical percentages times the person's body weight. TBW comprises approximately 60% of the body weight (50% in people with high body fat content); of the TBW, ICF makes up 67%, whereas ECF is 33% of total volume. Finally, within the ECF, interstitial fluid is 75% and plasma is 25% of the volume (Fig. 2-1 and Box 2-1).

III. BODY FLUID REGULATION

The factors that regulate total body solute and water homeostasis will be discussed in other chapters of this book. Here we will discuss the distribution of fluid among the compartments defined previously (Box 2-2 and Table 2-1).

A. Movement of Water between Intracellular Fluid and Extracellular Fluid Regulated by Osmotic Pressure

The principle of osmosis states that when a semipermeable membrane separates two fluid spaces, water will flow from an area of lower solute concentration to one of higher solute concentration to achieve equilibrium so that the osmotic pressures are balanced. In biologic systems, the cell membranes allow water to diffuse across them, but they are relatively impermeable to charged solutes (e.g., sodium, potassium) and large

> **Box 2-1.** Example: Body Fluid Composition Calculations
>
> 1. A 70-kg elderly woman has a high percentage of body fat.
>   Her total body water is $0.5 \times 70 = 35$ L.
>   Her intracellular fluid volume is $0.67 \times 35 = 23.5$ L.
>   Her extracellular fluid volume is $0.33 \times 35 = 11.5$ L.
>   Her interstitial fluid volume is $0.75 \times 11.5 = 8.6$ L.
>   Her plasma volume is $0.25 \times 11.5 = 2.9$ L.
> 2. A 90-kg muscular man has an average to low percentage of body fat.
>   His total body water is $0.6 \times 90 = 54$ L.
>   His intracellular fluid volume is $0.67 \times 54 = 36.2$ L.
>   His extracellular fluid volume is $0.33 \times 54 = 17.8$ L.
>   His interstitial fluid volume is $0.75 \times 17.8 = 13.4$ L.
>   His plasma volume is $0.25 \times 17.8 = 4.4$ L.

> **Box 2-2.** Key Points of Body Fluid Regulation
>
> The amount of solute in each space is a primary determinant of the fluid of that space. Sodium and the anions associated with it are the major solutes of the extracellular fluid (ECF) space, whereas potassium and organic solutes are the primary solutes of the intracellular fluid (ICF) space (see Table 2-1). Water moves *between* the ECF and the ICF according to differences in osmotic pressure, which are dictated by the relative concentration of these osmotically active solutes.
>
> The movement of water *within* the ECF (i.e., between the intravascular and interstitial spaces) depends on the hydrostatic and oncotic pressures as described by the Starling relationship.

organic molecules (e.g., glucose). Cell membranes have special transport systems (proteins or channels) that regulate the movement of these ions and molecules across the cell membrane. Small, uncharged molecules (e.g., urea, ammonia) diffuse across cell membranes quickly. The concentration of solutes in the compartment (molecules or ions dissolved in the water) determines the osmolality of the fluid, and this is expressed as mOsm/kg of water. In the steady-state condition,

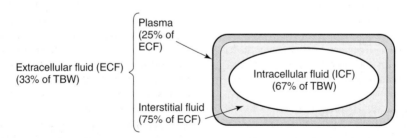

Figure 2-1. Diagrammatic representation of the distribution of water in the body's fluid compartments. The diagram is drawn to represent the relative percentage of total body water (TBW) that either the extracellular fluid (ECF) or intracellular fluid (ICF) compartments can accommodate under homeostatic conditions.

Table 2-1. Representative Ion and Solute Content of the Body Fluid Compartments Expressed in mmol/L (Note that, although the ionic composition is different from compartment to compartment, the overall osmolarity of each compartment is roughly equivalent.)

Electrolyte	Plasma	Interstitial fluid	Intracellular fluid
Cations			
Sodium	142	145	10
Potassium	4	4	160
Calcium	5	5	2
Magnesium	2	2	26
Anions			
Chloride	101	114	3
Bicarbonate	27	31	10
Phosphate	2	2	100
Sulfate	1	1	20
Organic acid	6	7	
Protein	16 (primarily albumin)	1	65

Data from Patlak J: *Ionic composition of body fluids* (website): http://physioweb.med.uvm.edu/bodyfluids/ionic.htm. Accessed February 20, 2008.

Referring to the case of the 70-kg woman (described in Box 2-1), assume that her serum osmolality is 280 mOsm/kg water. If a normal distribution of total body water is assumed, the solute content of each compartment can be calculated as follows:

Her total body solute content would be 280 mOsm/kg water × 35 L (1 L of water weighs 1 kg) = 9800 mOsm.

Her intracellular fluid solute content is 280 mOsm/kg water × 23.5 L = 6580 mOsm.

Her extracellular fluid solute content is 280 mOsm/kg water × 11.5 L = 3220 mOsm.

body water is distributed between ICF and ECF compartments so that the osmolality is the same in each compartment. Therefore, the plasma osmolality is a fairly accurate estimate of the total body osmolality.

The plasma osmolality can be measured directly or estimated from the following equation:

Plasma osmolality = 2 × (Sodium) + (Glucose in mg/dl)/18 + (Blood urea nitrogen in mg/dl)/2.8

The sodium concentration is doubled because each sodium ion is balanced, usually with a monovalent anion (e.g., chloride, bicarbonate). Although glucose and urea contribute to plasma osmolality, their contribution to the calculation is small compared with that of the plasma sodium concentration. Exceptions to this statement are the patient with hyperglycemia from uncontrolled diabetes mellitus and the patient with uremia (an extremely high blood urea nitrogen level).

Now we will consider the distribution of water between the intracellular and extracellular compartments. In the steady state, the osmolality of both compartments is the same, so the size of the compartment (or volume of fluid) is a function of how many dissolved solutes are in it (Box 2-3).

The solutes in each compartment generate the osmotic pressure. This pressure is created only by solutes that do not readily cross the membrane that defines the compartment. Solutes that freely cross the membrane (e.g., urea) cannot generate a gradient or osmotic pressure. When the solute concentration on one side of the membrane is different from the solute concentration on the other side and when the solutes cannot diffuse across the membrane, then an osmotic pressure gradient is established. Water will move quickly from the side of the lower osmotic concentration toward the side with the higher osmotic concentration until the osmotic gradient is abolished. Thus, the volume of a compartment reflects the percentage of osmotic solutes in that compartment and the total amount of water available (Fig. 2-2). In Section IV, the ways in which changes in compartment size occur will be discussed.

B. Movement of Water from Intravascular to Interstitial Space: The Starling Relationship

Fluid leaves the intravascular space as blood is forced through the capillary bed. This fluid bathes the cells and is picked up by the lymphatic system and delivered back into the bloodstream in the common thoracic duct. The capillary wall is the barrier between these two compartments, and the movement of fluid across this barrier is described by the relationship formulated by the physiologist Starling. This situation is different from the movement of water across the cell membrane. In a capillary, water and dissolved solutes move equally well across the capillary wall. The solutes do not generate any osmotic pressure because they flow with the water across the barrier. However, the plasma proteins (particularly albumin) do not move readily across the capillary wall. The plasma proteins, unlike the dissolved solutes, exert a force called *oncotic pressure* that retards the net movement of fluid out of the capillary.

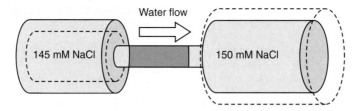

Figure 2-2. Diagrammatic representation of osmosis. When two compartments separated by a semipermeable membrane *(dark tube)* have unequal concentrations, only water can flow through the membrane to balance the concentrations of impermeant dissolved molecules. With this flow of water comes a subsequent change in compartment volume; thus, the two compartments that were once equal in size *(solid line)* have now shrunk or expanded on the basis of the presence of a lower or higher concentration, respectively *(dashed line)*.

The Starling relationship describes the net movement of fluid *(Q)* out of the capillaries by this relationship, which is known as the *Starling-Landis equation:*

$$Q = K_f\,[(P_C - P_i) - \sigma(\pi_C - \pi_i)]$$

In the previous equation, *P* is the hydrostatic pressure inside the capillaries *(c)* or the interstitial space *(i)*; π is the oncotic pressure; K_f is a permeability (filtration) coefficient that includes the porosity and surface area of the capillary; and σ is a reflection coefficient that relates the efficiency of the oncotic forces across this barrier. The forces that promote the movement of fluid out of the capillary are the hydrostatic pressure in the capillary and the oncotic pressure created by the tissue proteins in the interstitial space. The forces opposing this movement are the hydrostatic pressure of the interstitial fluid and the oncotic pressure created by the plasma proteins (Fig. 2-3). The coefficients vary depending on the location of the capillary bed and the presence of vasoactive substances that are present in certain disease states (e.g., septic shock).

In the next section are examples of how alterations in blood pressure and plasma protein content can affect the distribution of fluid in these two compartments.

IV. PATHOPHYSIOLOGY OF FLUID COMPARTMENT CHANGES

Before exploring the pathophysiologic situations that create changes in the distribution of body fluids, it is important to understand which clinical and laboratory techniques are employed to evaluate and monitor the contents of fluid compartments.

A. Methods of Monitoring Body Fluid Status and Distribution

To estimate the volumes of fluid in these compartments, the weight of the patient must be known. An estimate of the patient's body fat content is made and used to estimate the percentage of TBW (50% to 60%). This information and the assumptions outlined above are then used to calculate the compartment volumes. In patients with heart or kidney disease, the volume of the body fluid compartments may change dramatically in a relatively short time (days to weeks). In these

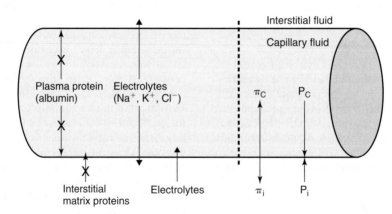

Figure 2-3. The Starling–Landis equation. The forces that dictate the movement of water between the intravascular *(c)* and interstitial *(i)* compartments within the ECF are determined by the forces generated by the impermeability of proteins (oncotic pressure, π) and by the space constraints inside and outside of the vasculature (hydrostatic pressure, *P*). The left side of the diagram highlights the permeability of the vasculature to small molecules and electrolytes and the impermeability of proteins. The right side shows the forces that promote and oppose the movement of fluid between the compartments.

patients, it is very important to know both the baseline weight as well as the current weight. Additionally, information from the patient's medical history is sought regarding the intake or loss of solutes and fluid. Together, this information gives clues to the volume status of the patient and establishes a comparison from baseline levels. However, more information is needed to determine how this actually affects water distribution in the various compartments.

To make use of body weight information, the concentrations of osmotic solutes in one of the body fluids must be known. Although body weight changes can indicate gross changes in volume distribution, the osmotic measurements give insight into which compartments are most affected. Remember that all body fluid compartments will be in osmotic equilibrium within a short time after perturbations. The osmolality of plasma is measured either directly or by calculating it from the plasma osmolality equation given previously. The plasma is sampled because it is easily obtained. The normal value is 285 ± 5 mOsm/kg of water. When this value is less than 280, there is an excess of water as compared with solutes in the fluid compartments. When the value is more than 290, there is a deficiency of water as compared with solutes in these compartments. Remember, these measurements provide information about the relative amount of solute and water in the body's compartments; they do not indicate whether the total volume of fluid or the solute content in the compartment is low, normal, or increased. Other pieces of information must be incorporated before that assessment can be made.

To assign meaning to changes in plasma solute concentration, it must be known whether the intravascular volume is adequate, decreased, or in excess. For this parameter, the physical examination of the patient is key. A patient with a strong pulse, warm extremities, and pink skin most likely has an adequate cardiac output and an adequate intravascular volume. A patient whose blood pressure is low or a patient who demonstrates orthostatic hypotension (i.e., whose blood pressure drops more than 10 mm Hg when the body position changes from lying to standing, with a compensatory increase in heart rate) probably has a decreased intravascular volume. The central venous pressure provides information regarding the volume of blood on the venous side of the circulation. By contrast, an elevation in blood pressure or the presence of pulmonary edema may be an indication of too much intravascular fluid and excessive amounts of ECF. One rapid test for this is checking for the presence of peripheral edema. This is best examined by pressing on the skin overlying a bony tissue (e.g., the shin in the lower extremities or the sacrum, depending on whether the patient is primarily sitting, standing, or lying down). A positive test depends on how long the skin remains indented after the application of pressure. It should be noted that edema in only one leg or foot is usually an indication of a defect in the venous or lymphatic circulation rather than of an excess of ECF.

B. Losing Fluid from the Body Compartments

Several things can happen when fluid is lost from the body compartments. One type of loss could be hemorrhage or bleeding from the intravascular compartment; this is the loss of isotonic fluid (salts and water) plus the loss of plasma proteins and blood cells. If the loss is large enough, there will be a tendency to lower the blood pressure (cardiac output drops), and, according to the Starling forces (i.e., a drop in capillary hydrostatic pressure [P_C]), ECF will move from the interstitial space to the intravascular space. Initially there is no change in oncotic pressure, but as ECF moves into the intravascular space, incoming fluid will diminish the concentration of plasma proteins, thereby decreasing the intravascular oncotic pressure (π_C). This will dampen the movement of ECF into the intravascular space. Note that, with blood loss, there is no change in the osmolality of the ECF, and there is no shifting of fluid between the intracellular and extracellular compartments. The fluid loss is therefore limited to the extracellular compartment.

Another type of fluid loss includes losses from the skin and gastrointestinal tract, such as from sweat, gastric tube drainage, diarrhea, and vomiting. In each of these cases, the individual loses fluid that contains both water and salts (predominately sodium), with lesser amounts of potassium (diarrhea) and protons (vomiting). The first consideration is whether the fluid lost is isotonic (the same ratio of salt to water as is found in normal body fluids) or hypotonic (relatively more water than salt as compared with normal body fluids). Sweat, for example, is almost always hypotonic, and it becomes more hypotonic (i.e., has less sodium in it) as the subject adapts to a hot environment. Losses from the lower gastrointestinal tract may be isotonic in the case of severe diarrhea (e.g., in a patient with cholera), but they are more likely hypotonic. The consequence of hypotonic fluid loss from the extracellular fluid compartment is that the depletion will immediately force the intravascular compartment to compensate, perhaps causing a reduction in hydrostatic pressure (i.e., lower P_C) and an increase in oncotic pressure (i.e., higher π_C). Similar to hemorrhaging or blood losses (as described previously), this will draw ECF from the interstitial compartment into the vascular compartment. However, because this type of fluid loss is hypotonic, the osmolality of the ECF (in both the intravascular and interstitial compartments) will tend to rise. As soon as it does, water from the intracellular compartment will flow into the extracellular compartment. Thus, both compartments (i.e., intracellular and extracellular) will share the water loss. The osmolality of the fluids will rise significantly (i.e., >5 mOsm/kg water) when total water loss exceeds 0.3% of TBW (Box 2-4).

A 90-kg man loses 2.0 L of sweat that contains 70 mmol/L of sodium and associated anions for a total loss of 280 mOsm. Before he replaces this fluid loss, what will be the size of his extracellular and intracellular fluid (ECF and ICF) compartments, and what will the serum osmolality be?

A 90-kg man has 54 L of total body water (see above). The fluid loss will come from this. Thus, the total body water content will become 52 L. The initial size of the ECF compartment is 17.8 L, and the ICF compartment volume starts at 36.2 L.

The osmolality of the body fluids will be the total initial total body solutes (280 mOsm/L × 54 L = 15,390 mOsm) minus the 280 mOsm lost in the sweat. The resulting total body solute is 15,110 mOsm. It is dissolved in 52 L of total body water, and the final osmolality is 15,110 divided by 52, which comes to 290.6 mOsm/L.

The total body sodium content will determine the size of this man's ECF compartment. He starts with a normal sodium concentration of 140 mmol/L multiplied by 17.8 L, for 2492 mmol of sodium. He loses 140 mmol (2 L × 70 mmol/L) and ends up with 2352 mmol. This is equivalent to 4704 mOsm (2 × sodium to account for the anions). Divide this figure by the final fluid osmolality of 290.6, and it will be found that the ECF volume is now 16.2 L.

The ICF compartment volume will be the difference between the total body water and ECF compartment volume (52 L − 16.2 L = 35.8 L).

Please note that the fluid loss is shared by all body compartments but that the ECF compartment takes a proportionally large share of the deficit as a result of the concomitant loss of sodium in the sweat.

C. Additions to the Body Fluid Compartments

Every day, fluids of the body must be replenished to counteract losses that occur throughout the day from excretion (urine and feces) as well as from the skin and the respiratory tract. Furthermore, the infusion of fluids may be necessary for gross losses, such as when hemorrhaging occurs. As an example (Fig. 2-4), what happens when a patient drinks "free water" or water without salt or solutes? Initially, the water is absorbed into the ECF, and this transiently lowers the osmolality of the fluid in the extracellular compartment. The decline in osmolality is transient because the water readily crosses the cell membranes until the osmolalities of the intracellular and extracellular fluid compartments are the same. The change in osmolality can be determined by measuring the plasma osmolality or by calculating the plasma osmolality from the known concentrations of sodium, glucose, and blood urea nitrogen (see the equation for plasma osmolality given previously). Because free water is being introduced in the absence of other electrolytes, one should see a reduction in the serum concentration of sodium. The net result is an increase in fluid volume in both compartments, with the ICF compartment accommodating 67% of the added free water and the ECF compartment accommodating 33%. An increase in the ICF volume will cause the cells to increase in size. If this increase in size is more than 5%, the swelling will disrupt cell function, particularly in the neurons. More severe swelling acutely will cause cells to lyse. Erythrocytes are particularly vulnerable to lysis in hypotonic environments. If the swelling persists, some cells regain their normal volume by expelling solute (potassium chloride) and water. The cells then become vulnerable to a sudden change in plasma osmolality from a low to a normal range (see Chapter 3; Box 2-5).

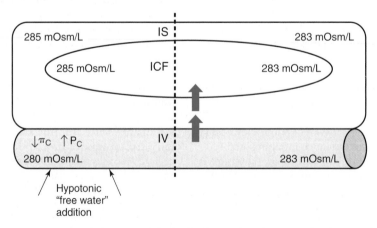

Figure 2-4. When free water is introduced, the intravascular *(IV)* fluid expands with water in the absence of solutes. *Left,* As a result, the water increases the capillary hydrostatic pressure *(P$_C$)* and dilutes the capillary oncotic pressure *(π$_C$)* and the osmolality. *Right,* The pressures rapidly equilibrate in the extracellular fluid by moving water and solutes *(arrows)* into the interstitial *(IS)* space. The osmolality equilibrates by shifting water into the intracellular fluid *(ICF)*.

Box 2-5. Example: Addition of Free Water

A 70-kg female drinks 2.0 L of diet soda in 1 hour without eating anything else. What happens to her fluid compartments and serum osmolality, assuming that, during this time period, the urinary loss of water is negligible?

Diet soda contains 2.0 L of free water and assorted artificial sweeteners and flavors. The free water will enter the extracellular fluid (ECF) and be distributed between the intracellular fluid (ICF) and the ECF: 1.3 L into the former and 0.7 L into the latter. There has been no change in the solute content of either compartment, so the water will follow the distribution of existing solutes.

According to the calculations given in Box 2-1, total body water was initially 35 L, and there is now 2.0 L more, for a total of 37 L. The ICF is 0.67 × 37 = 24.8 L, and the ECF is 0.33 × 37 = 12.2 L.

Let us assume that this woman's initial serum osmolality was 280 mOsm/kg water. Her total body solute content is 280 mOsm/kg × 35 L × 1 kg/L = 9800 mOsm. After adding the 2.0 L of soda, this amount of solute is now dissolved in 37 L. The resulting serum osmolality is (9800 mOsm/37 L) × 1 L/kg = 264.9 mOsm/kg. The serum sodium concentration will have fallen from near 140 to 132.5 mmol/L. This degree of change in serum osmolality would be associated with cell swelling, and it may be associated with neurologic symptoms (see Chapter 3).

Box 2-6. Example: Intravenous Infusion of Normal Saline

What happens to the body fluid compartments and the serum osmolality when a 90-kg man receives an intravenous infusion of 1.0 L of normal saline over the course of 1 hour?

From Box 2-1, it is known that this 90-kg man has initial total body water content of 54 L. His intracellular fluid (ICF) volume is 36.2 L, and his extracellular fluid (ECF) volume is 17.8 L. His initial serum osmolality is 280, and his total body solute content is 280 mOsm/kg × 54 L × 1 kg/L = 15,120 mOsm.

After the infusion of 1.0 L of normal saline, the total body fluid content is increased to 55 L. His total body solute content has increased by 280 mOsm and now equals 15,400 mOsm. The solute content of the ECF compartment was 280 mOsm/kg × 17.8 L × 1 kg/L = 4984 mOsm. Another 280 mOsm has been added to that because all of the solutes in the intravenous infusion will stay in the ECF compartment. Thus, the new solute content of the ECF compartment is 5264 mOsm. The percentage of solute in the ECF is now 5264/15,400 = 0.342 or 34.2% of the total body solute. This same percentage of total body water will now be in the ECF compartment: 0.342 × 55 L = 18.8 L. The ICF compartment will have the remaining 65.8% of body water: 0.658 × 55 L = 36.2 L.

In summary, the addition of normal saline by intravenous infusion added both solute and water to the ECF compartment, and it had no effect on the content of solute or water in the ICF compartment.

A different picture arises when a patient receives an intravenous infusion of normal or isotonic saline (0.9% saline; Fig. 2-5). Normal saline is an isotonic solution of sodium chloride that reflects normal plasma osmolality ($\cong$290 mOsm/kg). This addition increases the ECF volume. Unlike free water addition, however, the addition of an isotonic solution does not change the concentration of sodium and therefore does not create an osmotic gradient. As a result, there is no movement of water between the ICF and ECF compartments. Therefore, the addition of isotonic solution will expand the ECF compartment as a result of the increase in total body sodium while keeping the ICF volume unchanged. Other consequences of increasing the ECF compartment will be an increased blood pressure (i.e., increased P_C) caused by an increase in intravascular volume and, eventually, edema (i.e., an increase in interstitial fluid volume; Box 2-6).

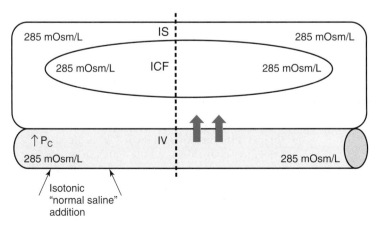

Figure 2-5. The infusion of isotonic fluids or normal saline into the body primarily affects the extracellular fluid volumes. *Left,* The increased volume in the capillary increases the hydrostatic pressure *(P$_C$),* but because the fluid is isotonic, it does not affect the overall osmolality. *Right,* As a result, the water and solutes *(arrows)* from the capillary *(IV)* rapidly equilibrate with the interstitial compartment *(IS)* and expand the extracellular fluid compartments. The intracellular fluid *(ICF)* remains spared because it does not need to equilibrate to any changes in osmolality.

D. Shifts in Fluid from One Compartment to Another

Glucose is another solute that is added to the ECF compartment in clinical conditions. It may come from the dietary intake, or it may be released from the liver's glycogen stores. In normal subjects, a rise in serum glucose concentration triggers the release of insulin, and the glucose is rapidly taken up and metabolized by cells. In patients with diabetes mellitus, the insulin response is absent or inadequate, and glucose cannot be transported out of the plasma. The glucose then stays in the ECF compartment and acts as an osmotic agent. In this case, the plasma osmolality is increased, and water shifts from intracellular to extracellular compartments. The serum concentration of sodium decreases as water moves into the ECF compartment and evens out the osmotic pressure. In this setting, glucose works as an osmotic agent; it will increase the intravascular volume, perhaps increase blood pressure, and increase renal perfusion and urine formation (Box 2-7).

Shifts in fluid volumes can also occur between the intravascular and interstitial compartments. These shifts result from changes in the Starling forces, which were discussed previously. The plasma proteins have an important role in determining the oncotic pressure of capillary fluid. A number of disease states (e.g., nephrotic syndrome, cirrhosis of the liver, severe protein malnutrition) can lower the level of plasma proteins, particularly albumin. In these states, the oncotic pressure in the capillaries is reduced, and the flow of fluid from the intravascular to interstitial space is enhanced. This condition leads to a shift of fluid in the ECF from the intravascular compartment to the interstitial one. The clinical manifestations of this fluid shift are edema (swelling, particularly of the legs) and lower blood pressure.

Increased amounts of interstitial fluid or edema may be expected in patients with hypertension, assuming that the increased blood pressure in the arteries is also present in the capillaries. However, this assumption is erroneous. The high blood pressure extends only as far as the arterioles. Elevated hydrostatic pressure in the capillaries occurs when the pressure on the venous side of the circulation is increased. Clinical situations such as cirrhosis, right-sided heart failure, and tricuspid valve insufficiency involve markedly elevated venous pressures. These conditions favor the expansion of the interstitial fluid compartment by promoting the filtration of fluid out of the capillaries and into the interstitial space and then dampening its return. In these clinical situations, peripheral edema is very pronounced, and it may be extremely difficult to treat.

V. SUMMARY

Water usually makes up 50% to 60% of the weight of a normal adult subject. This water is distributed between ICF and ECF spaces, with 67% in the ICF and

---

> **Box 2-7.** Example: Shifts in Fluids
>
> An elderly woman weighs 70 kg and has type 2 diabetes mellitus, and she develops a urinary tract infection. As a result, her serum glucose concentration rises from 100 to 300 mg/dL without any intake of fluid. Assume that her initial serum sodium concentration is 140 mmol/L. What happens to the composition and concentrations of her body fluids?
>
> From the data given, her initial total body water volume can be calculated at 35 L. Her intracellular fluid (ICF) volume is 23.5 L; her extracellular fluid (ECF) volume is 11.5 L; and her serum osmolality is 285.5 mOsm/kg.
>
> The addition of glucose to the ECF compartment raises the glucose concentration to 300 mg/dl (an increase of 11.1 mOsm/L). This change will raise the osmolality of the ECF, and water will flow from the ICF compartment to the ECF compartment. A decrease in the serum concentration of sodium should be seen.
>
> With the new equilibrium, it is found that the total body water is the same at 35 L but that the ICF volume is reduced slightly to 23.3 L. The ECF volume is increased to 11.8 L; the serum osmolality is increased to 289.2 mOsm/kg; and the serum sodium concentration is reduced to 136.4 mmol/L.
>
> **Calculation details:**
> 1. Determine the solute content in the ICF and ECF initially. For the ICF, $23.5 \times 285.5 = 6709.25$. For the ECF, $11.5 \times 285.5 = 3283.25$.
> 2. Add the additional glucose of $11.5 \times 11.1 = 127.65$ mOsm to the initial solute content of 3282.35 to get a new solute content of 3410.9 mOsm in the ECF.
> 3. The total solute content of $3410.9 + 6709.25 = 10,120.15$ mOsm is dissolved in 35 L of water. The new plasma osmolality is $10,120.15/35 = 289.15$ mOsm/kg water.
> 4. The new ECF volume is the ECF solute content (3410.9) divided by the plasma osmolality (289.15), for a result of 11.8 L. The new ICF volume is the ICF solute content (6709.25) divided by its osmolality (289.15), resulting in 23.2 L.
> 5. The new sodium concentration is the total sodium content ($140 \times 11.5 = 1610$ mmol) divided by the new ECF volume (11.8 L), for a total of 136.4 mmol/L.

33% in the ECF. The size of the ICF and ECF spaces are determined by their solute content. Sodium and its associated anions are the major solutes in the ECF, and potassium and organic compounds are the major solutes of the ICF. Water flows across cell membranes until the ECF and the ICF have the same osmolality (essentially until the equalization of osmotic pressure on both sides of the cell membrane occurs).

The ECF is divided into the intravascular and interstitial spaces, with 25% of the ECF being in the

intravascular space. The Starling forces of hydrostatic pressure and oncotic pressure determine the movement of fluid (water and dissolved solutes) across the capillary membranes into the interstitial space.

To assess the body fluid compartments, the patient's weight, the blood pressure in different positions, the tissue perfusion, the presence of edema, and the calculation or measurement of plasma osmolality must be known. It is also helpful to have information regarding the types and quantity of fluids and solutes taken in by the subject as well as about the quantity and types of fluid losses. The assessment of the patient's fluid compartments helps the physician to understand the physiologic basis for the perturbations and to develop an effective plan to correct them.

Clinical Case

A 55-year-old man has kidney failure and is receiving hemodialysis three times a week. He has negligible urine output, and he does not follow the prescribed dietary advice. He comes to the emergency department on the night before his next dialysis appointment with increased shortness of breath and the inability to lie flat. He has gained 6 kg since the last dialysis treatment. He has increased jugular venous pressure, rales in his lung bases, and pedal edema. His blood pressure is 160/90 mm Hg. His laboratory tests reveal a serum sodium level of 128 mmol/L, a blood urea nitrogen level of 80 mg/dl, and a blood glucose level of 98 mg/dl.

What do you think has happened to this patient's body fluid compartments since the last dialysis treatment to account for his symptoms and laboratory findings?

This patient has ingested excessive amounts of both water and salt since his last dialysis treatment. Because he has negligible kidney function, he is experiencing the expansion of his total body fluid compartments, as is noted by an increase of 6 kg in his weight. His difficulty breathing and his inability to lie flat are the result of an expanded ECF volume. This is confirmed by an increase in the jugular venous pressure, the blood pressure, and the pedal edema. The patient also has an increase in total body free water in both the ICF and the ECF compartments; this is demonstrated by a decrease in the serum sodium concentration.

Suggested Reading

Koeppen BM, Stanton BA: Physiology of body fluids. In Koeppen BM, Stanton BA (eds): *Renal Physiology*, 4th ed. Philadelphia, Mosby, 2006.

PRACTICE QUESTIONS

1. You have four types of intravenous solutions available to you. They are:

   A. Normal saline (0.9% sodium chloride in water)
   B. Half normal saline (0.45% sodium chloride in water)
   C. D5W (a solution of 5% glucose in water)
   D. D10W (a solution of 10% glucose in water)

   Select the best solution to use for each of the following patients. (Remember that, to restore the body's fluid compartments, what has been lost must be replaced.)

   A. An 80-year-old man with a recent cerebrovascular accident has been receiving tube feedings by nasogastric tube. Today it has been discovered that his serum sodium concentration is 148 mmol/L and that his blood pressure is 150/85 mm Hg.
   B. A 45-year-old man with alcoholism and cirrhosis has been bleeding from his gastrointestinal tract for the past 5 hours. His hematocrit is now 23%, and his blood pressure is 80/45 mm Hg. He is alert and responsive. His sodium concentration is 145 mmol/L. Packed red blood cells from the blood bank are on the way.
   C. An Army recruit from Wisconsin is undergoing basic training at a military base in Texas. After a day of conditioning exercises and drills, he passes out while standing at attention during inspection. No laboratory data is available, but the patient is quite sweaty, and his blood pressure is 90/60 mm Hg.

2. A 65-year-old woman has chronic congestive heart failure that involves both the right and left sides of the heart. Her normal weight was 85 kg, and it is now 95 kg. Her serum sodium was 140 mmol/L, and it is now 130 mmol/L. On clinical examination, the patient was found to have a normal blood pressure of 125/80 mm Hg, an elevated central venous pressure (by neck vein examination), and pitting edema (swelling) of her lower legs up to the knees.

   Select one of the following to indicate your assessment of the patient's fluid volumes and solute content.

   A. The ICF volume is increased/decreased/normal.
   B. The ECF volume is increased/decreased/normal.
   C. The interstitial fluid volume is increased/decreased/normal.
   D. The total body sodium content is increased/decreased/normal.

Disorders of Water Metabolism

3

Ryan Kipp
Peter C. Brazy

OUTLINE

I. Water Balance and Its Limits
   A. Input
   B. Output
II. Water Balance: The System
III. Assessment of the Patient
   A. Body Fluid Compartments
   B. Body Solute Concentration
   C. Renal Excretion of Solute and Water

D. Renal Excretion of Sodium
E. Water Deprivation Test
IV. Disorders of Water Metabolism
   A. Hyponatremia: Too Much Water Relative to Solute
   B. Hypernatremia: Too Little Water Relative to Solute
   C. Other Causes of Polyuria
V. Summary

Objectives

- Know the components of water balance (both input and output).
- Learn what controls the secretion of antidiuretic hormone.
- Understand how the kidneys make dilute or concentrated urine.
- Appreciate the interaction between circulating volume and plasma osmolality.
- Know the clinical conditions that are associated with excess or decreased antidiuretic hormone secretion.
- Be aware of the similarities and differences between a water diuresis and a solute diuresis.

I. WATER BALANCE AND ITS LIMITS

Human physiology depends on water. Water fills cells and bathes tissues, and water content and distribution are critical to the normal cellular function. Water removes wastes, cools the body, and facilitates secretions. A prime goal of physiologic systems is homeostasis, which is the constancy of body fluid volumes and composition. The processes that establish and maintain water balance are a key part of these homeostatic systems. In this chapter, normal water metabolism and clinically relevant disorders will be addressed.

A. Input

Consider the input of water into the human system. Fluids are taken in to quench the sensation of thirst. Sensors that detect an increase in plasma osmolality or a decrease in blood volume or blood pressure trigger the perception of thirst. Most humans also consume water and water-containing foods to satisfy taste, habit, and social custom. It should be noted that infants and those individuals who have a limited capacity to express or satisfy their thirst (e.g., those who are unconscious after surgery, those who have suffered a head injury, those with psychiatric illnesses) are more susceptible to disorders of water balance.

Daily water intake comes from beverages, from the water content of foods (approximately 50% of food weight is water), and from the metabolism of food (carbohydrates, proteins, and fats) into carbon dioxide and water. The intake of fluid is usually at least 500 mL per day, and it may exceed several liters per day. An average diet may contain 850 mL of water in the food itself, and it may generate another 350 mL of water from the metabolism of the food.

B. Output

The intake of water must be matched by its output to maintain homeostasis. The body excretes water as urine, sweat, water vapor in exhaled air, and gastrointestinal secretions. The amount of water that is excreted as urine each day can be seen and measured. The volume of urine produced depends on the amount of solute that must be excreted in the urine and how much the kidneys concentrate the urine. An average diet produces 600 mOsm of solute per day. If the urine is maximally concentrated at 1200 mOsm/kg, then it would take 0.5 L of water in the urine to carry away the 600 mOsm of solute. However, if the urine were extremely dilute at 100 mOsm/kg, then it would take 6.0 L of water to carry away the daily solute load. Thus,

the kidneys have a minimum amount of water that they must excrete each day to remove metabolic waste products and excess sodium. They also have an upper limit for the amount of water that they can excrete during a given period as a result of the limitations of the glomerular filtration rate and of the water that must be reabsorbed with solutes after filtration. The maximum amount in 24 hours has been estimated to be about 20 L of water for normal kidneys. If the rate of fluid ingestion exceeds that amount, the excess is retained within the body fluids, and an imbalance occurs (Table 3-1).

The other ways in which the body loses water are not measurable and are called *insensible losses*. The water vapor in the expired air of humans is estimated to contain 400 mL of water per day. The sweat from skin pores under normal indoor conditions is estimated at 500 mL per day. The fluid losses in sweat are quite variable and depend on body temperature (i.e., increased with fever) and the demands for body cooling during work or exercise. Additional water is lost from the gastrointestinal tract. This amount may be as low as 200 mL per day with normal bowel movements or as high as several liters per day with diarrhea or vomiting (Box 3-1).

Table 3-1. Urine Output

	Definition	Measurement
Polyuria	Too much urine	>3 L per day
Oliguria	Too little urine	<0.5 L per day
Anuria	No urine	<50 mL per day *100*

Box 3-1. Water Balance Sheet Example

A 90-kg man is eating a normal diet and producing 600 mOsm of solute. How much water must he drink to stay in balance if his urine is maximally concentrated (1200 mOsm/kg)?

Output	Intake
Perspiration: 500 ml	Free water: ?
Respiration: 400 ml	Food water: 850 ml
Stool: 200 ml	Food metabolism: 350 ml
Urine: 500 ml	
Total: 1600 ml	**Total:** 1600 ml

The intake of free water needs to be 1600 ml − 1200 ml = 400 ml.

If his intake of free water is 1000 ml, what would his urine osmolality be?

Total water intake would now be 2200 ml. His water losses other than urine would be 1100 ml; this would leave 1100 ml to be excreted in the urine. His urine osmolality would be 600 mOsm/1.1 L = 545 mOsm/kg.

II. WATER BALANCE: THE SYSTEM

A system of sensors, hormonal mediators, and the function of the tubules and blood vessels in the kidney combine to determine the amount of water that ends up in the urine each day. To understand the disorders of water balance, each of the components of the water regulatory system must be examined more closely. Alterations in one or more of these components cause the body to retain too much or too little water.

The osmoreceptors of the hypothalamus are one of the major regulators of antidiuretic hormone (ADH) secretion. They sense the sodium concentration and the osmolality of the extracellular fluid (ECF), and they stimulate the release of ADH (also known as vasopressin) when the osmolality of the ECF rises above 280 mOsm/kg. Above that osmolality, there is a steep positive relationship between ADH secretion and plasma osmolality. The system is very sensitive to small changes in plasma osmolality. Below 280 mOsm/kg, there is little or no ADH secreted by this pathway.

There are other sensors that affect ADH secretion. Primary among these are the baroreceptors in the carotid sinus. These receptors sense the "effectiveness" of the intravascular fluid volume. When the blood pressure is decreased by either heart failure or volume depletion, these receptors are activated. They stimulate ADH release via the parasympathetic afferent nerve network to the brain. ADH acts on a V1 receptor in blood vessels and thereby increases vascular resistance and blood pressure. Additionally, other stimuli of the central nervous system are associated with ADH secretion. Medical conditions that induce sustained nausea (e.g., chemotherapy) cause a release of ADH that is not mediated by demands for the regulation of plasma osmolality or volume. ADH secretion may be increased with lung disorders such as pneumonia or pulmonary embolism. These stimuli take precedent over those from the osmoreceptors so that ADH will be secreted in the setting of low intravascular volume, even when the plasma osmolality is less than 280 mOsm/kg (Box 3-2).

In the kidney, ADH acts on the collecting tubule via the V2 receptor to open channels in the tubule

Box 3-2. Antidiuretic Hormone Secretion

Factors that increase antidiuretic hormone secretion
1. Increases in extracellular fluid osmolality above 280 mOsm/kg as sensed by hypothalamic osmoreceptors
2. Decreases in actual effective intravascular fluid volume as sensed by the carotid sinus

Factors that inhibit antidiuretic hormone secretion
1. Increases in atrial natriuretic peptide levels
2. Alcohol intake

membrane. These channels, which are called *aqua-porins,* allow water to pass across the cell membrane (Fig. 3-1). This process can be altered by inherited disorders of the V2 receptor, by metabolic imbalances in calcium or prostaglandin production, or by the presence of specific pharmaceutical compounds that interfere with this process. Additionally, it is important to remember that ADH affects membrane permeability rather than the gradient for the movement of water. The effectiveness of ADH depends on the presence of an osmotic gradient for the movement of water from the urinary space to the interstitial space in the renal medulla. The loops of Henle and the vasa recta are responsible for the creation of high renal medullary tonicity and the maintenance of this gradient (Figs. 3-2 and 3-3).

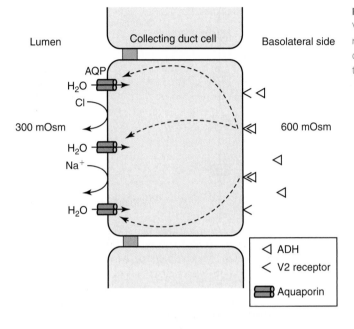

Figure 3-1. Upon activation by antidiuretic hormone, V2 receptors signal the placement of aquaporin channels into the apical surface of cells in the collecting duct. This allows water to flow down the concentration gradient, thereby concentrating the urine.

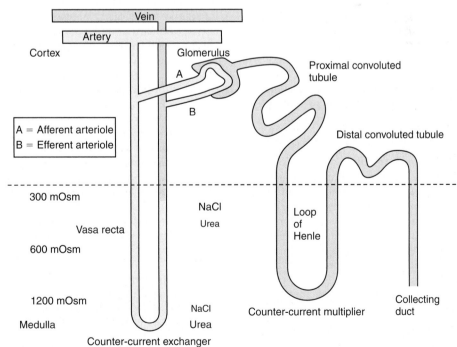

Figure 3-2. The concentrating mechanism of the kidney consists of the vasa recta, the loop of Henle, and the collecting duct. Sodium chloride and urea create the osmotic gradient in the medulla.

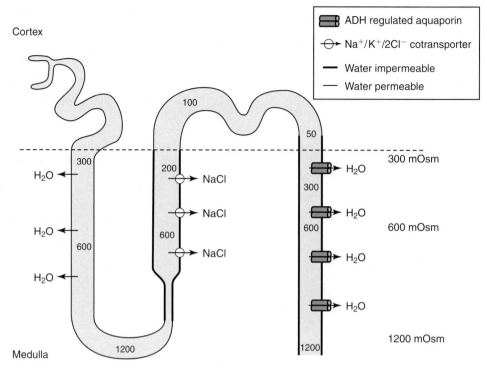

Cortex

ADH regulated aquaporin

Na$^+$/K$^+$/2Cl$^-$ cotransporter

— Water impermeable

— Water permeable

Figure 3-3. The counter-current multiplier of the thick ascending limb of the loop of Henle by reabsorbing sodium creates a hypotonic urine and maintains the medullary concentration gradient. The final urine can be concentrated by the action of antidiuretic hormones on the medullary collecting duct; the medulla is hypertonic.

III. ASSESSMENT OF THE PATIENT

As a physician approaches a patient with disordered water metabolism, it is very important to evaluate the components of the water regulatory system. This information is needed to make the correct diagnosis and to select the best therapy. It is key to determine the relative amounts of solute and fluid in the body compartments, the presence or absence of ADH, and the kidney's ability to respond to ADH.

A. Body Fluid Compartments

One of the first items that occurs during the assessment of water balance is the determination of the state of hydration of the patient; this assessment is discussed in Chapter 2. The object is to determine the adequacy of intravascular volume, the cardiac output, and whether the patient has too little, normal, or too much ECF volume. Knowledge of the ECF volume is combined with the measured plasma sodium concentration to determine whether total body sodium is too little, too much, or appropriate. The assessment of the adequacy of the cardiac output and the intravascular volume will provide a possible cause for ADH secretion. Remember, inadequate intravascular volume or cardiac output is a stimulus for ADH release.

B. Body Solute Concentration

Another early step is to determine the plasma osmolality. This parameter can be measured directly, and it can also be calculated from the equation given in Chapter 2 using measured values of serum sodium, glucose, and blood urea nitrogen (BUN) levels. The plasma osmolality indicates the relative amounts of water and solutes in the body (both ECF and intracellular fluid [ICF]). An osmolality of less than 280 mOsm/kg water means that water is present in excess of the available solutes. An osmolality of more than 290 mOsm/kg water means that water is deficient relative to available solutes. This measurement does not reflect total body water or total body solutes, only their relative amounts. Thus, this information is combined with the assessment of body fluid compartments to determine whether the patient needs more or less sodium. This assessment will be demonstrated in the examples that follow.

C. Renal Excretion of Solute and Water

The third step is to determine the urine osmolality. This parameter is measured in the laboratory. When the urine osmolality is less than the osmolality of plasma, the kidney is excreting dilute urine and getting rid of free water. By contrast, when the urine osmolality is greater than that of plasma, the kidney is excreting concentrated urine and generating free water.

The standard urinalysis measures the specific gravity of the urine. This determination gives data that roughly parallel urine osmolality. Dilute urine (i.e., with an osmolality less than that of normal serum) will have a specific gravity of less than 1.010. Urine that is similar to normal plasma osmolality will have a specific gravity of 1.010 to 1.015. Concentrated urine (i.e., with an osmolality greater than that of normal plasma) will have a specific gravity of more than 1.015. This correlation is upset by the presence of proteins and other substances in the urine that affect the specific gravity more than the osmolality.

D. Renal Excretion of Sodium

A fourth step is to determine the urinary sodium concentration or the fractional excretion of sodium. This factor is important if it is suspected that the patient has decreased ECF volume and the kidney is trying to retain sodium. A patient who has decreased ECF volume will have a very low urinary sodium excretion (often <20 mmol/L) and a very low fractional excretion of sodium. This information is important in cases of water imbalance, because these patients are also likely to have an elevated ADH level as the volume receptors activate the secretion of ADH.

E. Water Deprivation Test

A final maneuver is used to assess the possibility of the absence of ADH (central diabetes insipidus) or the lack of kidney response to ADH (nephrogenic diabetes insipidus). This assessment is the water deprivation test. The patient takes in no fluid or water after bedtime. The plasma and urine osmolality are measured with each voiding when the patient wakes up the next morning. The test looks for the maximal urine osmolality when there is a slight rise in plasma osmolality. When the urine osmolality stops rising, the patient is treated with an injection of ADH (vasopressin). The patient with central diabetes insipidus will have a limited rise in urine osmolality during the water deprivation and an increase in urine osmolality (>50 mOsm/kg water) after the ADH treatment. The patient with nephrogenic diabetes insipidus will have a marginal rise in urine osmolality with water deprivation and little or no response to the administered ADH.

IV. DISORDERS OF WATER METABOLISM

A. Hyponatremia: Too Much Water Relative to Solute

The normal balance between the water and solute contents of the body's fluids is disturbed when the rate of intake of water exceeds the output of water. In some cases, this is the result of the excessive intake of fluids in a manner that is not driven by thirst. For example, in cases of psychogenic polydipsia, patients have an uncontrollable urge to drink water, and the urge is not driven by the thirst mechanism or the need to correct plasma osmolality. Other times this sort of fluid disturbance occurs as a result of alterations in the kidney's normal physiology.

Hyponatremia is defined as a serum sodium level of less than 135 mmol/L. The drop in osmolality means that water is moving into cells and that they are swelling. If the hyponatremia develops slowly, the brain cells can correct their cell volume, and the patient may seem normal. Symptoms generally occur when the plasma osmolality falls to less than 240 mOsm/kg water (serum sodium concentration is usually less than 120 mmol/L). The special structural confinement of the brain within the skull does not allow the brain to expand when the brain cells swell, thereby leading to an increase in intracranial pressure and brainstem compression. The initial symptoms are changes in mental status with subsequent alterations in personality, lethargy, and confusion. If the plasma osmolality falls below 230 mOsm/kg, the patient will eventually develop stupor, neuromuscular hyperexcitability, convulsions, coma, and death. In clinical situations in which hyponatremia is likely to develop, the serum electrolytes must be monitored, with particular attention paid to the plasma sodium concentration and the calculated or measured serum osmolality.

The most common cause of hyponatremia is the presence of ADH, which blunts the excretion of excess water. ADH may be present for physiologic reasons, such as intravascular volume depletion (i.e., the activation of the baroreceptors), or it may be released for inappropriate reasons as a result of changes in the osmolality sensors or central nervous system responses to nonosmotic stimuli. When ADH is present, the kidney will produce urine that is not maximally diluted, and the retained water will lower the plasma osmolality.

When the laboratory evaluation indicates the presence of hyponatremia, the clinician needs to look for other solutes that may be maintaining the serum osmolality (e.g., glucose in the case of hyperglycemia) or the presence of an osmotic agent, which occurs with the intravenous infusion of mannitol. The osmotically active solute pulls water into the ECF space, thereby diluting the serum sodium concentration. At times when there is a great increase in the level of serum lipids (hypertriglyceridemia) or proteins (paraproteinemia), these compounds occupy much of the volume of the sample, so the sodium concentration in the serum may appear to be decreased if flame photometry is the method used in the laboratory. However, the serum sodium level in the aqueous phase of the plasma is within the normal range, so this condition is called

Hyponatremia with hypovolemia (decreased total body sodium)
- Gastrointestinal losses from vomiting or diarrhea
- Renal losses from diuretics or osmotic diuresis
- Aldosterone deficiency
- Fluid sequestration in third space in bowel obstruction, pancreatitis, peritonitis, burns

Hyponatremia with euvolemia (near-normal total body sodium)
- Hypothyroidism
- Glucocorticoid deficiency
- Primary polydipsia
- Syndrome of inappropriate antidiuretic hormone

Hyponatremia with hypervolemia (increased total body sodium)
- Cirrhosis of the liver
- Congestive heart failure
- Nephrotic syndrome
- Acute or chronic kidney disease

pseudohyponatremia. Other methods for serum sodium measurement (e.g., ion selective potentiometry) do not cause this difficulty.

Hyponatremia can be broken down into three separate categories on the basis of the volume status of the patient: hypovolemia, normovolemia, and hypervolemia (Box 3-3). The clinical cases presented in the following sections illustrate the pathophysiology, evaluation, and management of different types of hyponatremia.

1. Hyponatremia with Low Extracellular Fluid Volume
An elderly woman has a 5-day illness of nausea, vomiting, and fever. She is unable to keep much food down, and weak tea has been her predominant beverage. She comes to the emergency department weighing 67 kg (her usual weight is 70 kg), with a blood pressure of 110/70 mm Hg in the supine position and of 80/50 mm Hg in the standing position. Her pulse goes up from 110 beats per minute when supine to 130 beats per minute when standing. She is sleepy, but she can be aroused, and she makes appropriate responses to questions. Her blood studies show a serum sodium concentration of 128 mmol/L with a normal blood glucose level.

This patient has hyponatremia (sodium <135 mmol/L) and hypoosmolality (no compensating solutes). She has a low ECF volume documented by weight loss, orthostatic changes in blood pressure, and tachycardia.

To assess ADH activity in this patient, the osmolality of both serum and urine must be measured. In this example, the urine osmolality is found to be 550 mOsm/kg, and the serum osmolality is 260 mOsm/kg. The

patient is excreting concentrated urine in the setting of a low-serum osmolality. It is concluded that ADH is present and that the kidney is responding to it.

Why is ADH present in this clinical setting? The osmoreceptors in the brain should not be causing the release of ADH because the serum osmolality is low. However, the patient clearly has a decreased intravascular volume on the basis of the clinical demonstration of orthostatic hypotension and a decreased ECF volume on the basis of the change in weight. Thus, the volume receptors should be causing the release of ADH in this patient, although she has hyponatremia and a low osmolality. It is important to remember that demands for volume homeostasis take precedence over the need to maintain osmotic homeostasis.

With this information, it is clear that the depletion of ECF and intravascular volume should be corrected first with the intravenous infusion of normal saline (0.9% sodium chloride). Restriction of free water intake is also appropriate. This form of hyponatremia should be corrected in a few days.

2. Hyponatremia with High Extracellular Fluid Volume
A 47-year-old man has cardiomyopathy with severe congestive heart failure. He is on many medications, including drugs to improve cardiac muscle contractility and diuretics to enhance sodium excretion. His baseline weight is 90 kg, with a blood pressure of 115/80 mm Hg. He presents to the emergency department with shortness of breath for the past several days and swelling of both legs up to his knees. His weight has increased to 100 kg. His blood pressure is 100/60 mm Hg. Laboratory tests show a serum sodium level of 130 mmol/L, a BUN level of 75 mg/dl, and a serum creatinine level of 1.8 mg/dl. The osmolality of his serum and urine are 260 and 400 mOsm/kg, respectively. The urine sodium and creatinine concentrations are 15 mmol/L and 41 mg/dl, respectively.

The patient has increased his total body water by 10 L. His total body water content has increased more than his total body solute content because his serum osmolality has dropped from 280 to 260 mOsm/kg. However, he still has excess total body sodium because of the marked increase in ECF volume (edema of the legs). His effective intravascular volume (in the arterial side of the circulation) is low. His blood pressure is lower than normal, and the blood flow to the kidneys is reduced, resulting in an elevation in BUN and serum creatinine levels and decrease in urine sodium concentration. The retention of sodium leads to the expansion of the ECF volume.

The urine osmolality is higher than the serum osmolality. Therefore, ADH is present, and the kidneys are responding to it. Low blood pressure as a result of the congestive heart failure results in the activation of the baroreceptors in the carotid sinus, thereby causing the release of ADH and the retention of water.

The keys to managing this patient are to improve cardiac function and to restore effective blood pressure. An increase in the dose of stronger diuretics (e.g., furosemide) given by intravenous route can enhance sodium excretion. Restricting the intake of free water will help raise the serum sodium concentration. As in the other examples, this therapy requires close monitoring of the patient's water balance and of his cardiac and renal functions.

Recently, drugs that block the vasopressin receptors in the renal collecting duct and thus decrease the reabsorption of water (e.g., conivaptan) have been made available for clinical use in patients with heart failure and hyponatremia. They are effective for inducing aquaresis (increased water excretion by the kidney), and they are able to correct hyponatremia.

3. Hyponatremia with Normal Extracellular Fluid Volume

A 55-year-old man who weighs 100 kg presents to the emergency department with a 1-day history of confusion and being difficult to arouse. His blood pressure is 140/95 mm Hg in both the supine and upright positions. He has been eating and behaving normally up to the past 24 hours. A family member reports that he has smoked cigarettes for many years. The initial laboratory evaluation finds a lung mass on chest x-ray and a serum sodium concentration of 123 mmol/L.

Given the above information, it is likely that the patient has lung cancer. It is important to exclude a metastatic tumor to the brain as a cause for his altered mental status with the use of a computed tomography scan of the head. In this case, the computed tomography scan is found to be negative, so this patient's altered mental status is likely to be a consequence of hyponatremia. His urine osmolality is found to be 760 mOsm/kg, and his serum osmolality is 248 mOsm/kg. From these data, it can be concluded that the patient has an inappropriate level of ADH (or of an ADH-like molecule produced by some tumors) present, thereby resulting in water retention and hyponatremia. It is inappropriate because the patient has a normal intravascular volume and a low serum osmolality. This is an example of the syndrome of inappropriate ADH (Box 3-4). The rapid onset of hyponatremia is the likely cause of the changes in this patient's mental status.

The treatment of this condition can be challenging. The patient has excess total body water as a result of inappropriate water retention by the kidneys, although he has an appropriate amount of total body sodium. His symptoms of confusion suggest that he has cellular swelling in the brain. The goals for correcting the hyponatremia are to increase the serum Na concentration cautiously (less than 0.5 mmol/L/hr initially) and not to exceed an increase in the serum Na concentration of more than 8 to 10 mmol/L in the first 24 hours.

The main problem in this case is the inability to turn off ADH production. Therefore, the focus is on

Box 3-4. Disorders Associated with Syndrome of Inappropriate Antidiuretic Hormone

Malignancy
- Central nervous system
- Lung
- Gastrointestinal tract
- Lymphoma

Pulmonary disorders
- Lung abscess
- Pneumonia
- Positive-pressure ventilation

Central nervous system disorders
- Brain abscess
- Encephalitis
- Head trauma
- Meningitis
- Stroke
- Subdural or subarachnoid hemorrhage

Endocrine disorders
- Addison's disease
- Hypothyroidism

Miscellaneous causes
- Protein malnutrition
- Surgery

the kidney's response to ADH. The goal is to have the kidney excrete more free water (water in excess of isotonic saline) than the patient receives. To achieve this, the following is done: (1) the amount of free water that the patient gets by mouth or intravenous fluids is restricted, usually to between 700 and 1000 ml/day; (2) a diuretic (e.g., furosemide) is started intravenously to block the concentrating and diluting functions of the loop of Henle; and (3) the urinary fluid losses are replaced with normal saline.

Here's what happens. Furosemide blocks the sodium/potassium/chloride cotransporter on the thick ascending limb of the loop of Henle, thereby leading to water being retained in the lumen of the renal tubule and then excreted. This forced diuresis causes the concentration of solutes in the interstitium of the kidney's medulla to quickly decline until it has the same osmolality as the rest of the ECF. Then, even in the presence of ADH, the kidney produces urine with an osmolality that is the same as that of the glomerular filtrate (i.e., 248 mOsm/kg initially). Remember that ADH needs a concentration gradient across the collecting duct to reabsorb water. That amount of urine is replaced with normal saline, and this results in a fluid with osmolality of 290 mOsm/kg. In this way, the diuresis is sustained, and the osmolality of the body fluids is slowly raised. The serum osmolality is monitored every few hours to make sure that progress is being made but that it is not occurring too rapidly.

After the water balance is corrected, the second challenge is to maintain a normal serum osmolality in the setting of excess ADH. In mild cases, the same regimen of water restriction, furosemide (given intravenously for acute situations or orally in chronic ones), and a liberal salt intake may work. If that regimen is unsuccessful, the next step is to use drugs (e.g., demeclocycline) that block the action of ADH at the level of the collecting duct in the kidney. The drug blockade is usually not complete, and the drugs used may have untoward side effects. Thus, patients must be carefully monitored during this treatment. Specific inhibitors of V2 receptors (e.g., conivaptan) are now available, and they may be useful for counteracting the effect of excess ADH and inducing increased water excretion by the kidney.

It is generally considered safer to raise the serum sodium concentration slowly, especially if the hyponatremia has been present for some time and the patient does not have significant central nervous system symptoms. The too rapid correction of hyponatremia or the overcorrection of hyponatremia can be associated with permanent damage to cells in the central nervous system (i.e., the demyelination of the brainstem, including the pons); this condition is called *central pontine myelinolysis* or *osmotic demyelination syndrome*.

B. Hypernatremia: Too Little Water Relative to Solute

Hypernatremia is defined as an elevation in serum sodium concentration to more than 145 mmol/L that is caused by a deficit of intravascular water relative to intravascular solute. Hypernatremia is less common than hyponatremia, but it can be more serious. The symptoms of hypernatremia are similar to those of hyponatremia and involve central nervous system dysfunction. In hypernatremia, the shrinking of brain cells can at times result in the tearing of cerebral vessels with hemorrhage. The symptoms progress from confusion and increased neuromuscular excitability to coma and seizures. Hypernatremia occurs when the body loses water in excess of sodium and the subject does not have access to water. It can occur when both total body water and total body sodium are reduced or when total body water is decreased but total body sodium is normal or near normal (Box 3-5).

1. Hypernatremia with Low Total Body Water as well as Low Total Body Sodium

A 28-year-old woman ran a marathon and did not hydrate adequately. At the end of the race, she staggered and fell. She was taken to the nearby emergency department. Her body weight was reduced by 5% from 60 to 57 kg. Her serum sodium concentration was 151 mmol/L. Her urine sodium concentration was less than 10 mmol/L, and her urine osmolality

---

Box 3-5. Causes of Hypernatremia

Hypernatremia with hypovolemia (decreased total body sodium)
- Gastrointestinal losses from vomiting and diarrhea
- Burns or excessive sweating
- Renal losses from loop diuretics, renal disease, or osmotic diuresis

Hypernatremia with euvolemia (near-normal total body sodium)
- Central diabetes insipidus
- Nephrogenic diabetes insipidus
- Excessive sweating or fever
- Reset osmostat

Hypernatremia with hypervolemia (increased total body sodium)
- Hypertonic fluid administration
- Mineralocorticoid excess

---

was 900 mOsm/kg. She had a marked orthostatic drop in her blood pressure. Her pulse was 140 beats per minute.

It is determined that this is an acute onset of hypernatremia as a result of excessive water losses. The water losses are from sweating, which results in the loss of both water and salt. However, the loss is more water than salt. The woman's ADH system is activated by her hyperosmolality, which activates the osmoreceptors in the hypothalamus, and by her hypovolemia, which activates the baroreceptors in the carotid sinus. This results in the production of ADH, which causes the kidneys to retain water. This is evidenced by the kidneys producing concentrated urine.

The hypovolemia also affects the woman's kidneys, and this results in decreased renal perfusion. This leads to the retention of sodium in the kidneys, most likely through the renin–angiotensin–aldosterone system, and it is evidenced by the low urine sodium.

The treatment of acute hypernatremia and sodium depletion is twofold. The intravascular fluid compartment must be restored to maintain the circulatory system with isotonic saline, and the free-water deficit must also be replaced. Intravenous fluid (e.g., isotonic [0.9%] saline at a rate of 500 ml per hour) should be effective for correcting this patient's intravascular volume. After the first few liters of isotonic saline, if her blood pressure improves and her pulse rate falls, 0.45% saline would be given for the next few liters, and then treatment would continue with 5% dextrose in water. The patient's vital signs and electrolyte status would be closely monitored while watching for signs of electrolyte abnormalities or acid–base imbalances.

2. Hypernatremia with Normal Total Body Water and Sodium

A 55-year-old man has been taking lithium as a medication for bipolar disease for several years. He has required large doses, but he has achieved excellent control of the psychiatric symptoms. He now has problems with frequent urination and unquenchable thirst. He estimates that he drinks 4 to 6 L of fluid per day and that he goes to the bathroom every 2 or 3 hours. He presents to the clinic with these symptoms.

He has a normal blood pressure (130/80 mm Hg with no orthostatic changes), a normal pulse rate, and no peripheral edema. Blood tests show the following: a sodium level of 145 mmol/L, a potassium level of 3.7 mmol/L, a chloride level of 111 mmol/L, a bicarbonate level of 28 mmol/L, a calcium level of 9.5 mg/dl, a glucose level of 90 mg/dl, a creatinine level of 1.5 mg/dl, and a BUN level of 28 mg/dl. The evaluation of his urine shows an osmolality of 250 mOsm/kg and a sodium concentration of 33 mmol/L.

The physical evaluation of the patient indicates that his volume status is nearly normal. There is no evidence of decreased intravascular volume or increased ECF volume. The patient may have a slight decrease in intracellular fluid volume because his serum sodium is at the upper limit of normal. He does not have disorders of potassium or calcium metabolism or diabetes mellitus. Elevations in serum creatinine and BUN levels suggest that he has chronic kidney disease, perhaps as a result of lithium toxicity. The key element is the history of taking lithium, which is a known antagonist to ADH action at the collecting duct, as well as the frequent urination and thirst, which suggests dysfunction of the ADH system. The urine studies show that his urine is dilute, although the estimated serum osmolality is 305 mOsm/kg (sodium level of 145×2 + glucose [90/18] + BUN 28/2.8). This information is consistent with the absence of ADH action on the kidney (i.e., diabetes insipidus).

Diabetes insipidus can be divided into two categories: central and nephrogenic (Boxes 3-6 and 3-7). In central diabetes insipidus, there is decreased production of ADH from the pituitary gland. This may be the result of damage to the pituitary gland from trauma, compression of the pituitary gland from a malignancy (either primary or metastatic tumors), or a stroke. Nephrogenic diabetes insipidus results from either an inherited defect (X-linked recessive) in the V2 receptor in the collecting duct or from an acquired resistance to the action of ADH. The acquired form is associated with diseases that affect the tubule cells (e.g., polycystic kidney disease, pyelonephritis, postobstructive uropathy), electrolyte imbalances (e.g., hypokalemia, hypercalcemia), or medications (e.g., lithium). In the acquired cases, the defect may be incomplete or temporary. The signs and symptoms of diabetes insipidus (polyuria and polydipsia) may appear intermittently. Hypernatremia often develops when the patient is unable to drink sufficient water to replace renal losses.

A water deprivation test is useful to evaluate defects in ADH action. With this test, the maximum urinary concentrating ability of the kidney is assessed with and without the addition of exogenous ADH. First, the patient abstains from fluid intake overnight. In the morning, the serum and urine osmolality are measured every hour. When the maximum urine osmolality is reached (i.e., no further increase in osmolality is noted in urine samples or the patient has lost 3% to 5% of body weight), the patient is given a subcutaneous injection of 5 units of aqueous vasopressin (ADH). If the kidney can respond to ADH, a further rise in urine osmolality will be seen, and this indicates central diabetes insipidus. The lack of such a rise suggests nephrogenic diabetes insipidus.

One confounding variable is the role of the solute gradient in the medulla of the kidney. In some cases (e.g., patients with prolonged water diuresis [psychogenic polydipsia] or protein malnutrition), the kidney cannot generate a significant solute concentration of urea and sodium chloride in the medullary interstitium. Without these solutes in the medulla, the kidney's ability to concentrate the urine

---

Box 3-6. Causes of Central Diabetes Insipidus

Congenital
- Trauma
- Neurosurgery
- Malignancy; primary or metastatic tumors
- Granuloma (tuberculosis or sarcoidosis)

Idiopathic

Box 3-7. Causes of Nephrogenic Diabetes Insipidus

Inherited as an X-linked trait

Acquired with renal disease:
- Polycystic kidney disease
- Medullary cystic kidney disease
- Sickle cell nephropathy
- Medullary sponge kidney
- Amyloidosis/multiple myeloma

Temporary condition associated with the following:
- Postobstructive uropathy
- Hypokalemia
- Hypercalcemia
- Pyelonephritis
- Lithium toxicity

will be reduced. Hence, the increase in the urine osmolality will be less than maximal.

Although discontinuing lithium therapy may help with the recovery of the tubular response to ADH, other strategies could be used to reduce the volume of urine. The proximal tubule reabsorption of sodium and water can be enhanced by causing a slight degree of volume depletion with a low-sodium diet and the use of a low dose of thiazide diuretic. A change in the urine osmolality from 50 to 200 mOsm/kg implies a substantial decrease in urine volume. Patients with central diabetes insipidus may be treated with synthetic ADH (e.g., desmopressin) administered by injection or as a nasal spray.

C. Other Causes of Polyuria

The production of large amounts of urine (>3 L per day) is a symptom of diabetes insipidus. However, polyuria is a frequent manifestation of other conditions that arise when the kidney is excreting large amounts of solute or excess water. Polyuric states may be caused by water or solute diuresis.

Polyuria results, just as in patients with diabetes insipidus, when people habitually drink excessive quantities of fluids. This condition is referred to as *psychogenic polydipsia*. The ingestion of large quantities of free water will turn off the release of ADH, thereby resulting in a large volume of urine with a very low osmolality. The increased flow rate of fluid through the kidney leads to a reduced concentration gradient of solutes in the medulla. The patient will appear to have an incomplete form of nephrogenic diabetes insipidus when given a water deprivation test. If this condition is suspected, the patient should be kept on a modest fluid restriction and a normal diet for several days before a water deprivation test; the test will then yield a normal result.

Large urine volumes may be also be the consequence of the excretion of large amounts of solutes (e.g., glucose in patients with uncontrolled diabetes mellitus), the administration of exogenous substances (e.g., mannitol), or the use of excessive amounts of diuretics. Diuretic-induced diuresis would demonstrate significant amounts of sodium, potassium, and chloride in the urine, and it would quickly reduce the person's ECF volume and cause deficits in potassium levels.

V. SUMMARY

In most circumstances, people can maintain the balance of water in body compartments whether their fluid intake is unusually low or high. The body's system for handling water balance includes sensory mechanisms (osmoreceptors and baroreceptors), hormonal mediators (ADH), and an excretory organ (the kidney).

The assessment of the body's water metabolism requires knowledge of the status of the body's fluid compartments, the solute concentration in those compartments, the relative or absolute amount of sodium and water excretion by the kidney, and the kidney's ability to concentrate urine.

The two major disorders of water balance are hyponatremia (too much water relative to solute) and hypernatremia (too little water relative to solute). Each of these conditions may occur in the presence of low, normal, or high values of ECF volumes. Therefore, an assessment of the body's fluid compartments is key to sorting out these disorders.

Hyponatremia is caused by excessive fluid intake and/or by fluid retention. Excess ADH is frequently involved in fluid retention. ADH may be present for physiologic or nonphysiologic reasons. The latter cases are called the *syndrome of inappropriate ADH*.

Hypernatremia is caused by excessive fluid losses and the inability to take in sufficient water. The kidney is the source of excessive fluid losses in disorders called *diabetes insipidus*. If the pituitary does not make ADH, it is called *central diabetes insipidus*. If the kidney is unable to respond to ADH, it is called *nephrogenic diabetes insipidus*.

Polyuria (large amounts of urine) occurs whenever the kidneys are trying to excrete extra water (water diuresis), osmotic solutes such as glucose (osmotic diuresis), or sodium salts (diuretic-induced diuresis). These diuretic states are associated with losses of urea and potassium. By impairing the medullary concentration gradient, large urine volume impairs the kidney's ability to concentrate urine maximally.

Suggested Readings

Adrogue HJ, Madias NE: Hyponatremia. *N Engl J Med* 342:1581–1589, 2000.
Ellison DH, Berl T: The syndrome of inappropriate antidiuresis. *N Engl J Med* 356:2064–2072, 2007.

PRACTICE QUESTIONS

Conventional wisdom several years ago was that high school football players were to avoid drinking water during summer practice and to take salt (sodium chloride) tablets. This advice was given in the setting of workouts that induced voluminous amounts of sweat. The body's losses (sweat) contained more water than solutes (sodium), and the replacement contained more sodium than water.

1. What disorder of water metabolism is likely to occur at the end of a football practice session on a hot summer day?

   A. None
   B. Hyponatremia
   C. Hypernatremia
   D. Difficult to guess

2. What is the circulating concentration of ADH in an athlete who has just finished practice during a hot summer day?

   A. Absent
   B. Low
   C. Low normal
   D. Very high

3. What is the urine osmolality of this athlete likely to be?

   A. Zero (undetectable)
   B. Lower than that of plasma
   C. The same as that of plasma
   D. Higher than that of plasma

A 65-year-old man is admitted to the intensive care unit for increasingly difficult breathing. His family states that for the past couple of days he has been more confused than normal. He has a long history of cirrhosis of the liver, and he has been admitted in the past for gastrointestinal bleeding. A thorough physical examination reveals jaundiced skin and sclera, 3+ pitting edema in both legs, and ascites. His laboratory tests show a serum sodium level of 120 mmol/L and a creatinine level of 2.3 mg/dl.

4. Why does this patient have hyponatremia?

   A. Too much sodium retained within the cells
   B. Too little sodium in his ECF volume
   C. Laboratory artifact as a result of liver failure
   D. Excess fluid retention by the kidneys

5. What is the level of ADH in his serum?

   A. Decreased as a result of hyponatremia
   B. Low normal
   C. High normal
   D. High

6. What is happening to his kidneys?

   A. Decreased function because of chronic kidney disease
   B. Net sodium retention as a result of decreased kidney perfusion
   C. Cirrhosis of the kidney
   D. Excretion of excess sodium

Disorders of Sodium Metabolism

4

Claire Elliot Herrick
Jonathan B. Jaffery
Arjang Djamali

OUTLINE

I. Sodium Ion and Extracellular Fluid Volume
   A. Key Definitions
   B. The Importance of Salt
   C. Hypovolemia
   D. Hypervolemia
II. Sodium Transport in the Kidney
   A. Proximal Tubule
   B. Loop of Henle

C. Distal Convoluted Tubule
D. Collecting Duct
E. Tubuloglomerular Feedback (Autoregulation)
III. Mechanism of Action of Diuretics
IV. Regulation of the Extracellular Fluid Compartment

Objectives

To understand the following:

- The differences between salt and water content in the body
- Why the sodium ion determines the extracellular fluid volume
- How to evaluate total body sodium content
- Sodium transport in the nephron
- The mechanism of action of diuretics
- How the body regulates the sodium balance

Clinical Case

A 60-year-old man is admitted to the hospital after a syncopal episode. His wife says that he has been having diarrhea for the past 4 to 5 days. He has been taking lisinopril (an angiotensin-converting enzyme [ACE] inhibitor) to control his blood pressure for the past 5 years.

What is the most likely cause of syncope in this patient? How is his extracellular fluid (ECF) compartment as compared with his intracellular fluid (ICF) compartment? What about his urine sodium level? What is the best treatment approach?

I. SODIUM ION AND EXTRACELLULAR FLUID VOLUME

A. Key Definitions

Although salt and water balance problems are encountered almost daily in many clinical practices, few topics remain as frustrating for medical students.

Sodium ions are actively extruded from the cells toward the ECF compartment, which results in significantly greater extracellular concentrations as compared with intracellular concentrations of sodium (145 vs. 10 mmol/L, respectively). Therefore, total body sodium ions and the accompanying anions (chloride and bicarbonate) make up the large majority of solutes in the ECF space. This is why changes in salt content in the body manifest as changes in the ECF volume. Clinically, this is seen as volume depletion or volume overload. The assessment of volume status is a clinical assessment that is based mainly on the patient's history and physical examination (Box 4-1).

B. The Importance of Salt

Salt is vital for the support of the circulation and the perfusion of vital organs. Adequate amounts of salt in the intravascular space allow for the maintenance of blood pressure. Generally, in the healthy steady state, the body maintains a euvolemic condition, with neither too much nor too little intravascular volume. The kidney plays a major role in regulating this. In sensing inadequate volume (hypovolemia), the kidneys become sodium avid, aggressively reabsorbing sodium so that it is not lost in the urine. Alternatively, normally functioning kidneys will excrete excess salt in the urine as needed. Although most of the time the body manages volume status to achieve euvolemia readily, hypo- and hypervolemic states are among the most common problems faced by the clinician.

Total body sodium determines the extracellular fluid volume.

Total body salt and extracellular fluid are best assessed by physical examination and urine sodium concentration.

For example, volume/salt depletion is associated with the following:

- Orthostatic hypotension
- Tachycardia
- Low blood pressure
- Dry mucous membranes
- Weight loss (especially in children)
- Often a low-urine sodium concentration

C. Hypovolemia

In the absence of sufficient volume, tissues do not receive adequate nourishment. Clinically, patients may have low blood pressure (hypotension) or orthostasis (the blood pressure drops and the pulse rises on moving from a supine position to a sitting or standing position). In extreme cases, shock can ensue when underperfusion of tissues threatens to damage vital organs. Some common causes of hypovolemia include severe blood loss, profound gastrointestinal losses (i.e., vomiting, diarrhea), severe burns, and overdiuresis with pharmacologic agents. Hypovolemia, volume depletion, and low effective volume are commonly used to describe conditions that are associated with salt depletion and decreased effective circulating volume.

D. Hypervolemia

Excess volume can lead to tissue swelling, peripheral edema, and/or pulmonary edema. Excess salt in the intravascular space raises systemic blood pressure and can redistribute throughout the ECF space. Approximately 3/4 two thirds of the ECF volume is interstitial. Thus, in hypervolemic states, it is common for excess volume to end up in the interstitial space. Clinically, patients may have dependent edema (i.e., visible swelling of the tissues of dependent parts of the body, such as the ankles and legs when upright or the presacral area when supine). Patients typically describe this as being worse at the end of the day and improved or even resolved upon waking in the morning. In extreme cases, particularly if there is accompanying impairment of cardiac function, excess volume can accumulate in the lungs, which results in shortness of breath (dyspnea) on exertion, at rest, or when supine; crackles in the lungs on examination; and radiologic evidence of pulmonary edema. Some of the most common clinical scenarios include congestive heart failure, chronic kidney disease with proteinuria, and cirrhosis of the liver.

II. SODIUM TRANSPORT IN THE KIDNEY

The normal serum concentration of sodium is 140 mmol/L (range, 135 to 145 mmol/L). With the normal daily glomerular filtration rate (GFR) for adults at 180 L per day, this means that the kidneys filter more than 25,000 mmol (approximately 3 pounds of table salt) of sodium every day. This is more than 160 L of normal saline. If even a fraction of this were allowed to be excreted in the urine, the result would be profound hypovolemia or even shock. To avoid this, the kidney must reabsorb everything in excess of the dietary sodium intake minus what is spent on insensible losses. In general, tubules reabsorb the majority of sodium, and less than 1% of filtered sodium is excreted (fraction of excretion of sodium, <1%). Most (approximately two thirds) of the filtered sodium is reabsorbed in the proximal tubule. About 25% is reabsorbed in the medullary thick ascending limb of the loop of Henle, and approximately 5% to 10% of filtered sodium is reabsorbed in the distal convoluted tubule and the collecting ducts (Fig. 4-1).

The vectorial transport of sodium from the urinary lumen to the blood vessel via the tubular epithelial cell depends on two basic mechanisms:

1. The basolateral sodium/potassium (Na^+/K^+)-ATPase pump situated at the blood side of all nephron segments
2. The specific apical mechanisms in each nephron segment that allow sodium to move across the luminal membrane

Overall, active sodium chloride reabsorption by tubular epithelial cells is driven by the Na^+/K^+-ATPase pump that is present in all nephron segments. The activity of this pump is so important that it is responsible for the majority of renal oxygen consumption. The Na^+/K^+-ATPase pump uses metabolic energy that results from ATP hydrolysis to extrude sodium from the cells in the blood and to move potassium into the cell. The activity of this pump results in two

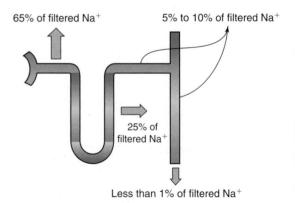

65% of filtered Na^+ 5% to 10% of filtered Na^+

25% of filtered Na^+

Less than 1% of filtered Na^+

Figure 4-1. Normally, nearly all filtered sodium is reabsorbed by the nephron.

mechanisms that facilitate sodium entry in the cell through the apical membrane: low cellular sodium concentration and negative cell voltage. Mechanisms that are specific to each nephron segment (described below) allow sodium to move from the lumen into the inside of the cell. The mechanism of action of diuretics is based on these segment-specific properties.

A. Proximal Tubule

The workhorse of the nephron, the proximal tubule (Fig. 4-2A), reabsorbs two thirds of the filtered sodium. Here, sodium is reabsorbed on the basis of its electrochemical gradient and coupled with other solutes, including bicarbonate, chloride, amino acids, and glucose. The overall reabsorption process is isotonic. The apical sodium/hydrogen exchanger plays an important role by moving sodium to the inside of the cell and extruding hydrogen into the lumen. The excreted hydrogen ion titrates the filtered bicarbonate, forming carbonic acid (H_2CO_3) in a reaction that is catalyzed by the luminal enzyme carbonic anhydrase. Sodium and bicarbonate are then functionally reabsorbed into the blood through basolateral Na^+/K^+-ATPase and the $Na^+/3HCO_3^-$ cotransporter. To this effect, intracellular carbonic anhydrase enzymes must first generate carbonic acid that then dissociates to form bicarbonate and hydrogen. The newly formed bicarbonate is reabsorbed by basolateral $Na^+/3HCO_3^-$ cotransporter, whereas the hydrogen ion is extruded into the lumen.

B. Loop of Henle

The loop of Henle (Fig. 4-2B) has several distinct parts. When learning about sodium and water balance, it is useful to think about the thin (descending) limb and the thick ascending limb (TAL). The thin limb has minimal sodium reabsorption, but allows for water reabsorption, resulting in a progressive increase in the osmolality of the tubular fluid. The TAL has different properties: first, it is impermeable to water. It also

contains the bumetanide-sensitive sodium/potassium/chloride ($Na^+/K^+/2Cl^-$) transporter. This protein reabsorbs all three electrolytes in an electroneutral manner, and this includes approximately 25% of the filtered sodium. By obligating the water-free reabsorption of electrolytes via the $Na^+/K^+/2Cl^-$ transporter (through a water-impermeable membrane), the fluid delivered to the distal tubule is dilute irrespective of the body's water balance. The remainder of the tubule is then able to adjust water reabsorption according to body's needs, as described in Chapter 3.

C. Distal Convoluted Tubule

This portion of the tubule (Fig. 4-2C), like the loop of Henle, reabsorbs more salt than water. Here, the sodium/chloride cotransporter reabsorbs as much as 5% to 10% of filtered sodium, with little water reabsorption. Consequently, tubular fluid that reaches the collecting duct remains dilute.

D. Cortical Collecting Duct

Under normal conditions, the collecting duct (Fig. 4-2D) sees only a small portion (2% to 5%) of filtered sodium. However, sodium reabsorption remains critical, because the loss of even a small percentage of the daily filtered sodium load could result in clinically significant volume depletion. To achieve this reabsorption, the basolateral membrane actively pumps sodium ions from the intracellular space into the blood, thereby creating a concentration gradient that drives sodium uptake from the tubular lumen into the cell.

Additionally, water permeability in this segment of the nephron is dependent on antidiuretic hormone. This allows for the excretion of dilute or concentrated urine, depending on the body's water balance (see Chapter 3). Remember, water balance is evaluated by measuring the serum sodium concentration.

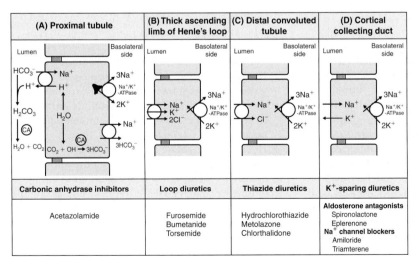

Figure 4-2. Sodium transport and the mechanisms of action of diuretics. *CA*, Carbonic anhydrase.

(A) Proximal tubule		(B) Thick ascending limb of Henle's loop	(C) Distal convoluted tubule	(D) Cortical collecting duct
Carbonic anhydrase inhibitors		Loop diuretics	Thiazide diuretics	K$^+$-sparing diuretics
Acetazolamide		Furosemide Bumetanide Torsemide	Hydrochlorothiazide Metolazone Chlorthalidone	**Aldosterone antagonists** Spironolactone Eplerenone **Na$^+$ channel blockers** Amiloride Triamterene

E. Tubuloglomerular Feedback (Autoregulation)

The goal of tubuloglomerular feedback refers to the regulation of the GFR in response to changes in the tubular fluid flow in the macula densa. When there is a decrease in GFR, the resultant decrease in tubular fluid flow to the macula densa will give a signal to the afferent arteriole for vasodilatation, which results in the increasing and restoring of the GFR. Thus, the role of autoregulation is to maintain not only the GFR but also the distal fluid flow. The consequence is to protect the body from excess sodium chloride losses. If proximal sodium reabsorption is decreased (i.e., diuretic medications block the tubular transport of sodium and other electrolytes), then distal sodium delivery increases. The distal nephron can increase the reabsorption of sodium in the face of increased distal delivery, but it has a limited capacity to do this. If this were to continue unchecked, vascular collapse could quickly ensue. To prevent this, cells in the macula densa sense changes in sodium and chloride delivery and signal the afferent arteriole to either constrict or dilate. This changes the GFR and thereby alters the filtered load of sodium. This feedback loop acts as a backup mechanism to prevent excess sodium chloride loss into the urine and to maintain the integrity of the vascular volume.

III. MECHANISM OF ACTION OF DIURETICS

Diuretics are medications that can increase sodium and water excretion in the urine. There are five primary types of diuretics:

1. Carbonic anhydrase inhibitors
2. Loop diuretics
3. Thiazide diuretics
4. Potassium-sparing diuretics
5. Osmotic diuretics

In general, diuretics act by inhibiting sodium reabsorption at various sites along the nephron, but each blocks a different mechanism for sodium transport.

1. **Carbonic anhydrase inhibitors.** Carbonic anhydrase inhibitors such as acetazolamide inhibit the activity of both luminal and cellular carbonic anhydrase enzymes in the proximal tubule (see Fig. 4-2A). This compound leads to sodium loss in the urine as well as to a loss of bicarbonate. Although the majority of filtered sodium is reabsorbed in the proximal tubule, blocking sodium reabsorption in this segment does not result in a very effective diuresis, because nonreabsorbed sodium is easily reabsorbed in later segments of the tubule. In addition, the resulting metabolic acidosis tends to abrogate the diuretic effect of the compound. These weak diuretics are used to treat metabolic alkalosis when chloride may not be given because of ECF expansion, and when the respiratory drive is compromised by metabolic alkalosis.

2. **Loop diuretics (see Fig. 4-2B).** The loop of Henle sees as much as a third of the glomerular filtrate, and it can avidly reabsorb sodium. The TAL, which is impermeable to water, reabsorbs sodium via the $Na^+/K^+/2Cl^-$ cotransporter on the tubular membrane. Intracellular sodium is extruded from the kidney epithelial cells into the blood via the energy-consuming Na^+/K^+-ATPase on the basolateral membrane. Loop diuretics (e.g., furosemide, bumetanide, torsemide) block the $Na^+/K^+/2Cl^-$ cotransporter. Although distal nephron segments may reabsorb some of the excess sodium that is not reabsorbed in the TAL as a result of the administration of loop diuretics, the general effect of loop diuretics is a robust natriuresis and diuresis. These medications are associated with an increase in urinary potassium, magnesium, and calcium loss.

3. **Thiazide or distal tubule diuretics (see Fig. 4-2C).** Compounds that inhibit sodium reabsorption in this portion of the nephron can have a significant effect, especially when used in combination with loop diuretics. In this part of the tubule, the thiazide-sensitive Na^+/Cl^- cotransporter reabsorbs sodium along with chloride and thus maintains electroneutrality. As in the TAL, excess intracellular sodium leaves the cell through the Na^+/K^+-ATPase on the basolateral membrane. Blockade of the thiazide-sensitive Na^+/Cl^- cotransporter is achieved by using a class of medications referred to as *thiazide diuretics.*

4. **Cortical collecting tubule (Fig. 4-2D).** Potassium-sparing diuretics—amiloride, triamterene, spironolactone, and eplerenone—act on the principal cells in the cortical collecting tubule. Sodium reabsorption in these cells occurs through an aldosterone-sensitive sodium channel. As noted, potassium secretion is needed in these cells to maintain electroneutrality. Thus, the inhibition of sodium reabsorption can lead to hyperkalemia. Amiloride and spironolactone decrease the number of open sodium channels. Triamterene also inhibits the sodium channel in the apical membrane of distal tubular and collecting duct cells. Amiloride is usually well tolerated clinically, with few side effects.

5. **Osmotic diuretics.** Mannitol is an osmotic diuretic. These agents are nonreabsorbable, and they inhibit sodium reabsorption in the proximal tubule and the TAL of Henle. Importantly, osmotic diuretics such as mannitol may lead to a water deficit because there is preferential water diuresis.

6. **The new steady state after diuretic use.** A new steady state commonly occurs after the initiation of diuretic therapy in which sodium intake and output are again equal but the extracellular volume has fallen as a result of the initial period of negative sodium balance. Diuretic-induced sodium losses are now counterbalanced by neurohormonal processes (mainly driven by angiotensin II and

aldosterone), which results in increases in the tubular reabsorption of sodium and water. Another counterbalancing mechanism is flow-mediated increases in tubular reabsorption distal to the site of action of the diuretic, because distal sodium delivery is enhanced. Of note is that loop diuretics lead to greater Na^+/K^+-ATPase activity in the distal and collecting tubules. Conversely, thiazide diuretics act in the distal tubule, and adaptation mechanisms are therefore limited.

IV. REGULATION OF THE EXTRACELLULAR FLUID COMPARTMENT

The regulation of total body salt and effective circulating volume is the most important function of the kidney. Effective circulating volume determines tissue perfusion and depends on plasma volume and blood pressure. Kidneys and neurohormonal mechanisms are closely involved in the regulation of effective circulating volume. The principal role of kidneys in this process is the regulation of urinary sodium excretion (Box 4-2).

1. **Renin–angiotensin–aldosterone system.** In the steady state, volume depletion is a major stimulus for renin release from juxtaglomerular cells. Increased circulating renin levels lead to the generation of angiotensin I, which is converted to angiotensin II through the actions of angiotensin-converting enzyme (ACE). Angiotensin II is a powerful vasoconstrictor that acts throughout the body, including in the efferent arteriole in the glomeruli. This leads to an increase in GFR. Angiotensin II also directly increases sodium reabsorption in the proximal tubule and stimulates the release of aldosterone (Fig. 4-3).
2. **Aldosterone.** The major effects of aldosterone are in the distal tubule, where it increases the reabsorption of sodium chloride (and the secretion of potassium) in the principal cells of the cortical collecting duct. Aldosterone stimulates sodium and potassium transport in these cells by increasing the number of open sodium and potassium channels

in the luminal membrane and the activity of Na^+/K^+-ATPase in the basolateral membrane. The main stimuli for aldosterone release are volume depletion (via renin and angiotensin II) and increased levels of plasma potassium.

3. **Atrial natriuretic peptide (ANP).** Atrial myocardial cells release ANP in response to stretch via volume expansion. ANP has two major volume regulatory actions: vasodilatation (leading to an increase in the GFR) and an increase in urinary sodium (by closing sodium channels in the luminal membrane of the papillary collecting duct) and water excretion.
4. **Arginine vasopressin (AVP).** Although its main role is to regulate osmolality via water balance, AVP also plays a part in volume regulation. Volume depletion serves as a nonosmotic stimulus for AVP secretion in an attempt to maintain volume in the vascular space, even at the expense of iso-osmolality.
5. **Aldosterone escape.** With high salt intake, aldosterone stimulates distal sodium reabsorption and potassium excretion. This initially leads to volume expansion and increased blood pressure. However, after a few days, natriuresis occurs as a result of volume expansion, which inhibits proximal sodium reabsorption and increases distal sodium delivery to overcome the distal aldosterone effect. A new steady state is then reached, at which point sodium intake equals sodium excretion and no edema develops. The result is a slightly hypervolemic clinical state, with a persistence of mild hypertension and hypokalemia.

In patients with congestive heart failure, two mechanisms may result in sodium and water retention by the kidneys. First, greater filling pressures in the ventricles result in increased venous pressure and the

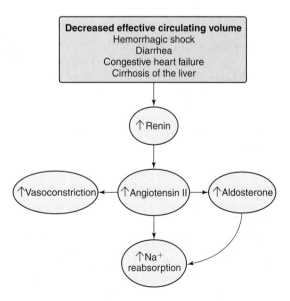

Figure 4-3. The effect of decreased effective circulating volume on the renin–angiotensin–aldosterone system.

movement of intravascular fluid to the interstitium. Second, the decreased cardiac output and arterial pressure and decreased effective circulating volume increases the renal reabsorption of sodium. The end result is identical with the development of edema.

In conclusion, the most important function of the kidney is to regulate the effective circulating volume by maintaining salt and water homeostasis. Total body salt content may be best assessed by clinical examination and urine sodium excretion rates. Nearly all filtered sodium molecules are reabsorbed in a steady state (fraction of excretion of sodium, <1%). Most of this reabsorption occurs in the proximal tubule, with the medullary TAL and distal tubules contributing to a lesser extent. Diuretics inhibit sodium reabsorption at the apical membrane, and they have specific sites of action in the nephron. A positive salt balance results in extracellular fluid volume expansion and edema, whereas severe sodium depletion results in a decreased effective circulating volume and hypotension.

Clinical Case

A 60-year-old man is admitted to the hospital after a syncopal episode. His wife says that he has been having diarrhea for the past 4 to 5 days. He has been taking lisinopril (an ACE inhibitor) to control his blood pressure for the past 5 years.

What is the most likely cause of syncope in this patient?

The patient may have syncope as a result of severe volume contraction (decreased circulating volume) caused by diarrhea.

How is his ECF compartment as compared with his ICF compartment?

The patient has lost isotonic fluid resulting from diarrhea. His ECF is decreased, and his ICF is probably normal.

What about his urine sodium level?

The urine sodium concentration reflects the total body salt content and is low (<10 mmol/L) as a result of increased tubular sodium reabsorption to conserve salt.

What is the best treatment approach?

The patient needs normal saline (isotonic fluid) to restore his hemodynamic status and to replace the isotonic fluid that he has lost.

Suggested Readings

Bichet DG, Fujiwara TM: Reabsorption of sodium chloride—lessons from the chloride channel. *N Engl J Med* 350:1281–1283, 2004.

Kumar S, Berl T: Sodium. *Lancet* 352:220–228, 1998.

Segal AS: Salty language is confusing. *Hosp Pract (Minneapolis)* 31:81–84, 1996.

PRACTICE QUESTIONS

A 63-year-old office worker with a history of congestive heart failure presents to your office with a chief complaint of shortness of breath. On physical examination, her blood pressure is 178/95 mm Hg, her pulse is 95 beats per minute, and her respirations are 22 breaths per minute. Her lungs exhibit bilateral basal crackles, and her extremities show 2+ pitting edema. Her laboratory tests reveal a sodium level of 132 mmol/L, a potassium level of 4.3 mmol/L, a chloride level of 92 mmol/L, a carbon dioxide level of 24 mmol/L, a blood urea nitrogen level of 11 mg/dl, and a creatinine level of 0.9 mg/dl.

1. The physical finding of pitting edema in the extremities is indicative of excess volume in which space?

   A. Intracellular
   B. Extracellular
   C. Intravascular
   D. All of the above

2. You are writing admission orders for the patient in the hospital. You can only block sodium reabsorption in one segment of the tubule. Which do you choose?

   A. Proximal tubule
   B. Descending limb of the loop of Henle
   C. Ascending limb of the loop of Henle
   D. Distal tubule

Pathophysiology of Potassium Metabolism

5

Kelly Ann Traeger
Sung-Feng Wen

OUTLINE

I. Physiology of Potassium Metabolism
   A. Potassium Intake
   B. Cellular Uptake of Potassium
   C. Excitability of Neuromuscular Tissues
   D. Kidney Handling of Potassium
   E. Potassium Balance
II. Hypokalemia
   A. Causes of Hypokalemia
   B. Consequences of Hypokalemia
   C. Treatment of Hypokalemia

III. Hyperkalemia
   A. Causes of Hyperkalemia
   B. Consequences of Hyperkalemia
   C. Treatment of Hyperkalemia

Objectives

To understand the following:

- The role of potassium, which is the major intracellular cation, in maintaining cell integrity, especially within the neuromuscular and cardiac systems
- The mechanisms that maintain potassium homeostasis
- The factors that lead to hypokalemia and hyperkalemia, including both nonkidney and kidney mechanisms, with special attention to potassium wasting and retention
- The pathophysiologic effects of potassium deficiency and excess on neuromuscular, cardiac, and kidney function
- The treatment of hypokalemia and hyperkalemia

Clinical Case

A 60-year-old man with a history of cardiac failure is hospitalized with increasing dyspnea, weight gain, and edema. He regularly takes digoxin, lisinopril (an angiotensin-converting enzyme [ACE] inhibitor), furosemide, and spironolactone. His blood pressure is 90/60 mm Hg, with a pulse of 90 beats per minute, and laboratory tests reveal an increase in blood urea nitrogen (BUN) to 60 mg/dl. His serum potassium level is 6.4 mmol/L. Previous serum BUN and creatinine values were 25 and 1.3 mg/dl, respectively, and serum potassium was 4.5 mmol/L.

Can you explain the increase in the serum potassium level in this patient at this time?

I. PHYSIOLOGY OF POTASSIUM METABOLISM

Potassium (K^+) is the major intracellular cation. Its total body content approximates 3000 to 4000 mmol (50 mmol/kg of body weight). Of the total body stores of potassium, about 98% is in the intracellular fluid (ICF) at concentrations of 140 to 150 mmol/L, whereas the extracellular fluid (ECF) contains only 2% of total body potassium, with the normal plasma potassium concentrations at 3.5 to 5.0 mmol/L (Box 5-1).

The ICF potassium concentration ([Ki]) is far greater than the ECF potassium concentration ([Ke]), which creates a steep gradient across the cell membrane. The potassium concentration gradient is maintained by the Na^+/K^+-ATPase pump, which actively transports sodium out of and potassium into the cell at a ratio of 3:2 (Box 5-2).

The ICF potassium participates in the regulation of many cell functions, such as protein synthesis and cell growth. The plasma potassium concentrations are maintained within a narrow normal range of 3.5 to 5.0 mmol/L through a balance of cellular uptake and the release of potassium, along with the regulation of kidney potassium excretion. As an example of the interactions between cellular potassium uptake on one hand and kidney potassium excretion on the other, in patients with diabetic ketoacidosis, ICF potassium depletion may be masked by normal plasma potassium as a result of a shift of potassium

---

Box 5-1. Distribution of Potassium in the Body Fluid Compartments

Total body potassium (100%): 3000–4000 mmol
(50 mmol/kg)
Intracellular fluid (98%): Close to 3000–4000 mmol
Concentration: 140–150 mmol/L
Extracellular fluid (2%): 60–80 mmol
Concentration: 3.5–5.0 mmol/L

Box 5-2. Key Facts about Potassium

1. Intracellular fluid potassium = 140–150 mmol/L
2. Extracellular fluid potassium = 3.5–5 mmol/L
3. Extracellular fluid to intracellular fluid gradient depends on 3 sodium/2 potassium-ATPase

---

out of the cells, which is caused by metabolic acidosis and hyperglycemia.

A. Potassium Intake

The average American diet contains 60 to 150 mmol of potassium daily ($\approx$1–2 mmol of potassium/kg of body weight daily). High-potassium–containing foods include citrus fruits, bananas, dried fruits (e.g., raisins), vegetables, and meat. Approximately 90% to 95% of ingested potassium is absorbed by the gastrointestinal tract and eventually excreted by the kidney within 6 to 8 hours. The remaining 5% to 10% is excreted in the stool.

B. Cellular Uptake of Potassium

In view of the small amount of potassium (60–80 mmol) in the ECF compared with the ICF, it may be surprising that a daily potassium intake of 60 to150 mmol does not cause a large surge in ECF and plasma potassium concentrations. This does not occur because ingested potassium is rapidly redistributed and taken up by the cells after absorption and eventually excreted in the urine to maintain potassium balance. Large changes in plasma potassium are initially blunted by the rapid cellular uptake of potassium through the action of the Na^+/K^+-ATPase pump at the cell membrane. This pump actively transports potassium into cells against a steep concentration gradient. There is also a passive potassium leak down the gradient through potassium channels as a counterregulatory mechanism. Factors that stimulate Na^+/K^+-ATPase activity to enhance potassium entry into the cells after the ingestion of potassium include a small rise in plasma potassium from gastrointestinal absorption, the release of insulin after dietary intake, and catecholamines (e.g., epinephrine) that may be released during stress. These factors promote the cellular uptake of potassium to

prevent a marked flux in plasma potassium levels. Other factors that also promote potassium uptake by the cells include aldosterone, alkaline pH, and cellular anabolic activity to incorporate potassium (Box 5-3). Because the cellular uptake of potassium only temporarily stabilizes potassium levels, the potassium load from dietary ingestion eventually needs to be excreted by the kidney to maintain potassium homeostasis (Box 5-4).

C. Excitability of Neuromuscular Tissues

The *resting membrane potential* is the voltage across a given cell membrane during the resting stage. In neuromuscular tissues (e.g., nerves, cardiac and skeletal muscle), it is determined primarily by the potassium concentration gradient across the cell membrane or the ratio of ICF to ECF potassium ([Ki]/[Ke]). The *threshold potential* is the potential at which an action potential is generated during depolarization. The excitability of the membrane is related to the difference between resting potential and threshold potential. Because the variations in plasma potassium will cause relatively large changes in the [Ki]/[Ke] ratio as a result of the smaller range of [Ke] as compared with [Ki], the abnormal plasma potassium levels are more likely to alter the excitability of the neuromuscular tissues, which leads to cellular dysfunction, changes in cardiac conductivity, and the weakness and paralysis of skeletal muscle. Therefore, the regulation of potassium homeostasis requires the maintenance of the proper amount of total body potassium and maintaining an optimal range for the [Ki]/[Ke]

Box 5-3. Factors Promoting the Cellular Uptake of Potassium

Plasma potassium
Insulin
Catecholamines (via β_2-adrenergic receptors)
Aldosterone
Alkaline pH of the blood
Cellular anabolism

Box 5-4. The Body's Handling of Potassium after Ingestion

Cellular uptake stimulated by the following:
Plasma potassium
Insulin
Catecholamines
Kidney excretion enhanced by the following:
Plasma potassium
Aldosterone
Distal sodium delivery
Vasopressin

ratio to protect the integrity of the neuromuscular function.

D. Kidney Handling of Potassium

Plasma potassium is freely filtered by the glomerulus, and most of the filtered potassium (about 90%) is subsequently reabsorbed in the first two segments of the nephron. Approximately 65% of the filtered potassium is passively reabsorbed along with the active reabsorption of sodium in the proximal convoluted tubule. Another 25% of the filtered potassium is actively reabsorbed in the thick ascending limb of the loop of Henle via the $Na^+/K^+/2\,Cl^-$ cotransporter. Thus, 90% of the filtered potassium is reabsorbed when the tubular fluid reaches the distal nephron. The eventual potassium excretion in the final urine (normal fractional excretion of potassium, 10% to 20%) is largely determined by potassium secretion undertaken by the principal cells of the cortical and outer medullary collecting tubules (Fig. 5-1). At these sites, active sodium reabsorption provides the driving force for the passive secretion of potassium. Sodium reabsorption leaves anions behind, thus creating a lumen-negative electrical potential. This negative potential promotes the passive secretion of cations (e.g., potassium) into the tubular lumen (Box 5-5).

Aldosterone, which is synthesized and released from zona glomerulosa of the adrenal cortex, also

> **Box 5-5.** The Kidney's Handling of Potassium
>
> Glomerular filtration (100%)
> Tubular reabsorption
>   Proximal tubule (65%)
>   Loop of Henle (25%)
> Distal delivery (<10%)
> Tubular secretion (passive, 10%–20%)
>   Cortical collecting tubule (principal cell)
>   Outer medullary collecting tubule (principal cell)
> Potassium conservation
>   Active reabsorption at the cortical collecting tubule and the outer medullary collecting tubule (intercalated cell)

plays an important role in the regulation of kidney tubular potassium secretion to maintain potassium homeostasis. The net effects of aldosterone are increased sodium reabsorption and potassium secretion in the distal tubule (Box 5-6). However, these effects depend on the adequate distal delivery of sodium. Aldosterone binds to mineralocorticoid receptors in the cells in the cortical collecting tubule to activate and increase the number of sodium channels at the luminal membrane. This in turn promotes sodium entry into the tubular cells. In addition, the permeability of the luminal membrane to potassium is increased through potassium channels, which results in potassium secretion in the lumen. Basolateral Na^+/K^+-ATPase synthesis and activity are also upregulated by aldosterone, thereby resulting in the intracellular movement of sodium from the luminal fluid, with potassium exchange (see Fig. 1-11). Overall, a favorable transepithelial, lumen-negative potential difference is generated by aldosterone to increase potassium secretion in the cortical collecting tubule.

A number of other factors also promote kidney potassium secretion (Box 5-7). Plasma potassium, when increased, can directly increase potassium secretion by providing more potassium to the tubular cells. It also stimulates aldosterone release to enhance potassium secretion. Distal sodium delivery and the rate of distal tubular fluid flow are also important factors that determine the rate of potassium secretion. When the distal tubular fluid flow rate is increased, secreted potassium is washed away more quickly, which helps to maintain the concentration gradient for passive potassium secretion. ECF volume expansion will deliver more sodium and

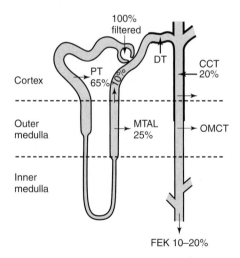

Figure 5-1. Kidney handling of potassium. Potassium excretion in the urine is largely derived from passive potassium secretion at the late distal tubule *(DT)*, the cortical collecting tubule *(CCT)*, and part of the outer medullary collecting tubule *(OMCT)*, indicated by the heavily lined segments. Active potassium reabsorption takes place during potassium conservation in the cortical collecting tubule and the outer medullary collecting tubule. *FEK,* Fractional excretion of potassium; *MTAL,* medullary thick ascending limb of the loop of Henle; *PT,* proximal tubule.

> **Box 5-6.** Aldosterone Actions on Electrolyte Excretion
>
> 1. An increase in potassium excretion
> 2. A decrease in sodium excretion

tubular fluid to the distal nephron to increase potassium secretion. However, ECF expansion also suppresses aldosterone release to limit the amount of potassium secretion. Therefore, the net effect will be an initial increase in kidney potassium excretion followed by a gradual decrease over time. Another factor that enhances lumen-negative potential and promotes tubular potassium secretion is the presence of poorly reabsorbable anions (e.g., sulfate, ketoanions) that remain unreabsorbed in the lumen of the cortical collecting tubule, thus creating a favorable transepithelial, lumen-negative potential difference for potassium secretion. In metabolic alkalosis, potassium enters cells and replaces hydrogen ions to maintain electroneutrality. This results in increased tubular potassium secretion. In addition, the delivery of unreabsorbed bicarbonate from the proximal tubule to the distal nephron during metabolic alkalosis also favors potassium secretion by promoting lumen-negative potential (see "Poorly reabsorbable anions/alkaline pH" later in this chapter).

E. Potassium Balance

Under physiologic conditions, potassium balance is maintained primarily by the regulation of urinary potassium excretion to match dietary intake. Fecal potassium excretion, which is 5% to 10% of ingested potassium, plays only a minor role under normal conditions; however, in patients with chronic kidney disease, colonic potassium secretion may increase to more than 30% of the dietary intake to maintain potassium balance. Normal kidneys have a large capacity to increase urinary potassium excretion to maintain potassium balance in response to increased potassium loads, helped by kaliuresis-promoting factors such as aldosterone and increased distal sodium delivery. Conversely, when potassium intake is reduced, potassium conservation by the kidneys may occur in 5 to 14 days, which is slower than that seen with sodium (2 to 3 days). Urinary potassium excretion is reduced to less than 20 mmol/24 hr, and urine potassium concentration falls below 20 mmol/L. This is achieved by reducing potassium secretion from principal cells and by increasing active potassium reabsorption by

H^+/K^+-ATPase pumps in intercalated cells of the cortical and outer medullary collecting tubules. Potassium conservation helps minimize the kidney potassium loss, but eventually hypokalemia and potassium depletion will develop if the reduced potassium intake continues.

II. HYPOKALEMIA

A. Causes of Hypokalemia

Hypokalemia is defined as a plasma potassium concentration of less than 3.5 mmol/L. The causes of hypokalemia in the clinical setting are listed in Box 5-8.

1. Transcellular Shifts of Potassium

The factors that promote the movement of potassium from the ECF to the ICF lower plasma potassium and lead to hypokalemia. These include alkalosis, insulin, and catecholamines. During metabolic or respiratory alkalosis, hydrogen ions move out of the cells in an attempt to correct the acid–base disturbance. This leaves an unbalanced negative charge within the cell. Because potassium is the major intracellular cation, it enters the cells to replace the reduced intracellular hydrogen ions to maintain electroneutrality (Fig. 5-2). This potassium shift into the cell may lead to mild hypokalemia. Insulin also plays a role in regulating plasma potassium levels. It is released in response to a rise in plasma potassium, and it stimulates Na^+/K^+-ATPase to increase

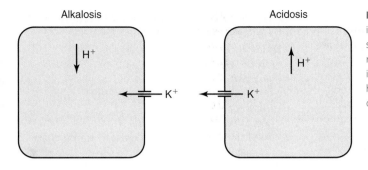

Alkalosis

Acidosis

Figure 5-2. Transcellular shifts of potassium during alkalosis and acidosis. During alkalosis, potassium enters the cell via potassium channels to replace hydrogen ion to maintain electroneutrality. During acidosis, as a result of the entrance of hydrogen ion into the cell, potassium leaves the cell to maintain electroneutrality.

the cellular uptake of potassium and to lower plasma potassium. Similarly, catecholamines (e.g., epinephrine) are released during stress. These act on β_2-adrenergic receptors to enhance potassium movement into the cells. Thus, the administration of insulin or β_2-agonists (e.g., albuterol) may lead to hypokalemia, and, indeed, these treatments are used for the medical management of hyperkalemia. In familial hypokalemic periodic paralysis, which is an inherited disorder, intermittent attacks of skeletal muscle paralysis occur with consequent hypokalemia caused by a shift of plasma potassium into cells.

2. Gastrointestinal Loss of Potassium

A severe reduction in dietary potassium intake, as is seen in patients with alcoholism or anorexia nervosa, leads to hypokalemia and potassium depletion. This cannot be compensated for completely by kidney potassium conservation, and hypokalemia ensues. During vomiting or gastric drainage, the route of potassium loss is more from the kidney than from the gastric juice. This is because the gastric juice contains only 5 to 10 mmol/L of potassium, and its loss during vomiting is relatively limited. The mechanisms of kidney loss of potassium during vomiting involve multiple factors. The development of metabolic alkalosis promotes kidney tubular potassium secretion directly by the entrance of potassium into tubular cells to enhance secretion and indirectly by delivering bicarbonate to the distal nephron for potassium secretion. Vomiting also leads to ECF volume contraction, which stimulates aldosterone release to increase kidney potassium secretion.

Although colonic fluid may contain up to 75 to 80 mmol/L from colonic potassium secretion, fecal potassium loss is minimal under normal conditions as a result of low fecal volume. With diarrhea, however, the increased fecal volume may lead to the significant excretion of potassium and other electrolytes. Laxative abuse induces hypokalemia through a similar mechanism. Moreover, aldosterone secretion resulting from decreased ECF volume will lead to an increase in potassium excretion.

3. Kidney Loss of Potassium

Kidney tubular potassium secretion is enhanced by factors such as sodium delivery to the distal nephron, aldosterone, poorly reabsorbable anions, and metabolic alkalosis. Therefore, the cases of hypokalemia as a result of kidney loss are usually based on these underlying mechanisms.

A. Increase in Distal Sodium Delivery

Diuretics such as thiazides and loop diuretics (e.g., furosemide, ethacrynic acid) inhibit sodium and chloride reabsorption at the distal convoluted tubule and at the ascending limb of the loop of Henle, respectively. Thiazides inhibit the Na^+/Cl^- cotransporter, and loop diuretics inhibit the $Na^+/K^+/2Cl^-$ cotransporter. Therefore, they increase the delivery of sodium and fluid to further distal nephron to enhance tubular potassium secretion, thus leading to hypokalemia. In addition, these diuretics also cause ECF volume contraction from sodium and fluid loss that stimulates aldosterone release to enhance kidney tubular potassium secretion. There are also hereditary clinical disorders that are related to the mutations of the transporters at these sites. Mutations in the $Na^+/K^+/2Cl^-$ cotransporter at the thick ascending limb of the loop of Henle are associated with Bartter syndrome. In Gitelman syndrome, the Na^+/Cl^- cotransporter at the distal convoluted tubule is impaired from mutations. These syndromes mimic the effects of loop diuretics and thiazide diuretics, respectively.

B. Mineralocorticoid Excess

In primary hyperaldosteronism, which is usually caused by an aldosterone-secreting adrenal adenoma, autonomous aldosterone production leads to hypertension from ECF volume expansion caused by aldosterone-stimulated distal sodium reabsorption. Hypokalemia is a common manifestation of primary hyperaldosteronism that is caused by enhanced kidney tubular potassium secretion by the action of aldosterone. In secondary hyperaldosteronism (e.g., renal artery stenosis), the renin–angiotensin–aldosterone system is stimulated in the affected kidney, which leads to renovascular hypertension and hypokalemia.

C. Poorly Reabsorbable Anions/Alkaline pH

The presence of bicarbonate and poorly reabsorbable anions (e.g., sulfate, ketoanions) in the lumen of the distal nephron promotes potassium secretion. They lead to the generation of a negative electrical potential from sodium reabsorption, with unreabsorbed anions left behind in the tubular lumen. In proximal renal tubular acidosis (type II RTA), filtered bicarbonate escapes reabsorption in the proximal tubule. The delivery of bicarbonate to the distal nephron leads to increased potassium secretion and hypokalemia in a type II RTA. In a type I RTA, reduced hydrogen ion secretion into the tubular lumen is compensated for by increased potassium secretion to maintain electroneutrality. In metabolic alkalosis, excess filtered bicarbonate exceeds the reabsorptive capacity of the proximal tubule and is delivered to the distal nephron to promote potassium secretion. In addition, metabolic alkalosis results in the movement of potassium into the tubular cells to replace the reduced intracellular hydrogen ion to maintain electroneutrality (see Chapter 6).

Acute metabolic acidosis reduces tubular potassium secretion by inhibiting basolateral Na^+/K^+-ATPase and lowering luminal potassium permeability. However, chronic metabolic acidosis is usually associated with increased kidney excretion of potassium. This is because most patients with chronic metabolic acidoses have additional kaliuresis-promoting factors evident. In diabetic ketoacidosis, a large quantity of poorly reabsorbable ketoanions are filtered by the glomerulus and delivered to the distal nephron, which results in increased kidney tubular potassium secretion from the lumen-negative potential. In addition, the osmotic diuresis from hyperglycemia and glycosuria also promotes kidney potassium loss by delivering more sodium and fluid to the distal nephron. The diuresis leads to volume depletion that stimulates aldosterone release, thereby furthering the kidney potassium loss. However, the potassium depletion common to these patients may be masked by metabolic acidosis, severe hyperglycemia, and insulin deficiency. Each of these leads to a shift of potassium out of the cells, and this may raise plasma potassium to normal levels, despite intracellular potassium depletion. Thus, plasma potassium may deviate from the true state of total body potassium in certain clinical conditions.

B. Consequences of Hypokalemia (Box 5-9)

1. Neuromuscular Function

Hypokalemia, especially when plasma levels are below 3.0 mmol/L, may be associated with symptoms of muscular weakness, fatigue, general malaise, and myalgia. In severe cases of potassium depletion, muscular paralysis and rhabdomyolysis may occur. The effect of hypokalemia on neuromuscular function is determined primarily by alterations in the membrane

---

Box 5-9. Consequences of Hypokalemia

Neuromuscular function
  Muscle weakness, myalgia
  Paralysis
  Rhabdomyolysis
Cardiac complications
  Electrocardiographic changes
  • ST-segment depression, flattened T waves, prominent U waves
  • Ventricular arrhythmias
Metabolic effects
  Carbohydrate intolerance
  Stimulated renin–angiotensin, low aldosterone
  Growth retardation
Kidney effects
  Thirst, polydipsia
  Concentrating defect, polyuria, nephrogenic diabetes insipidus
  Increased ammonia production, metabolic alkalosis
  Kidney potassium conservation
Kidney pathology
  • Vacuolization of the tubule
  • Chronic progressive kidney disease

---

potential. Hypokalemia results in the hyperpolarization of the membrane. These raise the threshold for initiating an action potential, thereby leading to muscular weakness. With more severe hypokalemia, sodium channels in the membrane may also be inactivated, which results in paralysis.

During exercise, local levels of potassium in skeletal muscle increase to maintain vasodilatation, which is a requirement for the adequate perfusion of the muscles. Therefore, potassium depletion may predispose an individual to the development of muscle ischemia during exercise. Muscle ischemia leads to the depletion of energy, the loss of cellular integrity, and, in severe cases, rhabdomyolysis.

2. Cardiac Complications

Plasma potassium levels of less than 3.0 mmol/L are frequently associated with changes in electrocardiograms (ECGs). Hypokalemia leads to the hyperpolarization of the cardiac cell membrane and delayed ventricular repolarization, which results in prominent U waves. The ECG changes of hypokalemia typically show ST-segment depression, flattened T waves, and prominent U waves (Fig. 5-3). The prominent U waves may appear as the apparent or actual prolongation of QT intervals. The prolonged QT intervals predispose hypokalemic patients to ventricular instability with arrhythmias such as premature ventricular beats and, in patients with preexisting cardiac diseases, potentially life-threatening ventricular tachycardia or fibrillation. An ECG should therefore be performed when severe

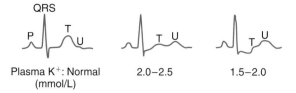

QRS

Plasma K+: Normal   2.0–2.5   1.5–2.0
(mmol/L)

Figure 5-3. Electrocardiographic changes in hypokalemia. Suppressed ST segments, flattened T waves, and prominent U waves are the characteristic patterns of hypokalemia.

hypokalemia is present. Hypokalemia also predisposes cardiac patients to digitalis toxicity and should be corrected in patients when initiating treatment with this medication.

3. Metabolic Effects

Patients with hypokalemia tend to develop carbohydrate intolerance. Hyperkalemia stimulates insulin release, whereas hypokalemia mildly inhibits insulin release. Therefore, hypokalemia blunts insulin secretion in response to the rise in blood glucose levels, which leads to carbohydrate intolerance. Hypokalemia also stimulates renin synthesis with an increase in angiotensin II, but with reduced aldosterone levels. This is because potassium directly stimulates aldosterone production, and therefore hypokalemia suppresses plasma aldosterone.

Because potassium is an important component of intracellular ions, it is an important element in tissue growth. Therefore, potassium depletion is associated with growth retardation and failure to thrive in children.

4. Kidney Effects

Potassium depletion stimulates thirst and impairs urinary concentrating mechanisms. This is manifested as polyuria, polydipsia, and, in severe cases, nephrogenic diabetes insipidus. The urinary concentrating defect is the result of the disruption of the countercurrent multiplier system of the loop of Henle. Hypokalemia also inhibits sodium chloride reabsorption at the thick ascending limb of the loop of Henle. Hypokalemia can induce metabolic alkalosis from increased kidney ammonia production. The latter is stimulated by intracellular acidosis in the proximal tubule where ammonia is produced, and this is caused by the cellular entry of hydrogen ion to replace potassium (see Chapter 6). Increased ammonia production leads to an increase in urinary ammonium and acid excretion and results in the development of metabolic alkalosis.

When hypokalemia is a result of nonkidney potassium loss, kidney conservation of potassium occurs after a period of 5 to 14 days. Urinary potassium excretion is reduced to less than 20 mmol/day or fractional potassium excretion to less than 6%. When

hypokalemia is a result of kidney losses, urinary potassium excretion will be more than 20 mmol/day and fractional excretion of potassium more than 10%. These parameters can be used to differentiate between kidney and nonkidney causes of potassium loss (Table 5-1).

Potassium depletion is associated with proximal and distal tubular cell degeneration with vacuolization. In patients with severe chronic potassium depletion, chronic progressive kidney disease may develop, and, in rare instances, kidney failure may ensue.

C. Treatment of Hypokalemia (Box 5-10)

In mild hypokalemia with plasma potassium at or slightly below 3.5 mmol/L, conservative management with the dietary supplementation of potassium-rich fruits and vegetables may suffice. However, potassium replacement with potassium salts is usually needed in patients with significant degrees of hypokalemia. Potassium replacement may be carried out using oral or intravenous routes. In cases of severe potassium depletion, potassium chloride may be given intravenously at a slow rate (not to exceed 10–20 mmol/hr), with ECG monitoring and frequent measurements of plasma potassium to avoid cardiac toxicity or overcorrection.

In patients with hypokalemia and hypochloremic metabolic alkalosis, potassium chloride should be used for the replacement of both potassium and chloride. Potassium bicarbonate and organic salts of potassium are a poor choice because the bicarbonate from these compounds will worsen alkalosis and

Table 5-1. FEK for Determining the Cause of Hypokalemia

FEK	Source of potassium losses
>10%	Kidney losses
<6%	Nonkidney losses

Box 5-10. Treatment of Hypokalemia

Dietary potassium supplement
Potassium salts used:
   Hypokalemia with metabolic alkalosis: potassium chloride
   Hypokalemia with metabolic acidosis: potassium bicarbonate, citrate, or other organic salts
   Intravenous rate of potassium chloride: up to 10–20 mmol/hr with electrocardiogram monitoring and frequent measurements of plasma potassium

increase the kidney loss of potassium. Alternatively, in patients with hypokalemia and hyperchloremic metabolic acidosis (e.g., patients with RTAs), potassium citrate or potassium bicarbonate is the preferred method of replacement to provide both potassium and bicarbonate.

III. HYPERKALEMIA

A. Causes of Hyperkalemia

Hyperkalemia is defined as a plasma potassium level of more than 5.0 mmol/L (Box 5-11). Pseudohyperkalemia needs to be ruled out before true hyperkalemia is considered. Hemolyzed blood and the tight or prolonged application of a tourniquet during a blood draw may result in a spuriously high plasma potassium level as a result of the release of potassium from the blood cells or the muscle. Whenever there is the potential for pseudohyperkalemia, the blood sampling should be repeated for confirmation.

1. Transcellular Shifts of Potassium

During metabolic or respiratory acidosis, hydrogen ions enter cells to increase plasma pH, and potassium moves out of the cells to maintain electroneutrality. This results in hyperkalemia (see Fig. 5-2). Hyperglycemia, which exerts a hyperosmotic effect in the plasma, also draws potassium out of the cells by shifting from ICF that is rich in potassium. In diabetic patients, insulin deficiency or resistance prevents the counterbalancing action of insulin on the

potassium shift that is caused by hyperglycemia and results in hyperkalemia. The use of drugs to block the β-adrenergic pathway (β-blockers) also increases potassium shift out the cells and may cause a modest rise in plasma potassium. Severe exercise, massive trauma, or tissue necrosis may also cause hyperkalemia from the cellular release of potassium, especially when there is an impairment of the kidney function. In familial hyperkalemic periodic paralysis, which is a hereditary disorder, intermittent attacks of skeletal muscle paralysis are associated with hyperkalemic episodes as a result of a shift of potassium out of the cells.

2. Increased Potassium Intake

The increased oral intake of potassium rarely causes hyperkalemia under normal conditions, unless an extremely large quantity (>150 mmol) is ingested in a short period of time to overwhelm the ability of the kidney to excrete potassium. However, with impaired kidney function, hyperkalemia may occur even with a modest increase in potassium intake. With the intravenous administration of potassium salts or potassium-containing drugs (e.g., penicillin G potassium), hyperkalemia may develop, depending on the rate of administration.

3. Kidney Retention of Potassium

A. Kidney Failure

Life-threatening hyperkalemia is most frequently seen in patients with acute oliguric kidney injury or failure. Impaired potassium excretion is the result of reduced kidney function (i.e., an extremely low glomerular filtration rate and a low functioning nephron population), with a consequent reduced delivery of tubular fluid to the distal nephron. This results in decreased potassium secretion. In addition, these patients are often catabolic with an increased potassium load (released from the catabolic tissues) that also increases the risk of hyperkalemia.

In chronic kidney disease, functional adaptation leads to increased potassium secretion per nephron. This results in maintaining the total kidney excretion of potassium at near-normal levels. Therefore, hyperkalemia is relatively uncommon in these patients until they reach kidney failure. However, these patients lack the kidney capacity to accommodate any change in the acute load of potassium, such as excessive dietary potassium intake, the use of potassium-containing or potassium-retaining drugs, or stresses such as infection or other catabolic states. Hyperkalemia may readily develop in patients with chronic kidney failure under such conditions.

B. Hypoaldosteronism

Aldosterone is a major regulator of kidney potassium secretion, and the conditions that involve reduced aldosterone production or the use of the drugs that

---

Box 5-11. Causes of Hyperkalemia

Pseudohyperkalemia
Hyperkalemia
  Transcellular shifts
  • Acidosis
  • Hyperglycemia (hyperosmolality)
  • β-Adrenergic blockade
  • Severe exercise, tissue breakdown
  • Hyperkalemic periodic paralysis
  Increased potassium intake
  • Dietary intake
  • Intravenous administration of potassium-containing substances
  Kidney retention of potassium
  • Kidney failure, both acute and chronic
  • Hypoaldosteronism
    Adrenal insufficiency (Addison disease)
    Hyporeninemic hypoaldosteronism/type IV renal tubular acidosis
    Potassium-retaining drugs: angiotensin-converting enzyme inhibitors, angiotensin receptor blockers, nonsteroidal antiinflammatory drugs, potassium-sparing diuretics

antagonize aldosterone action frequently lead to hyperkalemia. Hypoaldosteronism may be caused by adrenal insufficiency, an impaired renin–angiotensin–aldosterone axis as a result of kidney disease, and the use of aldosterone-antagonist drugs. *Addison disease* or *primary adrenal insufficiency* is a deficiency in both glucocorticoid and mineralocorticoid secretion. Hyporeninemic hypoaldosteronism is one of the common causes of hyperkalemia in patients with chronic kidney disease. It is usually seen in patients with diabetic nephropathy or chronic interstitial nephritis. Renin production by the juxtaglomerular apparatus is suppressed as a result of the underlying disease process, and this results in low renin and reduced aldosterone production. Hyperkalemia is caused by the reduced kidney secretion of potassium from low aldosterone levels. About half of the patients with hyporeninemic hypoaldosteronism also have metabolic acidosis, and they are classified as having a type IV RTA. Type IV RTA is distinguished from type I and type II RTA by its hyperkalemia. In type IV RTA, hyperkalemia suppresses kidney ammonia production and reduces urinary ammonium excretion, thereby resulting in low urinary acid excretion and metabolic acidosis. Type IV RTA is frequently seen in patients with obstructive nephropathy and sickle cell nephropathy.

The drugs that reduce aldosterone secretion or release are frequent causes of hyperkalemia. These drugs include ACE inhibitors, angiotensin receptor blockers, and nonsteroidal antiinflammatory drugs. Another group of drugs that may cause hyperkalemia are potassium-sparing diuretics, including spironolactone, triamterene, and amiloride. Spironolactone competitively inhibits the action of aldosterone on kidney tubular potassium secretion. Triamterene and amiloride block the luminal sodium channels to inhibit sodium reabsorption at the cortical collecting tubule to reduce potassium secretion. Hyperkalemia is more prevalent in patients who are on the potassium-retaining or potassium-sparing medications and who also have impaired kidney function. Therefore, these drugs should be used with caution in these patients, and the dosage of these drugs should be reduced according to the degree of kidney insufficiency to avoid hyperkalemia.

B. Consequences of Hyperkalemia
1. Neuromuscular Function
Hyperkalemia, like hypokalemia, may also cause skeletal muscle weakness and paralysis (Box 5-12). However, severe paralysis is not commonly seen in hyperkalemic patients because cardiac toxicity unfortunately predominates. Hyperkalemia exerts subthreshold depolarization, which activates sodium channels at the neuromuscular junction transiently. However, persistent inward sodium current from activated sodium channels sustains membrane depolarization, thereby inactivating sodium channels. This

> **Box 5-12.** Consequences of Hyperkalemia
>
> Neuromuscular function
>   Muscle weakness
>   Paralysis
> Cardiac effects: electrocardiographic changes
>   Peaked T waves
>   Flattening and loss of P waves
>   Widening of QRS complexes
>   Ventricular tachycardia, ventricular fibrillation
>   Cardiac arrest
> Metabolic effects: normal anion gap metabolic acidosis
>   (type IV renal tubular acidosis)

results in a loss of electrical excitability with the manifestation of weakness.

2. Cardiac Effects
Cardiac effects are the most serious complications of hyperkalemia and can be fatal. Hyperkalemia leads to sustained subthreshold depolarization, which causes a delay in atrial and ventricular depolarization during an action potential. On an ECG, this is manifested by the flattening and loss of P waves and the widening of QRS complexes. The early ECG changes of hyperkalemia include increases in the conductance of potassium channels, which leads to enhanced ventricular repolarization manifested by peaked T waves. As hyperkalemia becomes severe, ventricular arrhythmias (e.g., ventricular tachycardia, fibrillation) develop, with merging of the widened QRS complexes with T waves and eventually a classic sine-wave pattern (Fig. 5-4). If untreated, cardiac arrest may ensue. Thus, an ECG should be performed in patients with severe hyperkalemia.

3. Metabolic Effects
Hyperkalemia may be associated with a normal-anion-gap (hyperchloremic) metabolic acidosis. Hyperkalemia suppresses kidney ammonia production and reduces urinary acid excretion. This occurs because hyperkalemia promotes the cellular uptake

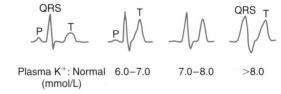

Plasma K^+: Normal 6.0–7.0   7.0–8.0   >8.0
  (mmol/L)

Figure 5-4. Electrocardiographic changes in hyperkalemia. Peaked T waves, flattening and lost P waves, and widened QRS complexes are the characteristic patterns of hyperkalemia. The widened QRS complexes may merge with peaked T waves to present a sine-wave pattern in severe hyperkalemia.

of potassium and creates intracellular alkalosis with potassium entering the cells to replace hydrogen ion. The hydrogen ion leaves the cells to maintain electroneutrality. The intracellular alkalosis suppresses kidney ammonia production in the proximal tubule, which leads to a decrease in urinary ammonium and acid excretion and a type IV RTA.

C. Treatment of Hyperkalemia

The treatment of hyperkalemia depends on the degree of hyperkalemia and the patient's general and cardiac conditions, especially with regard to ECG changes (Box 5-13). Because the severe hyperkalemia may be life threatening, swift therapeutic measures under close ECG monitoring must be undertaken to effectively correct severe hyperkalemia.

1. Temporary Measures to Stabilize Plasma Potassium

With the ECG showing significant hyperkalemic changes, calcium gluconate or chloride should be administered intravenously to antagonize the toxic effects of potassium on the cardiac muscle. Hyperkalemia lowers the excitability of the cardiac muscles, and the administration of calcium restores it and stabilizes the cardiac myocyte cell membrane. This helps to prevent potentially fatal arrhythmias. In addition, insulin should be administered to lower the plasma potassium concentration; this works by driving potassium into the cells. To avoid hypoglycemia, glucose solution should be concurrently administered. The administration of sodium bicarbonate may also lower the plasma potassium level by raising the plasma pH to increase the movement of potassium into the cells. However, sodium bicarbonate is less effective than insulin in this regard, and it may cause volume overload. Its

use is usually limited to hyperkalemic patients with coexisting metabolic acidosis. The administration of β_2-adrenergic agonists (e.g., albuterol) by nebulizer stimulates the cellular uptake of potassium and can help to lower the plasma potassium level within 30 to 60 minutes. This is most effective for individuals with chronic kidney disease or kidney failure.

2. Removal of Potassium from the Body

A. Cation Exchange Resins

The preceding measures do not remove excess potassium from the body. Sodium polystyrene sulfonate (Kayexalate) is a cation exchange resin that takes up potassium in the gut in exchange for sodium. It is usually administered orally with sorbitol, to enhance bowel movement, for the fecal excretion of potassium. Because the bowel route takes a longer time for potassium excretion, it is used for less-severe degrees of hyperkalemia or in conjunction with the previously mentioned corrective measures.

B. Dialysis

For the treatment of severe hyperkalemia, especially in patients with kidney failure, hemodialysis is the most effective therapeutic modality. With the use of a low-potassium concentration in the dialysate (bath solution) and a high dialysate flow rate, the rapid removal of potassium can be achieved during hemodialysis. Peritoneal dialysis may also be used to remove potassium and to correct hyperkalemia, but, as a result of the limited volume of dialysate, its efficiency is low, and it is not suited for acute hyperkalemic emergency.

3. General Measures

Whenever possible, the correction of the underlying causes of hyperkalemia should be attempted. For patients with a tendency toward chronic accumulation of potassium (e.g., patients with hyporeninemic hypoaldosteronism), a low-potassium diet and loop diuretics with sodium bicarbonate or citrate may be useful. For patients with a tendency toward salt wasting (e.g., those with Addison disease), the use of mineralocorticoid agents (e.g., fludrocortisone) may be efficacious. However, the use of fludrocortisone may be problematic in patients who are hypertensive or who have a tendency to retain fluid. When necessary, the intermittent use of cation exchange resins with sorbitol may help to correct hyperkalemia in resistant cases.

Clinical Case

A 60-year-old man with a history of cardiac failure is hospitalized with increasing dyspnea, weight gain, and edema. He regularly takes digoxin, lisinopril (an ACE inhibitor), furosemide, and spironolactone. His blood pressure is 90/60 mm Hg, with a pulse of 90 beats per

---

Box 5-13. Treatment of Hyperkalemia

Treatment of life-threatening hyperkalemia
- Close electrocardiogram monitoring
- Intravenous administration of calcium gluconate or chloride
- Insulin with glucose
- Sodium bicarbonate to correct metabolic acidosis
- β_2-Adrenergic agonists
- Cation exchange resin with sorbitol for milder cases or in combination with other treatments
- Hemodialysis for kidney failure patients

General measures
- Low-potassium diet
- Loop diuretics
- Sodium bicarbonate
- Fludrocortisone
- Cation exchange resin with sorbitol

minute, and laboratory tests reveal an increase in BUN to 60 mg/dl. His serum potassium level is 6.4 mmol/L. Previous serum BUN and creatinine values were 25 and 1.3 mg/dl, respectively, and serum potassium was 4.5 mmol/L.

Can you explain the increase in the serum potassium level in this patient at this time?

This elderly man shows the symptoms of congestive heart failure with increasing dyspnea, weight gain, and edema despite the use of diuretic furosemide. This indicates that his urine output has substantially decreased as a result of the hypoperfusion of the kidney, which is associated with congestive heart failure as shown by low blood pressure and an increase in the BUN level from 25 mg/dl to 60 mg/dl. The use of potassium-retaining drugs, including lisinopril (ACE inhibitor) and spironolactone (aldosterone inhibitor), decreases the tubular secretion of potassium. This is superimposed on decreased perfusion to the kidney and decreased urine output. All of these have led to hyperkalemia. In addition, digoxin, which is an inhibitor of Na^+/K^+-ATPase, also interferes with the cellular uptake of potassium.

Suggested Readings

Faubel S, Topf J: Introduction to potassium. Hypokalemia. Hyperkalemia. In Faubel S, Topf J (eds): *The Fluid, Electrolyte and Acid-Base Companion*. San Diego, Alert and Oriented, 1999.

Preston RA: Hypokalemia. Hyperkalemia. In Preston RA (ed): *Acid-Base, Fluids, and Electrolytes Made Ridiculously Simple*. Miami, MedMaster, 1997.

Peterson LN, Levi M: Disorders of potassium metabolism. In Schrier RW (ed): *Kidney and Electrolyte Disorders*, 6th ed. Philadelphia, Lippincott Williams & Wilkins, 2003.

PRACTICE QUESTIONS

1. A 26-year-old woman is seen in the kidney clinic for fatigue and generalized weakness. She denies a history of hypertension or the use of medications. On physical examination, she appears undernourished. Her blood pressure is 105/60 mm Hg and her pulse rate is 72 beats per minute in the supine position; when standing, her blood pressure is 90/50 mm Hg, and her pulse rate is 96 beats per minute. Her laboratory results include a blood urea nitrogen level of 30, a creatinine level of 1.2 mg/dl, a sodium level of 133, a potassium level of 2.6, a chloride level of 85, and a bicarbonate level of 38 mmol/L. Her urine electrolyte levels include a sodium level of 15 mmol/L, a potassium level of 44 mmol/L, and a chloride level of less than 10 mmol/L. In this patient, hypokalemia is a result of potassium loss that occurs mainly from which of the following routes?

   A. Fecal loss from diarrhea
   B. Kidney loss from increased tubular potassium secretion
   C. Via the gastric juice as a result of vomiting
   D. From profuse sweating

2. A 32-year-old woman with a history of type 1 diabetes mellitus comes to the emergency department as a result of nausea and vomiting. She has not taken her last insulin dose because she has had a poor appetite. She also complains of polyuria and polydipsia, and she has lost 6 lb in weight during the previous week. Her laboratory studies reveal the following: a blood urea nitrogen level of 35, a creatinine level of 1.5, a glucose level of 875 mg/dl, a sodium level of 127, a potassium level of 4.2, a chloride level of 88, and a bicarbonate level of 10 mmol/L. Her plasma ketones are positive. Her urine shows 3+ glucose, positive ketones, a sodium level of 65 mmol/L, and a potassium level of 53 mmol/L. Which of the following statements regarding the potassium status of the patient's body is correct?

   A. Normal serum potassium indicates adequate body potassium content.
   B. Serum potassium is normal as a result of the hemoconcentration caused by dehydration.
   C. The patient's potassium deficit is mild and not enough to cause hypokalemia.
   D. Intracellular potassium is likely depleted, and hypokalemia is masked by acidosis and hyperglycemia.

3. A 48-year-old man is involved in a motor vehicle accident and sustains crush injuries with multiple fractures. He has a history of hypertension, and he has been taking the ACE inhibitor lisinopril. Forty-eight hours later, his urine volume declines to 310 mL/24 h. His laboratory results show a worsening of kidney functional parameters, with his BUN rising from 30 to 95 and his creatinine rising from 1.5 to 3.8 mg/dL in 2 days. Other laboratory values include a sodium level of 138, a potassium level of 6.1, a chloride level of 98, a bicarbonate level of 12 mmol/L, and a creatine kinase level of 35,000 IU/L. Urinalysis shows many granular casts and tubular epithelial cells high per field. All of the following factors contribute to the development of hyperkalemia except which one?

   A. Metabolic acidosis
   B. Acute kidney injury
   C. Increased aldosterone as a result of ECF volume contraction
   D. The potassium-retaining effect of an ACE inhibitor

Acid–Base Homeostasis and Metabolic Alkalosis

6

Kelly Ann Traeger
Frederick J. Boehm III
Arjang Djamali

OUTLINE
I. Kidney and Acid–Base Homeostasis
   A. Introduction
   B. Acids and Bases
   C. Understanding Buffering: The Henderson-Hasselbalch Equation
   D. The Role of the Kidney in Acid–Base Regulation
   E. Factors That Regulate Renal Hydrogen Excretion

II. Metabolic Alkalosis
   A. Introduction
   B. Pathogenesis
   C. Diagnostic Approach to a Patient With Metabolic Alkalosis
   D. Treatment Approach in Metabolic Alkalosis

Objectives

- Understand the role of the kidney in acid–base handling.
- Recognize the factors that regulate kidney hydrogen excretion.
- Understand the underlying pathogenesis of metabolic alkalosis in the generation phase and the maintenance phase.
- Understand the diagnostic approach to metabolic alkalosis.
- Understand the principles of therapy for metabolic alkalosis.

Clinical Case

A 40-year-old man with a history of chronic duodenal ulcer develops increased abdominal pain and black stools. In the outpatient clinic, his physical examination is normal except for epigastric tenderness; his blood pressure is 140/85 mm Hg. There is blood in his stool. Laboratory findings show a blood urea nitrogen level of 56 mg/dl, a creatinine level of 0.8 mg/dl, a hematocrit level of 36%, a sodium level of 142 mmol/L, a potassium level of 4.2 mmol/L, a chloride level of 104 mmol/L, and a bicarbonate level of 28 mmol/L. Urinalysis shows a specific gravity of 1.024; the results are negative for protein and glucose. A week later, the patient develops persistent vomiting as a result of a small bowel obstruction, and he is admitted to the hospital. His blood pressure is 135/80 mm Hg without postural change. His laboratory values include the following: blood urea nitrogen, 48 mg/dl; creatinine, 1.0 mg/dl; hematocrit, 34%; sodium, 138 mmol/L; potassium, 2.9 mmol/L; chloride, 80 mmol/L; and bicarbonate, 45 mmol/L. His blood pH is 7.57, and his partial pressure of carbon dioxide is 45 mm Hg. Gastric suction is initiated, and the patient is found to be losing gastric fluid at a rate of 500 ml/hour; the fluid contains 100 mmol/L hydrogen chloride and 10 mmol/L potassium chloride; the sodium content is negligible.

How does vomiting result in metabolic alkalosis? At what rate is bicarbonate being generated in the blood by the gastric fluid loss? What is the most important urine electrolyte in this patient? Why? What is it expected to be? How will the extracellular fluid volume be affected? What effect would this eventually have on renal bicarbonate reabsorption? Give the important reasons for the low plasma potassium level.

I. KIDNEY AND ACID–BASE HOMEOSTASIS

A. Introduction

A basic understanding of the mechanisms that control acid–base regulation and a systematic approach to acid–base disorders can save hours of frustration.

The goal of acid–base homeostasis is to keep hydrogen ion concentrations ($[H^+]$) within the normal range (40 ± 2 nmol/L) in the plasma. This extremely small concentration range demonstrates the importance of hydrogen ion physiology. Free hydrogen ions can be destructive particles that alter the function and structure of proteins. Therefore, assessing the hydrogen concentration is important in the clinical setting. This is accomplished by measuring the plasma

pH, which is defined as the negative base 10 logarithm of $[H^+]$:

$$pH = -\log[H^+]$$

Therefore, with an arterial $[H^+]$ level of 40 nmol/L, normal plasma pH is 7.40:

$$7.40 = -\log(40\text{ nmol/L})$$

Thus defined, acidemia is characterized by plasma $[H^+]$ concentrations of more than 42 nmol/L (or pH <7.38). Alkalemia occurs with $[H^+]$ levels of less than 38 nmol/L (or pH >7.42) (Fig. 6-1).

B. Acids and Bases

Acids are molecules that donate hydrogen, whereas bases are molecules that accept hydrogen ions. Examples of several important acids and their corresponding physiologic bases are shown in Table 6-1.

C. Understanding Buffering: The Henderson-Hasselbalch Equation

The body's first defense is to buffer against changes in acid–base status. Bicarbonate is the major buffer for the free hydrogen ions. The concentrations of hydrogen, bicarbonate, and carbon dioxide are tied together by the association constant (Ka) of bicarbonate:

Water (H_2O) + Carbon dioxide (CO_2) ↔ Carbonic acid (H_2CO_3) ↔ Hydrogen (H^+) + Bicarbonate (HCO_3^-)

However, because the carbonic acid concentration is very small as a result of the rapid breakdown caused by carbonic anhydrase and the rapid dissociation to its conjugate base and a proton, carbonic acid may be dropped from the equation, thus leaving the following:

$$H_2O + CO_2 \leftrightarrow H^+ + HCO_3^-$$

Thus defined, the Ka of bicarbonate may be represented as follows:

$$Ka = \frac{\left[H^+\right]\left[HCO_3^-\right]}{\left[H_2O\right]\left[CO_2\right]}$$

Table 6-1. Common Acids and Corresponding Bases in Physiology

Acid name	Acid	Base	H^+ ion
Carbonic acid	H_2CO_3 ↔	HCO_3^-	$+H^+$
Hydrochloric acid	HCl ↔	Cl^-	$+H^+$
Ammonium	NH_4^+ ↔	NH_3	$+H^+$
Phosphate (dibasic)	$H_2PO_4^-$ ↔	HPO_4^-	$+H^+$
Sulfate (dibasic)	$H_2SO_4^-$ ↔	HSO_4^-	$+H^+$

Because the concentration of water in the body is stable, this formula may be simplified:

$$Ka' = \frac{\left[H^+\right]\left[HCO_3^-\right]}{\left[CO_2\right]}$$

This may be rewritten as the following:

$$\left[H^+\right] = Ka'\frac{\left[CO_2\right]}{\left[HCO_3^-\right]}$$

or:

$$pH = pKa' + \log\frac{\left[HCO_3^-\right]}{\left[CO_2\right]}$$

Because carbon dioxide is normally measured in partial pressure, a conversion factor is used. This is presented in the Henderson-Hasselbalch equation as follows:

$$pH = 6.1 + \log\frac{\left[HCO_3^-\right]}{0.03 * PCO_2}$$

This equation defines acid–base status in the body. Note that the association constant (pKa') for plasma is 6.1, which is an experimentally determined value. The Henderson-Hasselbalch equation demonstrates that plasma pH can be determined by the partial pressure of carbon dioxide and the bicarbonate levels.

The regulation of the bicarbonate concentration is accomplished primarily by the kidneys, whereas the partial pressure of carbon dioxide is regulated

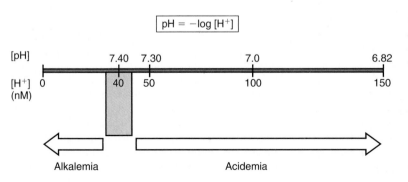

Figure 6-1. Acidemia and alkalemia are defined by plasma pH or hydrogen ion concentrations. Note that the pH normal range is centered around 7.40.

primarily by the lungs. This combined effort results in the tight control of [H⁺] around 40 nmol/L ± 2 (plasma pH = 7.40 ± 0.02).

For example, if plasma bicarbonate levels fall, the pH will fall as well, which results in metabolic acidosis. Acidemia will stimulate a compensatory fall in the partial pressure of carbon dioxide. This is achieved by hyperventilation, which is a physiologic response that is aimed at normalizing plasma hydrogen concentrations and pH levels.

Four primary acid–base disorders can thus be defined, each of which is accompanied by a physiologic, compensatory effort: (1) metabolic acidosis prompting respiratory alkalosis (hyperventilation); (2) metabolic alkalosis prompting respiratory acidosis (hypoventilation); (3) respiratory acidosis with a compensatory metabolic alkalosis; and (4) respiratory alkalosis that results in metabolic acidosis (Fig. 6-2).

D. The Role of the Kidney in Acid–Base Regulation

Body acids are generated in large part from dietary intake and from the metabolism of amino acids. The average American diet results in a net acid excess of approximately 1 mmol/kg/day. The body's response to this acid load is to excrete the excess [H⁺] through the kidneys. The kidneys also maintain the internal acid–base homeostasis.

The overall kidney handling of acid–base can be summarized by two principal mechanisms:
1. Bicarbonate reabsorption (near total reabsorption of filtered bicarbonate)
2. Acid excretion (eliminating the dietary acid load: 70 mmol/day of hydrogen)
   a. Titratable acid formation ($H_2PO_4^-$), which occurs at a relatively constant rate
   b. Formation of urinary ammonium by renal tubular epithelial cells (the major adaptive response)

Titratable acid formation and ammonium excretion both result in bicarbonate regeneration and

enable the buffering of excess acid. *Net acid excretion* (NAE) is defined by the sum of ammonium (NH_4^+) and dibasic phosphate ($H_2PO_4^-$) minus the bicarbonate in the urine. Because urine bicarbonate concentrations are usually negligible (because there is a near-total reabsorption of filtered bicarbonate), approximately 40 mmol/24 hr of ammonium and 30 mmol/24 hr of phosphate are eliminated to offset the daily acid burden (Fig. 6-3, Box 6-1).

NAE reflects the net acid–base status of the urine and therefore the urine pH. In healthy subjects with a normal plasma pH of 7.4, urine pH is approximately 5.6. If acidemia is present, the appropriate renal response to eliminate the excess acid load should result in an increased NAE and a decreased urine pH.

1. Bicarbonate Reabsorption by Tubular Epithelial Cells

Nearly all filtered bicarbonate is reabsorbed by the kidneys. Most (approximately 80%) of the reabsorption occurs in the proximal tubules, whereas the thick ascending limb and the distal nephron each reabsorb 10% of the filtered bicarbonate. In fact, it is not the same filtered bicarbonate ion that is reabsorbed (Fig. 6-4). Instead, each filtered molecule is transformed stepwise to carbon dioxide and water as it combines with the hydrogen secreted by the apical sodium/hydrogen exchanger (proximal tubule) or the hydrogen/ATPase pump (collecting tubule). The resulting carbonic acid molecule is then transformed into water and carbon dioxide by the enzyme carbonic anhydrase in the lumen. Water and carbon dioxide are reabsorbed within the cell and generate carbonic acid again, this time through the action of intracellular carbonic anhydrase. Carbonic acid generates bicarbonate molecules that are excreted in the interstitial space (and later in the peritubular capillaries) via basolateral sodium/bicarbonate cotransporters. Thus, for each filtered

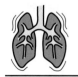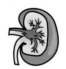

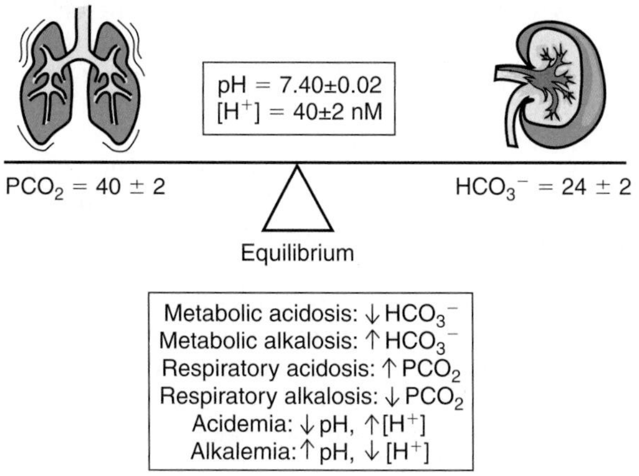

pH = 7.40±0.02
[H⁺] = 40±2 nM

$PCO_2 = 40 \pm 2$ Equilibrium $HCO_3^- = 24 \pm 2$

Metabolic acidosis: ↓HCO_3^-
Metabolic alkalosis: ↑HCO_3^-
Respiratory acidosis: ↑PCO_2
Respiratory alkalosis: ↓PCO_2
Acidemia: ↓pH, ↑[H⁺]
Alkalemia: ↑pH, ↓[H⁺]

Figure 6-2. Acid–base homeostasis is maintained by the balance in function of the lungs and the kidneys. When there is a disturbance either in carbon dioxide (CO_2) levels, which are primarily regulated by the lungs, or in bicarbonate (HCO_3) levels, which are primarily regulated by the kidneys, there is a compensatory change in the other component. For example, the retention of CO_2 by the lungs, which is an example of a respiratory acidosis, is compensated for by the increased retention of HCO_3^- by the kidneys.

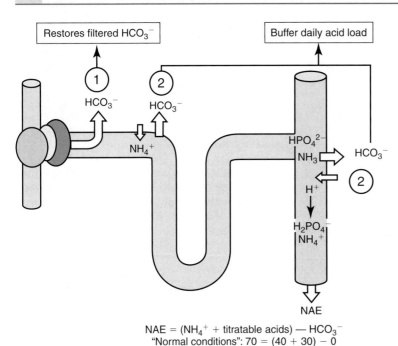

Figure 6-3. Kidney regulation of acid–base. Most of the kidney's processing of acid and base occurs in the proximal tubule and the collecting duct. The proximal tubule cells absorb bicarbonate and secrete ammonium. The absorbed bicarbonate enters the bloodstream and ultimately buffers the daily acid load. There is a net secretion of protons by the epithelium of the collecting duct. These protons react with several chemical species, including ammonia (NH_3) and phosphoric acid (HPO_4^{2-}). Net acid excretion (NAE) can be calculated as the difference between the concentrations of acids (namely ammonium [NH_4^+] and other titratable acids) and the concentration of base (namely bicarbonate [HCO_3^-]).

$$NAE = (NH_4^+ + \text{titratable acids}) - HCO_3^-$$
"Normal conditions": $70 = (40 + 30) - 0$

Box 6-1. Roles of the Kidney in Acid–Base Regulation

To reabsorb filtrated bicarbonate
To regenerate bicarbonate by the excretion of
    ammonium and titratable acids

---

bicarbonate molecule, there is a bicarbonate ion that is reabsorbed into the peritubular capillaries. This is facilitated by the $Na^+/3\ HCO_3^-$ cotransporter in the basolateral membrane of proximal tubular epithelial cells (see Fig. 6-4). The same applies to the distal collecting tubule. However, here a basolateral chloride/bicarbonate exchanger facilitates reabsorption.

2. Titratable Acid Formation by Tubular Epithelial Cells

Titratable acid formation is responsible for the excretion of 30 to 40 mmol of acid per day. Titratable acid excretion is maintained at a relatively constant rate, and it does not significantly contribute to the excretion of an additional acid load. Titratable acid formation occurs principally in the distal collecting tubule, although the proximal tubule may contribute to a lesser extent. Filtered buffers such as major urinary buffer HPO_4^-, creatinine, and others bind to the secreted hydrogen ions and form titratable acids that are eliminated. For each hydrogen ion that is buffered in the lumen, there is a bicarbonate ion that is reabsorbed in the peritubular capillaries (Fig. 6-5).

3. Formation of Urinary Ammonium by Tubular Epithelial Cells

Ammoniagenesis is normally responsible for excreting 30 to 40 mmol/day. This rate can increase to >300 mmol/day in the face of an acid load. Ammonium is generated primarily from the breakdown of amino acids. Glutamine is first metabolized to ammonium and α-ketoglutarate in the cytosol. Ammonium then enters the urine via one of two mechanisms, depending on the segment of the tubule. In proximal tubules, ammonium uses the sodium/hydrogen exchanger by taking the place of hydrogen. In distal tubules, ammonia passively diffuses into the lumen, where it combines with hydrogen to form ammonium. Ammonium, which is a charged ion, is lipid insoluble and cannot back-diffuse out of the lumen. In tubular epithelial cells, α-ketoglutarate serves as a new substrate for the formation of "new" bicarbonate ions that will be reabsorbed in the peritubular capillaries via the sodium/3 bicarbonate cotransporter (Fig. 6-6). Overall, for each ammonium ion excreted, there is a bicarbonate ion reabsorbed in the peritubular capillaries.

In summary, the net acid–base status of the urine is represented by the NAE and, therefore, the urine pH. In healthy subjects with a normal plasma pH (7.4), urine pH is approximately 5.6. If acidemia is present, the appropriate renal response to eliminate excess acid load should result in an increased NAE and a decreased urine pH (as low as 4.5–5). This may happen through increased bicarbonate reabsorption and the excretion of acid via titratable acid formation and ammoniagenesis.

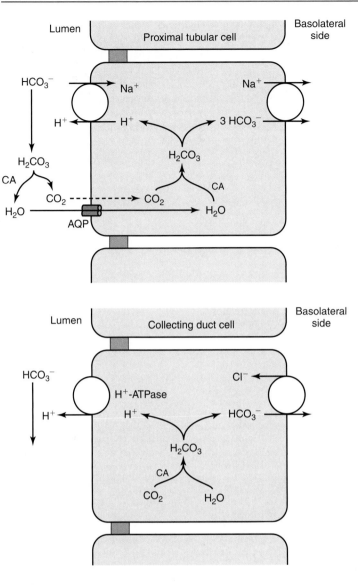

Figure 6-4. Kidney bicarbonate reabsorption. Bicarbonate handling occurs in the proximal tubule and the collecting duct. In the proximal tubule lumen, a bicarbonate ion combines with a proton to form carbonic acid, which then breaks into one molecule of carbon dioxide (CO_2) and one of water (H_2O). Both molecules enter the proximal tubule epithelial cell, where they recombine to form carbonic acid, which rapidly dissociates to bicarbonate (HCO_3^-) and a proton. The proton can reenter the tubule lumen, whereas the bicarbonate can be transported with sodium ions into the interstitium and ultimately to the bloodstream. In the collecting duct epithelium, CO_2 combines with H_2O to form carbonic acid, which then dissociates to a proton and bicarbonate. The bicarbonate is transferred to the interstitium, whereas the proton is pumped in an ATP-dependent manner into the collecting tubule lumen. *AQP,* Aquaporin; *CA,* carbonic anhydrase.

E. Factors That Regulate Renal Hydrogen Excretion

There are four factors that regulate hydrogen excretion:
1. Plasma pH
2. Effective circulating volume
3. Aldosterone
4. Plasma potassium concentrations

1. Plasma (Extracellular) pH

The overall goal of the kidney is to "match" urine pH to extracellular or plasma pH. The human body is designed to lower urine pH through increased hydrogen excretion when plasma pH is low (acidemia) and to increase urine pH by reducing hydrogen excretion in the case of alkalemia (pH >7.42).

For example, in the proximal tubule, acidemia directly stimulates the activity and synthesis of sodium/hydrogen exchangers in the apical membrane, increases ammoniagenesis, and results in the increased activity of basolateral sodium/bicarbonate cotransporters.

In the cortical tubules, acidemia leads to the insertion of preformed, cytoplasmic hydrogen/ATPase pumps into the apical membrane and to the trapping of ammonium in the urinary lumen. Together, these mechanisms increase urinary hydrogen excretion and bicarbonate reabsorption.

Therefore, the net effects of acidemia on kidney acid–base handling are an increase in net acid excretion, an increase in bicarbonate reabsorption, a decrease in urine pH, and a normalizing plasma pH.

2. Effective Circulating Volume

Decreased effective circulating volume contributes to the generation and maintenance of metabolic alkalosis. Volume contraction is often associated with the

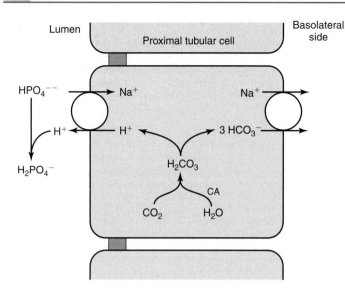

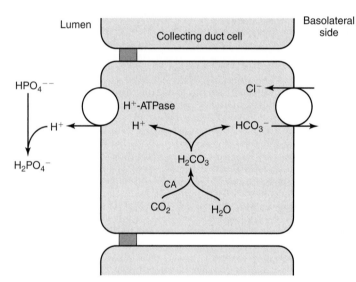

Figure 6-5. Kidney titratable acidity formation. Both the proximal tubule cells and the collecting duct cells can provide protons to partially neutralize the phosphoric acid (HPO_4^{2-}) ions in the tubule lumen. Note that, as in Figure 6-4, the protons are generated from a carbonic acid molecule which, in turn, is generated from the combination of one molecule of water (H_2O) and one of carbon dioxide (CO_2).

activation of the renin–angiotensin–aldosterone system (RAAS) and chloride depletion. Both of these can result in increased tubular hydrogen excretion. Angiotensin II increases hydrogen excretion in the proximal tubule by increasing the activity of apical sodium/hydrogen exchangers and basolateral sodium/bicarbonate cotransporters. Chloride depletion and aldosterone both result in greater hydrogen secretion through both sodium-dependent and sodium-independent mechanisms.

3. Aldosterone
Aldosterone is a primary regulator of sodium balance. However, hyperaldosteronism results in metabolic alkalosis through its effect on distal tubules via sodium-dependent and sodium-independent factors:

Sodium-dependent factors. In principal cells (collecting tubules), aldosterone-mediated sodium reabsorption creates a lumen-negative potential difference that promotes hydrogen and potassium secretion, thus potentiating metabolic alkalosis and hypokalemia.

Sodium-independent factors. Aldosterone directly stimulates the apical hydrogen/ATPase pump (increased hydrogen excretion) and activates the basolateral chloride/bicarbonate exchanger (increased bicarbonate reabsorption) in the distal tubules.

4. Plasma Potassium Concentrations
Hypokalemia results in a transcellular shift of potassium ions from cells to plasma in an attempt to restore the plasma potassium concentrations toward normal. To maintain electroneutrality, hydrogen ions enter the cell, thereby lowering the intracellular pH. This, in turn, can lead to the following:

- Increased bicarbonate reabsorption in both the proximal and distal tubules through the

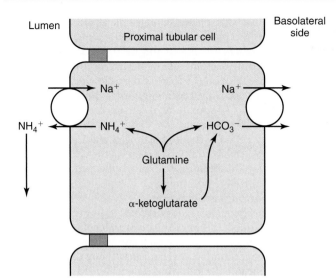

Lumen

Proximal tubular cell

Basolateral side

Figure 6-6. Kidney ammonium excretion. Glutamine is absorbed by the proximal tubule cells and broken down to α-ketoglutarate and ammonium ions. The α-ketoglutarate is metabolized to bicarbonate ions, which subsequently enter the interstitium. The ammonium ions enter the lumen, and, by changing the transmembrane electrochemical gradient, they promote sodium absorption by the proximal tubule cells. In the collecting duct, the newly generated protons enter the lumen via the ATP-dependent transporter and protonate ammonia to generate ammonium, which is excreted in the urine.

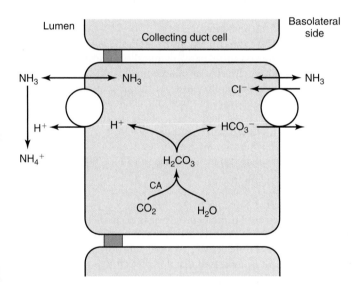

increased activity of apical sodium/hydrogen exchangers and basolateral sodium/bicarbonate cotransporters

Increased ammoniagenesis in proximal (mainly) and distal tubules

Hypokalemia can therefore result in metabolic alkalosis. Conversely, hyperkalemia may result in the inhibition of ammoniagenesis and subsequent metabolic acidosis (see Chapter 7). The relationship between potassium and acid–base is demonstrated in Figure 6-7.

In summary, the kidneys and the lungs regulate acid–base balance through the tight control of plasma bicarbonate concentrations and partial pressure of carbon dioxide levels, respectively. Whereas lungs require a short time to respond, the kidneys are slower, requiring up to 3 days to complete their adaptive response. Kidney regulation of acid–base

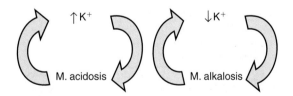

Figure 6-7. Changes in serum potassium concentration in acid–base disturbances.

occurs through the reabsorption of filtered bicarbonate in concert with ammonium and titratable acid elimination. There are four principal factors that regulate kidney hydrogen excretion (Box 6-2): (1) plasma pH; (2) effective circulating volume; (3) aldosterone; and (4) plasma potassium ion concentrations.

Box 6-2. Factors That Increase Urine Hydrogen Excretion

Decreased effective circulating volume
Decreased plasma pH
Decreased plasma potassium
Increased aldosterone activity

II. METABOLIC ALKALOSIS

A. Introduction

Metabolic alkalosis is a systemic disorder that is defined by a primary rise in plasma bicarbonate levels (i.e., >26 mmol/L) associated with a rise in plasma pH (>7.42). Alkalemia triggers a compensatory rise in partial pressure of carbon dioxide levels by hypoventilation (respiratory acidosis; Fig. 6-8). In primary metabolic alkalosis, the plasma pH is often increased (i.e., >7.42).

B. Pathogenesis

Under normal conditions, there is no bicarbonate excreted in the urine. However, when the threshold for bicarbonate reabsorption is exceeded, the kidney fails to recapture all of the filtered bicarbonate, and bicarbonate is excreted in the urine. Thus, greater levels of plasma bicarbonate result in greater filtration and ultimately greater bicarbonate excretion. This threshold for the excretion of excess bicarbonate provides relative protection against metabolic alkalosis. Therefore, persistent metabolic alkalosis requires some "participation" by the kidneys, which involves their inability to excrete the appropriate amount of bicarbonate when plasma bicarbonate levels are increased.

The pathogenesis of metabolic alkalosis can be split into two phases: generation and maintenance.

1. *Generation* is the inciting disturbance. This phase involves an increase in plasma bicarbonate as a result of one or more of the following:
   a. Plasma hydrogen ion loss via the following:
      (1) Gastrointestinal secretions
      (2) Urine
      (3) Movement of hydrogen ions into cells
   b. Plasma bicarbonate gain via the administration of bicarbonate or a compound that is metabolized to bicarbonate
   c. Volume contraction
2. *Maintenance* is the paradoxic response of the kidney. This phase involves an insufficient excretion of bicarbonate for a given plasma bicarbonate concentration. Mechanisms driving this response include the following:
   a. Effective circulating volume depletion
   b. Hypokalemia
   c. Hypochloremia

Thus, the correction of metabolic alkalosis may require volume expansion and the administration of sodium chloride or potassium chloride. Here we will review the pathogenesis of the generation and maintenance phases of metabolic alkalosis.

1. Generation of Metabolic Alkalosis

The generation phase can result from a loss of plasma hydrogen ions, a gain of bicarbonate, or volume contraction with constant bicarbonate content.

A. Hydrogen Loss in the Urine
Increased urine hydrogen loss occurs when adequate distal salt delivery is combined with increased aldosterone activity. As noted, aldosterone can result in increased distal hydrogen loss through

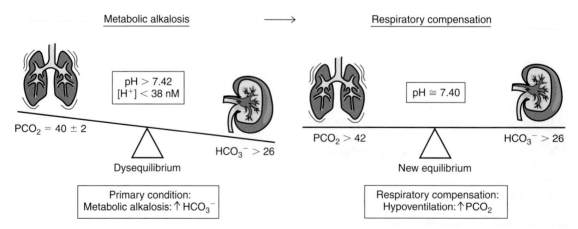

Figure 6-8. Metabolic alkalosis can induce respiratory compensation and lead to an increase in the partial pressure of carbon dioxide. The figure on the left represents the state after the initial disturbance, whereas the figure on the right represents the state after the compensation has occurred.

sodium-dependent and sodium-independent mechanisms. In principal cells (collecting tubules), aldosterone-mediated sodium reabsorption creates a lumen-negative potential difference that promotes hydrogen and potassium secretion. In the distal tubules (intercalated cells), aldosterone directly stimulates apical hydrogen/ATPase activity (increased hydrogen excretion) and results in bicarbonate reabsorption. The end result is metabolic alkalosis with hypokalemia. The conditions described in the following present with increased urine hydrogen loss.

Loop or thiazide diuretic administration. Loop diuretics inhibit the $Na^+/K^+/2Cl^-$ cotransporter that is located in the thick ascending limb of the loop of Henle. Thiazide diuretics inhibit the Na^+/Cl^- cotransporter that is located in the early distal tubule. This inhibition decreases sodium reabsorption, thereby increasing the distal delivery of sodium to the collecting tubule. The initial volume loss caused by low-sodium reabsorption stimulates increased aldosterone secretion and results in metabolic alkalosis (Fig. 6-9).

Bartter and Gitelman syndromes. These disorders produce electrolyte abnormalities that mimic those demonstrated with diuretic therapy. This is not surprising, because they are associated with genetic defects in the transporters in the loop of Henle and distal tubule—the very ones inhibited by loop and thiazide diuretics, respectively. The most common phenotype of Bartter syndrome is associated with a mutation in the gene for the bumetanide-sensitive $Na^+/K^+/2Cl^-$ cotransporter on the apical membrane in the thick ascending limb of the loop of Henle, whereas Gitelman syndrome is caused by a mutation in

the gene that encodes the thiazide-sensitive Na^+/Cl^- cotransporter in the distal convoluted tubule.

Primary mineralocorticoid excess. Primary mineralocorticoid excess (congenital, tumor) can lead to metabolic alkalosis along with hypertension and hypokalemia. By contrast, patients with secondary hyperaldosteronism usually do not present with metabolic alkalosis because the effect of aldosterone is balanced by the decreased distal delivery of sodium.

Posthypercapnic alkalosis. Chronic respiratory acidosis results in an appropriate increase in hydrogen secretion and a rise in the plasma bicarbonate concentration. The rapid lowering of a chronically elevated partial pressure of carbon dioxide (mechanical ventilation) causes metabolic alkalosis as a result of the persistently high plasma bicarbonate concentration. The fall in the partial pressure of carbon dioxide will acutely raise the cerebral intracellular pH, potentially resulting in serious neurologic complications, including death.

Hypercalcemia and the milk-alkali syndrome. Hypercalcemia increases renal bicarbonate reabsorption by an unknown mechanism. Patients with increased alkaline load (as a result of the ingestion of calcium carbonate or antacids) develop the milk-alkali syndrome, which is characterized by hypercalcemia, metabolic alkalosis, and kidney failure.

B. Gastrointestinal Hydrogen Loss
Each millimole of hydrogen lost in the gastrointestinal tract generates 1 mmol of bicarbonate in the plasma. Therefore, when there is excessive acid loss, there is a parallel increase in plasma bicarbonate levels. This can occur in the following situations.

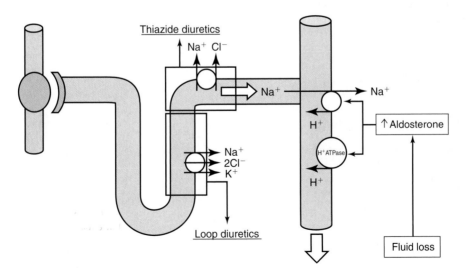

Figure 6-9. Diuretics and metabolic alkalosis. The use of loop or thiazide diuretics leads to increased levels of intraluminal sodium that reach the collecting duct. With greater sodium levels in the lumen of the collecting duct, there will be a higher level of sodium absorption by collecting duct cells, which, in turn, promotes increased proton secretion. The increased proton secretion leads to metabolic alkalosis.

Removal of gastric secretions (Fig. 6-10). Normally, for each hydrogen ion secreted into the stomach, there is one bicarbonate ion generated by the gastric parietal cells that is reabsorbed in the blood. In the duodenum, chemoreceptors detect the low pH and stimulate the pancreas to secrete bicarbonate and neutralize acid secretions locally (the stomach can tolerate high acid contents, but the rest of the gastrointestinal tract cannot). This secretion of bicarbonate into the duodenum is accompanied by the secretion of hydrogen into the blood to neutralize the bicarbonate that is released into circulation by parietal cells. In the presence of vomiting or gastric suctioning, the acid content of the stomach does not reach the duodenum. Therefore, there is no production of bicarbonate into the duodenum and no hydrogen release into the circulation to neutralize the bicarbonate production from the parietal cells. This will result in the generation of metabolic alkalosis.

During the early phase (i.e., the first 3 days) after vomiting or nasogastric suctions, the rise in plasma bicarbonate concentrations results in greater bicarbonate filtration by the kidneys, increased urine bicarbonate loss, and a high urine pH. However, there is sodium and potassium wasting because urine sodium and potassium follow bicarbonate to conserve electroneutrality (despite hypovolemia). However, urine chloride excretion is decreased (<25 mmol/L) because chloride is the only reabsorbable anion (it can be reabsorbed with sodium), and there is volume and chloride depletion. During the late phase (>3 days), all bicarbonate is reabsorbed if volume and chloride depletion are still present. This is the result of increased bicarbonate reabsorptive capacity. Urine pH decreases (paradoxic aciduria) because all of the bicarbonate is reabsorbed, and urine sodium, potassium, and chloride

concentrations all decrease as a result of volume and chloride depletion (Table 6-2).

In summary, in cases of vomiting and gastric suctioning, for each millimole of hydrogen loss, there is one of bicarbonate generation in the blood. This will soon become a vicious circle if there is no volume expansion by normal saline.

Loss of intestinal secretions. Intestinal secretions contain relatively high levels of bicarbonate, and the loss of these secretions typically leads to metabolic acidosis (diarrhea). However, patients with a villous adenoma or factitious diarrhea (laxative abuse) can develop metabolic alkalosis.

C. Intracellular Shift of Hydrogen
Metabolic alkalosis can also be induced by the shift of hydrogen ions into the cells. Hypokalemia induces a transcellular shift in which potassium leaves the cells toward the plasma, and hydrogen enters the cells to maintain electroneutrality. The movement of hydrogen into the cells increases the plasma bicarbonate concentration and lowers the intracellular pH. The lower intracellular pH in the epithelial cells promotes hydrogen secretion and bicarbonate reabsorption, thereby further contributing to a metabolic alkalosis.

D. Alkali Administration
Metabolic alkalosis can occur if very large quantities of bicarbonate are given acutely or if the ability to excrete bicarbonate is impaired. Metabolic alkalosis can be induced by the following:
- The use of sodium bicarbonate to treat lactic acidosis or ketoacidosis
- The ingestion of sodium bicarbonate
- The administration of large quantities of citrate by the infusion of more than eight units of banked blood (anticoagulated with acid–citrate–dextran)

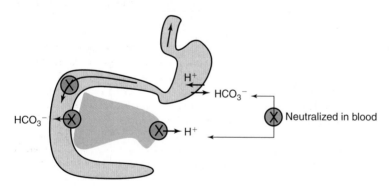

Vomiting: No pancreatic secretion of HCO_3^- in the gut
No pancreatic secretion of H^+ in blood
Persistent gastric HCO_3^- secretion in blood
Generation of metabolic alkalosis (equimolar to HCl loss)

Figure 6-10. The removal of gastric secretions and metabolic alkalosis. In a healthy state, the protons that are ordinarily secreted by the stomach's parietal cells would be neutralized in the duodenum by bicarbonate ions that are secreted by the pancreas. Note also that the bicarbonate pumped into the bloodstream from the stomach is neutralized by protons from the pancreas. However, when gastric secretions are lost externally, there is a continuous secretion of bicarbonate ions into the blood that results in metabolic alkalosis.

Table 6-2. Urine Tests during the Early and Late Phases of Vomiting or Gastric Suction

	Bicarbonate (plasma)	U_{HCO3^-}	U_{Na^+}	U_{K^+}	U_{Cl^-}	U_{pH}
At 1 to 3 days	Increased	Increased	Increased	Increased	Decreased	Increased (>6.5)
At 3 or more days	Increased	Decreased	Decreased	Decreased	Decreased	Decreased (5.5; paradoxic aciduria)

- The use of citrate rather than heparin as an anticoagulant in hemodialysis patients who are at high risk for bleeding
- The administration of fresh frozen plasma as a replacement fluid during plasmapheresis

E. Contraction Alkalosis
Contraction alkalosis occurs when there is loss of relatively large volumes of bicarbonate-free fluid. The plasma bicarbonate concentration rises because there is a contraction of the extracellular volume around a relatively constant quantity of extracellular bicarbonate. Loop diuretics inducing rapid fluid removal in markedly edematous patients are the most common cause of a contraction alkalosis.

2. Maintenance of Metabolic Alkalosis
The number one priority for the kidneys at all times is to preserve intravascular volume. This and other factors described later in this chapter contribute to the maintenance phase of metabolic alkalosis. These factors create a "vicious circle" that results in bicarbonate reabsorption despite already increased plasma bicarbonate levels.

A. Effective Circulating Volume Depletion
This is the most common cause of metabolic alkalosis. Decreased effective circulating volume results in a fall in the glomerular filtration rate and in the amount of filtered bicarbonate. Volume contraction is often associated with salt avidity, the activation of the RAAS, and chloride depletion. These conditions increase urinary hydrogen loss and prevent sodium bicarbonate excretion. Most of the increase in net bicarbonate reabsorption occurs in the collecting tubules, in part under the influence of the resulting hyperaldosteronism. The following factors contribute to the maintenance of metabolic alkalosis when volume contraction is present:
1. **Angiotensin II.** Angiotensin II increases hydrogen excretion in the proximal tubule by increasing the activity of apical sodium/hydrogen exchangers and basolateral sodium/bicarbonate cotransporters.
2. **Secondary hyperaldosteronism.**
   a. *Sodium-independent mechanisms.* Aldosterone directly enhances acidification in distal intercalated cells by increasing the activity of the hydrogen/

ATPase pumps in the luminal membrane. This promotes the secretion of hydrogen ions into the tubular lumen.
   b. *Sodium-dependent mechanisms.* Aldosterone-stimulated sodium reabsorption in the principal cells (collecting tubules) makes the lumen electronegative as a result of sodium loss. This results in a greater urinary excretion of hydrogen and potassium to maintain electroneutrality.
3. **Chloride depletion.** Decreased chloride delivery diminishes bicarbonate secretion in type B intercalated cells, which is thought to be an important component of the normal kidney response to a bicarbonate load.

B. Chloride Depletion
Hypochloremia can contribute to the maintenance of metabolic alkalosis by increasing the reabsorption of and reducing the secretion of bicarbonate in the distal tubule.
   Increased distal reabsorption of bicarbonate. Bicarbonate reabsorption in the outer medullary collecting tubules and type A intercalated cells is mediated by hydrogen secretion through the hydrogen/ATPase pumps in the luminal membrane. There is a passive cosecretion of chloride along with hydrogen to maintain electroneutrality. A decline in the tubular fluid chloride concentration will enhance both chloride and hydrogen secretion and result in bicarbonate reabsorption by the basolateral chloride/bicarbonate exchanger.
   Decreased distal secretion of bicarbonate. Type B intercalated cells in the cortical tubules are able to directly secrete bicarbonate by reversing the location of transporters during alkalemia. The chloride/bicarbonate exchangers are located in the luminal membrane here and lead to bicarbonate secretion into the tubular lumen. This is a response to excrete the excess bicarbonate. However, decreased tubular chloride concentration will decrease the favorable inward gradient for chloride and reduce bicarbonate secretion.

c. Hypokalemia
Hypokalemia directly increases bicarbonate reabsorption. Hypokalemia results in a transcellular shift of potassium ions from cells to plasma in an attempt to restore the plasma potassium concentrations toward

normal. To maintain electroneutrality, hydrogen ions enter the cell, resulting in intracellular acidosis in all cells. Intracellular acidosis can result in the following:
1. Increased bicarbonate reabsorption in both proximal and distal tubules by increased activity of apical sodium/hydrogen exchangers and basolateral sodium/bicarbonate cotransporters
2. Increased ammoniagenesis in proximal (mainly) and distal tubules

Hypokalemia can therefore result in metabolic alkalosis. Conversely, hyperkalemia may result in the inhibition of ammoniagenesis and subsequent metabolic acidosis (see Fig. 6-7 and Chapter 7). Thus, both hypokalemia and aldosterone can have a potentiating effect on distal hydrogen secretion and therefore on the development and maintenance of metabolic alkalosis.

C. Diagnostic Approach to a Patient with Metabolic Alkalosis
The diagnosis of metabolic alkalosis is usually evident from the history, which may include emesis, nasogastric suction, and diuretic therapy. However, all entities do need to be considered. A thorough history and physical in combination with appropriate laboratory tests often leads to the differential diagnosis of metabolic alkalosis.

1. Urine Sodium in Metabolic Alkalosis
Metabolic alkalosis represents one of the conditions in which volume depletion may not lead to a low urine sodium concentration, because the attempt to retain sodium is offset by the need to excrete bicarbonate. Therefore, sodium wasting occurs during the first few days of emesis as the plasma bicarbonate concentration and the filtered bicarbonate load are increased (see Fig. 6-10).

2. Urine Chloride in Metabolic Alkalosis
This is the most important ancillary test in metabolic alkalosis. The presence of underlying hypovolemia can be detected more accurately by finding a urine chloride concentration of less than 25 mmol/L. The appropriate chloride conservation in this setting is the result of both volume depletion and hypochloremia induced by chloride loss in gastric secretions (see Figs. 6-10 and 6-11).

3. Differential Diagnosis of Metabolic Alkalosis
This list—together with Figure 6-11—attempts to provide both a diagnostic and therapeutic approach to metabolic alkalosis.
1. Sodium chloride responsive
   a. Gastrointestinal losses of hydrogen
      (1) Emesis/gastric suctions
      (2) Villous adenomas
      (3) Chloride diarrhea
   b. Kidney losses; diuretic therapy
   c. Posthypercapnic
   d. Severe potassium depletion
2. Sodium chloride resistant
   a. Primary hyperaldosteronism
   b. Cushing syndrome
   c. Bartter syndrome
   d. Steroids
   e. Excess licorice intake
   f. Hypokalemia
3. Other
   a. Alkaline administration
   b. Milk-alkali syndrome

D. Treatment Approach in Metabolic Alkalosis
Metabolic alkalosis is characterized by a primary rise in the plasma bicarbonate concentration, and the condition persists because the kidney is unable to excrete the excess bicarbonate, usually as a result of effective

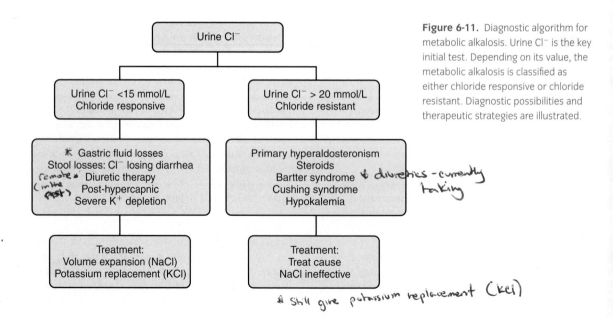

Figure 6-11. Diagnostic algorithm for metabolic alkalosis. Urine Cl⁻ is the key initial test. Depending on its value, the metabolic alkalosis is classified as either chloride responsive or chloride resistant. Diagnostic possibilities and therapeutic strategies are illustrated.

volume depletion, hypokalemia, and hypochloremia. Therefore, the therapy of metabolic alkalosis requires the correction of the underlying cause, volume expansion, potassium, and chloride repletion.

Clinical Case

A 40-year-old man with a history of chronic duodenal ulcer develops increased abdominal pain and black stools. In the outpatient clinic, his physical examination is normal except for epigastric tenderness; his blood pressure is 140/85 mm Hg. There is blood in his stool. Laboratory findings show a blood urea nitrogen level of 56 mg/dl, a creatinine level of 0.8 mg/dl, a hematocrit level of 36%, a sodium level of 142 mmol/L, a potassium level of 4.2 mmol/L, a chloride level of 104 mmol/L, and a bicarbonate level of 28 mmol/L. Urinalysis shows a specific gravity of 1.024; the results are negative for protein and glucose. A week later, the patient develops persistent vomiting as a result of a small bowel obstruction, and he is admitted to the hospital. His blood pressure is 135/80 mm Hg without postural change. His laboratory values include the following: blood urea nitrogen, 48 mg/dl; creatinine, 1.0 mg/dl; hematocrit, 34%; sodium, 138 mmol/L; potassium, 2.9 mmol/L; chloride, 80 mmol/L; and bicarbonate, 45 mmol/L. His blood pH is 7.57, and his partial pressure of carbon dioxide is 45 mm Hg. Gastric suction is initiated, and the patient is found to be losing gastric fluid at a rate of 500 ml/hour; the fluid contains 100 mmol/L hydrogen chloride and 10 mmol/L potassium chloride; the sodium content is negligible.

How does vomiting result in metabolic alkalosis?

Vomiting produces metabolic alkalosis by two mechanisms: generation and maintenance. The generation mechanism is the more important one.

Generation: The loss of hydrogen-rich hydrochloric acid (HCl) gastric fluid generates metabolic alkalosis. The pH of gastric juice is 1.0, which represents a hydrogen concentration that is 1 million times the concentration of hydrogen seen in the blood. Of all causes of metabolic alkalosis, vomiting can result in the most dramatic rise in serum pH. Normally, for each hydrogen ion secreted into the stomach, there is one bicarbonate ion generated by gastric parietal cells that is reabsorbed in the blood. In the duodenum, chemoreceptors detect the low pH and stimulate the pancreas to secrete bicarbonate and to neutralize acid secretions locally (the stomach can tolerate high acid contents, but the rest of the gastrointestinal tract cannot). This secretion of bicarbonate into the duodenum is accompanied by the secretion of hydrogen into the blood to neutralize the bicarbonate that is released into circulation by parietal cells. In vomiting or gastric suctioning, the acid content of the stomach does not reach the duodenum. Therefore, there is no production of bicarbonate into the duodenum and no hydrogen release into the circulation to neutralize the bicarbonate production from the parietal cells. This will result in the generation of metabolic alkalosis.

Maintenance: Volume contraction will result in the activation of the renin-angiotensin-aldosterone system (RAAS), which will in turn reabsorb sodium in the distal tubule in exchange of potassium and hydrogen, thereby leading to more alkalosis. Other maintenance factors are hypokalemia and hypochloremia.

At what rate is bicarbonate being generated in the blood by the gastric fluid loss?

In vomiting and gastric suctioning, for each millimole of hydrogen loss, there is 1 mmol of bicarbonate generation in the blood. This will soon become a vicious circle if there is no volume expansion by normal saline.

What is the most important urine electrolyte in this patient? Why? What is it expected to be?

Urine chloride is the most important electrolyte in this case. During the early phase (first 3 days) after vomiting or nasogastric suctions, the rise in plasma bicarbonate concentrations results in greater bicarbonate filtration by the kidneys, increased urine bicarbonate loss, and high urine pH. However, there is sodium and potassium wasting, because urine sodium and potassium follow bicarbonate to conserve electroneutrality, despite hypovolemia. However, urine chloride excretion is decreased (<25 mmol/L) because chloride is the only reabsorbable anion (it can be reabsorbed with sodium), and there is volume and chloride depletion. During the late phase (>3 days), all bicarbonate is reabsorbed if volume and chloride depletion are still present. This is the result of increased bicarbonate reabsorptive capacity. Urine pH decreases (paradoxic aciduria) because all the bicarbonate is reabsorbed, and urine sodium, potassium, and chloride concentrations all decrease because of volume and chloride depletion (see Table 6-2).

How will the extracellular fluid volume be affected? What effect would this eventually have on renal bicarbonate reabsorption?

Extracellular fluid volume will be decreased, thereby resulting in greater urine bicarbonate reabsorption; this is described in more detail earlier in this chapter.

Give the important reasons for the low plasma potassium level.

Plasma potassium is low mainly as a result of the activation of RAAS. RAAS activation will lead to the reabsorption of sodium in exchange of potassium. In addition, metabolic alkalosis creates a shift of potassium into the cells. Finally, there is some potassium lost in the gastric fluid, although it is minimal

Suggested Readings

Galla JH: Metabolic alkalosis. *J Am Soc Nephrol* 11:369–375, 2000.

Gluck SL: Acid-base. *Lancet* 352:474–479, 1998.

PRACTICE QUESTIONS

A 50-year-old man presents to the emergency department with severe metabolic acidosis as a result of diabetic ketoacidosis. He is hypotensive, hypokalemic,
and obtunded.

1. The regulation of acid–base by the kidneys
   requires all except which one of the following?

   A. Bicarbonate reabsorption (near-total reabsorp-
      tion of filtered bicarbonate)
   B. Titratable acid formation ($H_2PO_4^-$)
   C. The formation of urinary ammonium by tubu-
      lar epithelial cells
   D. Healthy lungs

2. In cases of acidemia (diabetic ketoacidosis, in this
   case), what is the appropriate renal response?

   A. Increased net acid excretion
   B. Decreased urine pH
   C. Decreased ammoniagenesis
   D. Both A and B

3. In this case, net acid excretion may be increased
   by which of the following?

   A. Hypokalemia
   B. Hyperaldosteronism
   C. Decreased effective circulating volume
   D. All of the above

Metabolic Acidosis and Approach to Acid–Base Disorders

7

Frederick J. Boehm III
Kelly Ann Traeger
Arjang Djamali

OUTLINE
I. Metabolic Acidosis
  A. Introduction
  B. Pathogenesis
  C. Differential Diagnosis of Metabolic Acidosis
  D. Approach to a Patient with Metabolic Acidosis
  E. Treatment of Metabolic Acidosis

II. Approach to Patients with Acid–Base Disorders
  A. Required Data
  B. Stepwise Approach to Acid–Base Analysis

Objectives

- Understand the pathogenesis of metabolic acidosis.
- Understand the notion of the anion gap.
- Differentiate anion gap and normal anion gap metabolic acidosis.
- Most importantly, learn a stepwise approach to acid–base disorders.

Clinical Case

A 30-year-old African-American woman with a history of type 1 diabetes presents after 1 week of illness. Her husband reports that she had some fevers at the beginning of the week and that she was unable to eat because of intense nausea and vomiting during the past 3 days. The patient is confused during the examination. Her blood pressure is 80/40 mm Hg, her heart rate is 128 beats per minute, and her respiration rate is 22 breaths per minute. Her laboratory values include the following: pH, 7.15; partial pressure of carbon dioxide (PCO$_2$), 22 mm Hg; sodium, 132 mmol/L; potassium, 5.8 mmol/L; bicarbonate, 5 mmol/L; chloride, 80 mmol/L; blood urea nitrogen, 155 mg/dl; creatinine, 2.2 mg/dl; and glucose, 650 mg/dl. Her urine pH is 5.6, sodium is 5 mmol/L, and potassium is 10 mmol/L. There are white blood cell clumps, many bacteria, and ketones present.

What is the current water and salt status of this patient? What is the underlying acid–base status? What is the principal cause of this acid–base disorder? How should this patient be managed? What is the underlying cause of the hyperkalemia?

I. METABOLIC ACIDOSIS

A. Introduction

Metabolic acidosis is a systemic disorder that is defined by a primary fall in bicarbonate that can lead to acidemia if left unopposed. Metabolic acidosis triggers a predictable respiratory compensation through hyperventilation that lowers the partial pressure of carbon dioxide (PCO$_2$) level. In metabolic acidosis, each 1 mmol decrease of plasma bicarbonate concentration correlates to a 1 to 1.5 mm Hg decrease in PCO$_2$ levels (Fig. 7-1). This response begins during the first hour and is complete by 12 to 24 hours. The presence of an inappropriate respiratory response leads to a mixed acid–base disorder.

B. Pathogenesis

Metabolic acidosis can be produced by three major mechanisms.

1. Bicarbonate loss
   a. Kidney: proximal renal tubular acidosis (RTA type II)
   b. Gastrointestinal: diarrhea
2. Bicarbonate consumption in response to excessive endogenous acid production or exogenous acid intake
3. Decreased acid excretion with failure to regenerate bicarbonate
   a. Acute kidney injury or chronic kidney disease
   b. Distal RTA (types I and IV)

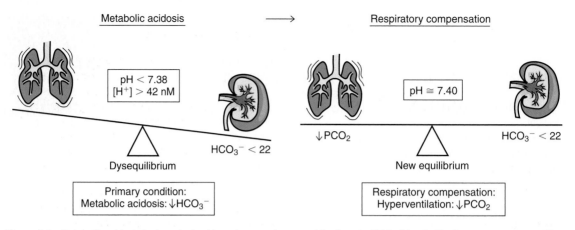

Figure 7-1. Metabolic acidosis is characterized by a decrease in serum bicarbonate (HCO_3^-) levels. The lungs compensate with a decrease in partial pressure of carbon dioxide (PCO_2). The pulmonary compensation defends the pH and raises it closer to 7.40.

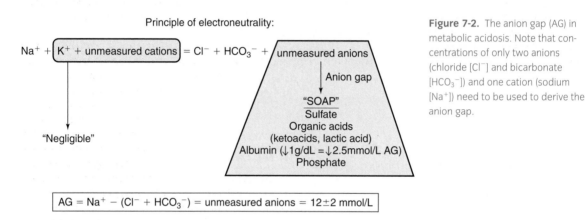

Figure 7-2. The anion gap (AG) in metabolic acidosis. Note that concentrations of only two anions (chloride [Cl^-] and bicarbonate [HCO_3^-]) and one cation (sodium [Na^+]) need to be used to derive the anion gap.

$$AG = Na^+ - (Cl^- + HCO_3^-) = \text{unmeasured anions} = 12 \pm 2 \text{ mmol/L}$$

C. Differential Diagnosis of Metabolic Acidosis

1. Anion Gap

The determination of the plasma anion gap (AG) is an important step in approaching the differential diagnosis of metabolic acidosis. AG calculation is based on the principle of electroneutrality. The sum of the positively charged particles (cations) equals the sum of the negatively charged particles (anions) in the plasma. The AG is the sum of unmeasured anions (Fig. 7-2). These unmeasured anions are usually defined by plasma sulfate, organic acids (i.e., lactic acid and ketoacids), albumin, and phosphate. Thus, in hypoalbuminemia, a correction of 2.5 mmol/L in the AG is made for every 1 g/dl reduction in albumin below 4.

The addition of a nonchloride-containing acid (e.g., lactic acid) to the plasma results in an equimolar increase in the AG as compared with the decrease in plasma bicarbonate levels (Fig. 7-3).

Similarly, the addition of a chloride-containing acid (e.g., hydrochloric acid) to the plasma results in an equimolar increase in chloride concentrations as compared with the decrease in plasma bicarbonate levels (Fig. 7-4).

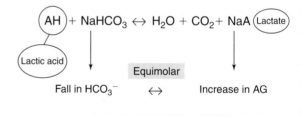

Figure 7-3. In cases of anion gap metabolic acidosis (AGMA), the fall in the serum bicarbonate (HCO_3^-) level as a result of its buffering of the acid moiety is equivalent to the increase in anion gap.

Therefore, the first step in the approach to the differential diagnosis of metabolic acidosis is the determination of the AG. This will distinguish high AG metabolic acidosis (AGMA; AG >14 mmol/L) from normal AG metabolic acidosis (NAGMA; AG = 12 ± 2 mmol/L; Fig. 7-5). It is important to realize that the normal value of AG may vary from laboratory to laboratory.

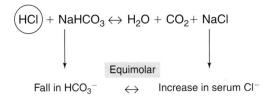

$$HCl + NaHCO_3 \leftrightarrow H_2O + CO_2 + NaCl$$

Equimolar

Fall in HCO_3^-   ↔   Increase in serum Cl^-

$$\downarrow HCO_3^- = \uparrow Cl^- \ (NAGMA)$$

Figure 7-4. In normal anion gap metabolic acidosis (NAGMA), the fall in the plasma bicarbonate (HCO_3^-) level is balanced by an equivalent increase in the level of serum chloride (Cl^-).

2. High Anion Gap Metabolic Acidosis

A. Categories

AGMA can be divided in two categories (see Fig. 7-5):

1. Low acid output, where there is decreased net acid excretion and failure to regenerate bicarbonate:
   a. Acute kidney injury
   b. Chronic kidney disease
2. High acid input, where bicarbonate is consumed to titrate endogenous or exogenous acids:
   a. Increased acid generation
      (1) Lactic acidosis as a result of shock or tissue hypoperfusion
      (2) Ketoacidosis:
         (a) Diabetic ketoacidosis (DKA)
         (b) Alcoholic ketoacidosis
         (c) Fasting ketoacidosis
   b. Increased acid intake, typically as a result of the following:
      (1) Aspirin overdose
      (2) Ethylene glycol overdose

(3) Alcohol overdose
(4) Methanol overdose

B. Causes of Anion Gap Metabolic Acidosis

Lactic acidosis. Normally, lactate is formed in the cell cytosol from pyruvate in a reaction that is catalyzed by the enzyme lactate dehydrogenase. The rates of lactic acid regeneration and use are usually equal in physiologic conditions (10–20 mmol/day). Most of the lactic acid metabolism occurs in the liver and, to a lesser extent, in the kidney, where it is converted to pyruvate and glucose, respectively. Lactic acidosis is observed in severely ill patients with marked tissue hypoxia as a result of hypoperfusion with or without hypoxia (type A lactic acidosis). Patients with liver failure or malignancies with no evidence of tissue hypoperfusion may also present with lactic acidosis (type B). In either case, lactic acid production exceeds its use, and AGMA ensues.

Ketoacidosis. DKA is characterized by hyperglycemia and AGMA that results from the overproduction of ketoacids (i.e., acetoacetic and β-hydroxybutyrate). The diagnosis is made on the basis of hyperglycemia, AGMA, and ketonemia or ketonuria. Most patients with this condition present with severe volume contraction (osmotic diuresis as a result of hyperglycemia). The overproduction of ketoacids results from low insulin levels. In this condition, fatty acids generated by lipolysis are used as an alternative source of energy and are delivered to the liver, where they are converted to ketoacids. The precipitating factor in DKA is often an infection or a cardiovascular event. This is a severe condition with potentially high mortality rates, and

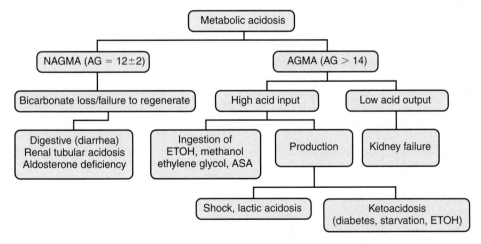

Figure 7-5. The diagnostic approach to metabolic acidosis. The first step is to determine whether the patient's metabolic acidosis is characterized by an elevated anion gap (AG; >14). In normal anion gap metabolic acidosis (NAGMA), the loss of bicarbonate is either from the gastrointestinal tract (e.g., in patients with diarrhea) or from the kidneys (e.g., in patients with renal tubular acidosis or aldosterone deficiency). Anion gap metabolic acidosis (AGMA) can occur in many situations, such as after ingestion of ethylene glycol, methanol, alcohol (ETOH), or acetyl salicylic acid (ASA); when there is the increased production of lactic acid or ketoacids; or in cases of kidney failure.

therefore, diabetic patients with DKA need prompt diagnosis and treatment. Alcohol and fasting may also result in ketoacidosis in which β-hydroxybutyrate is the primary unmeasured anion.

Acute kidney injury or chronic kidney disease. In patients with acute kidney injury or chronic kidney disease, there is the retention of both hydrogen and anions such as sulfate, phosphate, and urate. This is the result of the decreased filtration of acids and the inability of the remaining nephrons to regenerate enough bicarbonate. Therefore, these patients present with AGMA. However, depending on the level of kidney dysfunction and the underlying cause of the kidney disease, a component of NAGMA may also be present.

Ingestions. The major retained anions are formate with methanol, glycolate and oxalate with ethylene glycol, and ketones and lactate with aspirin.

3. Normal Anion Gap Metabolic Acidosis

NAGMA, which is also called *hyperchloremic metabolic acidosis,* often results from a loss or lack of the generation of plasma bicarbonate (Box 7-1).

A. Kidney Causes of Normal Anion Gap Metabolic Acidosis

The ingestion of an average protein-containing diet generates a net acid excess of approximately 1 mmol/kg/day. The kidneys regulate the acid–base balance via two mechanisms:

1. Reabsorption of the entire filtered bicarbonate (proximal tubule)
2. Acid excretion through ammonium (NH_4^+) excretion and titratable acid formation ($H_2PO_4^-$), both of which occur in the distal tubules

The kidneys may fail to provide an adequate net acid excretion balance because of either decreased acid excretion (i.e., distal RTAs, chronic kidney disease) or increased alkali wastage (i.e., proximal RTA). There are three forms of RTA: types I, II, and IV. There is no type III RTA. It may be more appropriate to use the terms proximal, distal hypokalemic, and distal hyperkalemic, because they are more descriptive (Table 7-1).

Distal hypokalemic RTA (type I). In patients with type I RTA, there is decreased hydrogen secretion in the collecting tubules, often as a result of hydrogen/ATPase pump failure. This leads to decreased ammonium excretion, which results in decreased distal bicarbonate regeneration and NAGMA. Urine pH is always greater than 5.6 (usually >6), and hypokalemia may be a consequence of secondary hyperaldosteronism and accelerated potassium secretion in the distal nephron. Both hereditary and acquired cases of distal hypokalemic RTA have been described. In addition, several medications induce type I RTA, including amphotericin B and lithium.

Proximal RTA (type II). Urine bicarbonate concentration is normally very low (<1 mmol/L). Most of the filtered bicarbonate is reabsorbed in the proximal tubule so that plasma bicarbonate concentrations stay higher than 24 mmol/L. In proximal RTA, a large fraction of the filtered load of bicarbonate is excreted because the kidney threshold of proximal bicarbonate reabsorption is "reset" at values less than 20 mmol/L (normal is 24–25 mmol/L). The regulation of bicarbonate reabsorption remains the same except for this lower threshold. Therefore, after plasma bicarbonate concentrations are below the new bicarbonate threshold, urine pH falls to levels that would be seen in normal subjects (≈5.6). An example is the Fanconi syndrome, which involves a generalized defect in proximal tubular transport that is manifested by glycosuria, aminoaciduria, phosphaturia, uric aciduria, and NAGMA.

Distal hyperkalemic RTA (type IV; see Table 7-1). Type IV RTA is characterized by hyperkalemic hyperchloremic metabolic acidosis associated with hypoaldosteronism and the preserved ability to lower urine pH to approximately 5.6. Decreased aldosterone activity results in impaired distal sodium reabsorption and potassium and hydrogen secretion. This is the most common form of RTA, and it generally results from decreased ammonia (NH_3) formation in the distal tubules. Genetic causes, hyperkalemia, and aldosterone deficiency may lead to type IV RTA. These findings are commonly associated with the syndrome of hyporeninemic hypoaldosteronism that is observed in diabetic patients.

Chronic kidney disease. At advanced stages of chronic kidney disease (i.e., a glomerular filtration rate of <20 ml/min), there may be a mixed AGMA and NAGMA as the kidneys fail to regenerate bicarbonate (NAGMA) and also fail to excrete titratable acids, including sulfate and phosphate (AGMA).

Box 7-1. Causes of Nonanion Gap Metabolic Acidosis

1. Increased input of chloride-containing acids
   a. Hydrochloric acid
   b. Ammonium chloride
2. Increased bicarbonate loss
   a. Renal
      (1) Proximal renal tubular acidosis (type II)
      (2) Urinary tract diversions to the intestine
   b. Digestive
      (1) Diarrhea
      (2) Ileus
      (3) Fistula
3. Decreased bicarbonate regeneration
   a. Distal hypokalemic renal tubular acidosis (type I)
   b. Distal hyperkalemic renal tubular acidosis (type IV)
   c. Aldosterone deficiency
   d. Kidney failure (glomerular filtration rate <20 ml/min)
   e. Hyperkalemia

Table 7-1. Common Causes of Renal Tubular Acidosis

	Renal tubular acidosis I	Renal tubular acidosis II	Renal tubular acidosis IV
Also called	Distal hypokalemic renal tubular acidosis	Proximal renal tubular acidosis	Distal hyperkalemic renal tubular acidosis
Pathophysiology	Decreased distal acidification	Decreased bicarbonate reabsorption	Decreased aldosterone
Cause, hereditary	Autosomal dominant; autosomal recessive	Cystinosis; Wilson disease	Primary aldosterone deficiency
Cause, acquired	Amphotericin B; lupus; Sjögren's syndrome; rheumatoid arthritis	Heavy metals; multiple myeloma; amyloidosis *Fanconi syndrome*	Potassium-sparing diuretics; angiotensin-converting enzyme inhibitors; nonsteroidal antiinflammatory drugs; cyclosporine A; hyporeninemic hypoaldosteronism
Serum bicarbonate	Sometimes <10 mmol/L	12–20 mmol/L	≥16 mmol/L
Serum potassium	Decreased	Decreased	Increased
Urine pH	Always >5.6	May be lowered	May be lowered

B. Gastrointestinal Causes of Normal Anion Gap Metabolic Acidosis

Bicarbonate concentration in the stool is between 50 and 70 mmol/L. Diarrhea may result in a significant bicarbonate loss and therefore NAGMA.

4. Mixed Cases

There may be overlap between the causes of AGMA and NAGMA. Diarrhea is most often associated with NAGMA. In some patients, however, there is an increase in the AG as a result of volume contraction and hypoperfusion. The same observation was made previously when it was noted that chronic renal failure may cause both AGMA and NAGMA together.

D. Approach to a Patient with Metabolic Acidosis

The diagnostic approach to a patient with metabolic acidosis includes a history and physical examination, the calculation of the AG (see Fig. 7-5), and the determination of the urine pH and arterial blood gases. The urine AG and the plasma ormolu gap are other diagnostic tools that may be used in complex acid–base disturbances.

E. Treatment of Metabolic Acidosis

The treatment of metabolic acidosis may vary markedly with the underlying disorder. However, the general principles outlined here may be applied to all causes of metabolic acidosis.

The aim of therapy in metabolic acidosis is the restoration of a normal extracellular pH. The normal renal response in this setting is to markedly increase acid excretion, primarily as ammonium. Thus, exogenous alkali may not be required if the acidemia is not severe (i.e., arterial pH >7.20), if the patient is asymptomatic, and if the underlying process can be controlled (e.g., diarrhea). In cases in which the plasma pH is less than 7.20, however, correction of the acidemia can be achieved more rapidly by the administration of sodium bicarbonate. The initial aim of therapy is to raise the systemic pH to higher than 7.20; this is the level at which the major consequences of severe acidemia should not be observed. Few available formulae can estimate the bicarbonate deficit on the basis of patient weight (lean body mass), plasma bicarbonate concentrations, and the estimated space of distribution for bicarbonate.

II. APPROACH TO PATIENTS WITH ACID–BASE DISORDERS

The approach to the patient with an acid–base disturbance needs to be thorough. Only a systematic strategy can ensure that the student, resident, or physician omits nothing.

A. Required Data

There are four sets of data that are required to fully analyze acid–base disorders:

1. **A thorough history and physical examination** will clarify whether there has been a history of kidney disease (acute or chronic), lung disease (acute or chronic), vomiting, diarrhea, toxic drug intake,

and so on. It will determine whether the patient is volume contracted, and it will enable the health care provider to determine the primary disorder (metabolic vs. respiratory) and to use the appropriate compensation formulae (see Box 7-1).

2. **Arterial blood gases** are a critical step in acid–base analysis because they will define the problem and provide the values for measured plasma pH, PCO_2, partial pressure of oxygen, and oxygen saturation and calculated bicarbonate levels (Fig. 7-6).

3. **Plasma electrolytes** will help to determine measured bicarbonate levels, the AG, and plasma potassium concentrations, all of which are important players in acid–base regulation. The physician should obtain arterial blood gases and electrolytes simultaneously.

4. **Urinalysis and urine pH** will guide the physician toward potential underlying renal disease (e.g., proteinuria, hematuria, casts) and the appropriateness of urine pH as compared with plasma pH (e.g., low urine pH when acidemia is present and increased urine pH with alkalemia).

B. Stepwise Approach to Acid–Base Analysis

After the appropriate data are acquired, a stepwise approach will help with the complete analysis of the acid–base disturbance (Box 7-2). A stepwise approach will prevent mistakes and ease the anxiety of analyzing a patient's acid–base status. The first step is to use the pH to determine whether acidemia or alkalemia is present. Next, examine the plasma bicarbonate level. If metabolic acidosis is present, determine the AG to help with the differential diagnosis. Next, examine the PCO_2 to determine whether respiratory acidosis or alkalosis is present. Steps 5 and 6 are key steps that examine the physiologic response (e.g., hyperventilation by the lungs and respiratory alkalosis if underlying metabolic acidosis is present) using various formulae. First, one needs to determine the primary disorder. Then, the appropriate formula must be applied to estimate the physiologic response. For example, if the bicarbonate level has moved in the same direction as the pH, then a metabolic disturbance is in play (i.e., pH = 7.35 with bicarbonate = 19 → metabolic acidosis). The history and physical examination should also help

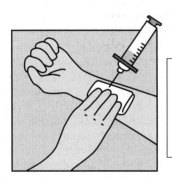

Arterial blood gases (ABGs)

pH = 7.40±0.02
PCO_2 = 40±2 mm Hg
HCO_3^- = 24±2 mmol/L
O_2 = 90 − 100 mm Hg
O_2 Saturation = 95 − 100%

Figure 7-6. Normal arterial blood gas values.

Box 7-2. Stepwise Approach to Acid–Base Analysis	
1. pH = 7.40	Acidemia or alkalemia
2. Bicarbonate (HCO_3^-) (25 ± 2)	Metabolic acidosis or alkalosis
3. Anion gap (12 ± 2)	Measure if metabolic acidosis present or chloride level is low
4. Partial pressure of carbon dioxide (PCO_2) (40 ± 2)	Respiratory acidosis or alkalosis
5. Primary disorder	History and serum pH: primary disorder usually defines pH
6. Physiologic response	Use compensation on the basis of the primary disorder
a. Metabolic acidosis	$\Delta PCO_2 = 1.25\Delta HCO_3^-$ (±2)*
	or Winter's formula: $PCO_2 = (1.5 \times HCO_3^-) + 8$ (±2)
b. Metabolic alkalosis	$\Delta PCO_2 = 0.7\Delta HCO_3^-$ (±2)
c. Respiratory acidosis	Acute: $\Delta HCO_3^- = 0.2\Delta PCO_2$ (±2)
	Chronic: $\Delta HCO_3^- = 0.4\Delta PCO_2$ (±2)
d. Respiratory alkalosis	Acute: $\Delta HCO_3^- = 0.2\Delta PCO_2$ (±2)
	Chronic: $\Delta HCO_3^- = 0.4\Delta PCO_2$ (±2)
7. Final diagnosis	Simple vs. mixed acid–base disorder

Other sources may present slightly different constant coefficients than those presented here. This should not be a source of distress. In most cases, no significant difference is found in the final result.

to determine the underlying primary disorder (e.g., a young patient with type 1 diabetes with urinary tract infection and vomiting suggests DKA and therefore a metabolic disorder). After the compensation formulae are used, the physician can determine if a simple or a mixed acid–base disturbance is present.

Clinical Case

A 30-year-old African-American woman with a history of type 1 diabetes presents after 1 week of illness. Her husband reports that she had some fevers at the beginning of the week and that she was unable to eat because of intense nausea and vomiting during the past 3 days. The patient is confused during the examination. Her blood pressure is 80/40 mm Hg, her heart rate is 128 beats per minute, and her respiration rate is 22 breaths per minute. Her laboratory values include the following: pH, 7.15; partial pressure of carbon dioxide (PCO_2), 22 mm Hg; sodium, 132 mmol/L; potassium, 5.8 mmol/L; bicarbonate, 5 mmol/L; chloride, 80 mmol/L; blood urea nitrogen, 155 mg/dl; creatinine, 2.2 mg/dl; and glucose, 650 mg/dl. Her urine pH is 5.6, sodium is 5 mmol/L, and potassium is 10 mmol/L. There are white blood cell clumps, many bacteria, and ketones present.

What is the current water and salt status of this patient?

She is hypertonic because her serum osmolality is increased.

$$2\,Sodium + Blood\ urea\ nitrogen/2.8 + Glucose/18 = 355\ mOsmol/kg$$

She is hypovolemic as a result of low blood pressure, low urine sodium, a history of low food and fluid intake, increased gastrointestinal output, and osmotic diuresis (high glucose levels).

What is the underlying acid–base status?

This is a case of mixed metabolic and respiratory acidosis. Using the stepwise approach, the following is determined:

    pH = 7.15: acidemia
    Bicarbonate = 5: metabolic acidosis
    AG = Sodium – (Bicarbonate + Chloride) = 47: increased significantly; this is a case of AGMA (ketone bodies in urine)
    PCO_2 = 22: respiratory alkalosis
    The primary disorder is metabolic for two reasons. First, bicarbonate is low (metabolic acidosis) and pH is

low (acidemia), and both are going in the same direction (acidosis). Furthermore, the history of a diabetic patient with ketone bodies in the urine and acidosis makes for the diagnosis of DKA, which is a metabolic disorder.

Next, the physiologic respiratory response will be examined. According to Winter's formula, $PCO_2 = 1.5 \times$ Bicarbonate + 8 (±2), which, in this case, is $1.5 \times 5 + 8 = 15.5$ (±2). However, PCO_2 is at 22 here, which is higher than the expected physiologic response. Thus, there is a component of respiratory acidosis.

The final diagnosis is mixed metabolic and respiratory acidosis. The reason for respiratory acidosis is that the patient cannot hyperventilate enough to compensate for the level of metabolic acidosis. She is getting confused and tired.

What is the principal cause of this acid–base disorder?

There is mixed metabolic and respiratory acidosis. From the metabolic standpoint, diabetic ketoacidosis (DKA), acute kidney injury, hypotension, and the increased production of fatty acids and the resulting organic acids (ketone bodies) are all responsible for the low bicarbonate levels. The patient also hypoventilates for the level of metabolic acidosis to compensate appropriately.

How should this patient be managed?

For patients with DKA, the mainstays of treatment are the treatment of the cause (in this case, antibiotics for urinary tract infection) and a combination of insulin and normal saline with potassium chloride. Therapy with sodium bicarbonate is not needed because volume expansion with normal saline and insulin therapy together will progressively correct the underlying metabolic acidosis.

What is the underlying cause of the hyperkalemia?

Hyperkalemia is only a response to severe acidemia. In fact, in this patient, body potassium is likely to be significantly decreased, and there is an increased risk for cardiac arrhythmias and death if potassium supplements are not provided. Poor oral intake, gastrointestinal losses, and osmotic diuresis are responsible for decreased potassium pools.

Suggested Readings

Boron W: Acid-base transport by the renal proximal tubule. *J Am Soc Nephrol* 17:2368–2382, 2006.
Gluck SL: Acid-base. *Lancet* 352:474–479, 1998.

PRACTICE QUESTIONS

A 50-year-old man with a medical history that includes bipolar disorder presents to the emergency department with increasing confusion and sleepiness of 2 days' duration. The physician learns that the patient's psychiatrist recently increased his lithium dose. His plasma pH is 7.30, his PCO_2 level is 30 mm Hg, his sodium level is 135 mmol/L, his bicarbonate level is 9 mmol/L, and his chloride level is 116 mmol/L.

1. Which acid–base disorder is most likely to be present in this patient?

   A. Metabolic acidosis
   B. Metabolic alkalosis
   C. Respiratory acidosis
   D. Respiratory alkalosis

2. Which class of RTA is most likely to be present in this patient?

   A. I
   B. II
   C. III
   D. IV

3. Which of the following is least likely to be associated with this patient's distal hypokalemic RTA?

   A. Urine pH <5
   B. Increased potassium secretion in the distal nephron
   C. Hydrogen-ATPase pump failure (or inhibition) in the collecting duct
   D. Elevated serum aldosterone level

Glomerular Diseases

8

A. Vishnu Moorthy
Byram H. Ozer
Terry D. Oberley
Weixiong Zhong

OUTLINE
I. Introduction to Glomerular Disease
  A. Basic Terminology
  B. Review of Glomerular Physiology
II. Methods of Evaluating Kidney Disorders
  A. Clinical Findings in Glomerular Disease
  B. Urinalysis in Glomerular Disease
  C. Laboratory Studies in Glomerulonephritis
  D. Microscopic Evaluation of Glomeruli in Renal Biopsy
III. Mechanisms of Glomerular Injury
IV. Pathology of Glomerular Diseases
  A. Primary Nephrotic Syndrome Glomerular Pathology

  B. Secondary Nephrotic Syndrome Glomerular Pathology
  C. Primary Nephritic Syndrome Glomerular Pathology
  D. Secondary Nephritic Syndrome Glomerular Pathology
V. Mechanisms of Vascular Injury
  A. Systemic Vasculitis
  B. Thrombotic Microangiopathies
VI. Summary

Objectives
- Review important glomerular physiology.
- Recognize the clinical manifestations of the major categories of glomerular disease.
- Understand the pathophysiology of the various forms of glomerular injury.
- Know the underlying morphology of some common types of glomerular injury.

Clinical Case

A 7-year-old girl is referred to a kidney specialist by her pediatrician for lower extremity and periorbital edema of a few weeks' duration. Her physical examination is normal aside from the edema. Blood chemistries are significant for an albumin level of 2.5 g/dl, a serum creatinine level of 0.6 mg/dl, and a cholesterol level of 270 mg/dl. Urinalysis reveals no blood, but 4+ protein by the dipstick and the microscopy of the sediment shows hyaline casts and several fat globules. A Maltese-cross shape is noted when the urine sediment is viewed under polarized light, and protein excretion is more than 8 g in a 24-hour urine collection.

Is this a nephrotic or a nephritic presentation? What should the physician expect to see on renal biopsy under light microscopy and under electron microscopy? What is the proposed site and mechanism of this disease?

I. INTRODUCTION TO GLOMERULAR DISEASE

Diseases of the glomeruli can be caused by diverse mechanisms. Although some of these mechanisms are well understood at the present time, the causes of many other glomerular diseases and their respective mechanisms of tissue injury remain obscure. The symptoms and signs of glomerular disease for which the patient comes to see the physician are highly variable. Although one patient may be symptomatic and present with many classic symptoms, others may remain asymptomatic until their glomerular disease has advanced to such a degree that they require dialysis or transplantation. Despite this wide range of presentations, in many cases, clinical signs and symptoms can be correlated with a histologic presentation after the biopsy of the kidney. The study of the kidney tissue often reveals not only the type of disease but also lends insights into its cause. Therefore, knowledge of the clinical symptoms and signs in the patient, as well as the histologic appearances in the kidney tissue, are vital to approaching patients with glomerular diseases and to understanding the underlying pathologies. After studying this chapter, the reader should be able to identify some of the better-characterized glomerular

diseases and to think critically about the effects that these diseases have on the patient.

A. Basic Terminology
The following definitions are used to describe histologic findings in glomerular disease. These serve to illustrate the location, extent, and appearance of glomerular injury without necessarily reflecting the mechanism:

Focal: Lesions involving less than 50% of the glomeruli noted on light microscopy.

Diffuse: Lesions involving more than 50% of the glomeruli noted on light microscopy.

Segmental: Lesions involving a portion of the glomerular tuft (often these lesions are also focal).

Global: Lesions involving the entire glomerular tuft (often these lesions are also diffuse).

Membranous: Thickening of the glomerular capillary wall as a result of deposits on the epithelial side of the glomerular capillary basement membrane.

Proliferative: An increased number of cells in the glomerulus, either proliferating glomerular cells or infiltrating inflammatory cells (the term *exudative* is used when these infiltrating cells are neutrophils).

Mesangiopathic: Disease process that is confined to the mesangium of the glomerulus and that does not affect the outer capillary wall. The mesangium may have increased cells, matrix, or both.

Membranoproliferative: Evidence of thickening of the capillary wall, expansion of the mesangium, and proliferative changes to the glomeruli.

Crescent: An accumulation of cells in the Bowman's space (frequently monocytes and Bowman's capsule cells).

Glomerulosclerosis: Segmental or global capillary collapse with scarring.

Glomerulonephritis: Any condition associated with inflammation of the glomerulus.

B. Review of Glomerular Physiology
Renal histology and physiology have already been reviewed in Chapter 1 of this text, and the reader may wish to review some of the important concepts discussed there before proceeding with this chapter.

The primary function of the glomerulus is to filter the components of the plasma. Specifically, the glomerulus separates the cellular components of the blood and plasma proteins from water and a range of waste products to be excreted in the urine. The glomerular capillary wall is composed of three layers that are collectively known as the filtration barrier (Box 8-1):

1. The inner fenestrated glomerular endothelium
2. The central glomerular basement membrane (GBM)
3. The foot processes and slit diaphragms of the outer epithelial cell, which is known as the *podocyte*

Filtration by these three layers occurs either by size or charge exclusion. The inner fenestrated endothelium

---

Box 8-1. Filtration Layers of the Glomerulus

1. Inner endothelium: charge exclusion (i.e., exclusion of anions)
2. Middle glomerular basement membrane: charge exclusion (i.e., exclusion of anions)
3. Outer podocyte: charge and size exclusion (i.e., exclusion of anions and large molecules)

---

contains openings that are approximately an order of magnitude larger than most plasma proteins. However, its negatively charged surface anions (e.g., heparan sulfate) help to repel the largely anionic macromolecules (e.g., proteins) that are contained in the circulating plasma. Similarly, the GBM contains proteins with negative charges that further serve to exclude anions from the glomerular filtrate. Consistent with this hypothesis is that the glomerular filtration of anions is very limited at values of more than a molecular weight of 70,000, whereas cations are much more permeable and can be filtered at a size of nearly an order of magnitude larger.

By contrast, the outer podocyte filters both by charge and size exclusion. This epithelial cell attaches to the GBM via discrete cytoplasmic appendages called *foot processes*, which interdigitate in a fencelike mesh that makes up the slit diaphragms. This effectively allows smaller solutes (e.g., electrolytes, water, urea) to pass into the filtrate while excluding cells and larger biomolecules.

The example given in Box 8-2 applies the terminology from this section and introduces clinical reasoning, which will be discussed in more detail in the next section.

II. METHODS OF EVALUATING KIDNEY DISORDERS

A. Clinical Findings in Glomerular Disease
The most important step in establishing any diagnosis is to obtain a good clinical history and physical examination. However, the usefulness of this is particularly challenging in patients with glomerulonephritis because their symptom presentation is widely variable: some patients may have the classic signs of chronic kidney disease or other obvious symptoms, whereas many others can be completely asymptomatic. Therefore, it is essential for the clinician to understand this spectrum of presentation and to further define the overarching syndromes by which glomerular diseases can manifest themselves.

1. Asymptomatic Glomerulonephritis
Some patients, as mentioned previously, may be clinically asymptomatic and yet have urinary abnormalities such as minimal proteinuria or microscopic

Box 8-2. Example A.

A 43-year-old woman presents with concerns about her urine turning dark brown. The physician orders a dipstick test to confirm hematuria (blood in urine) as well as a minimal amount of proteinuria (protein in urine). The urine sediment reveals many dysmorphic red blood cells (RBCs) and RBC casts. In the process of the clinical workup, the physician makes note of the elevated blood pressure and kidney failure, which is reflected in an elevated serum creatinine level. Suspecting a kidney disorder, the physician orders a kidney biopsy. The results indicate a segmental necrosis of the glomerular capillaries under light microscopy as well as the presence of cellular crescents in many glomeruli. Immunofluorescence microscopy reveals the linear deposition of immunoglobulin G along the glomerular basement membrane (GBM). A radioimmunoassay confirms the presence of circulating anti-GBM antibodies in the serum. The physician concludes that the patient suffers from anti-GBM disease.

Anti-GBM disease is an uncommon condition that causes a very severe and rapidly progressive kidney failure. The primary damage is in the GBM as evidenced by both the disruption in light microscopy and the immunofluorescence studies. With a disruption of the GBM and an injury to the filtration apparatus, the presence of hematuria with dysmorphic RBCs and RBC casts is noted. The crescent pattern results from the proliferation of the podocytes as well as from the accumulation of monocytes, and it is a common finding among patients with anti-GBM disease.

The segmental disruption of the GBM suggests that only portions of any individual glomerulus are affected. Therapy with immunosuppressive agents, along with plasmapheresis with the removal of antibodies from the serum, is beneficial for recovery from the kidney failure.

a large-scale movement of protein into the urine that causes the massive proteinuria. One of the primary losses is of albumin, which results in low blood albumin levels (hypoalbuminemia). As a result of the loss of this oncotically active component from the plasma (see Chapter 4), there is a movement of fluid to the interstitial space that results in edema. The decrease in plasma volume causes a decrease in perfusion of the kidneys that, in turn, leads to greater sodium retention by the kidneys and the exacerbation of the edema. The patient can have considerable weight gain and swelling as well as ascites and pleural effusion in severe cases. Finally, an increase in the production of lipoproteins by the liver in nephrotic patients causes hyperlipidemia, although the exact mechanism for this is unknown. This carries increased risks for atherosclerosis and cardiovascular disease with it, which can complicate the renal insult. Other common findings reflect urinary losses of circulating anticlotting factors. The loss of antithrombin III can lead to hypercoagulability and thromboembolic complications. An increased incidence of infection (e.g., pneumococcal peritonitis) may be noted from losses of antibodies and opsonization factors in the urine.

3. The Nephritic Syndrome
In some types of glomerular diseases, hematuria is the predominant finding in a urinalysis, and it is accompanied by RBC casts. In extreme cases, the urine is visibly darkened and adopts a smoky or cola-colored hue from the effects of acidic urine on hemoglobin. This is a classic description of the nephritic syndrome, the hallmark feature of which is an "active" urine sediment that contains RBCs and RBC casts. Other findings include oliguria (small amounts of urine) and edema as well as hypertension and increased blood urea nitrogen and serum creatinine levels. At times there is acute kidney injury that may require dialysis. Massive proteinuria is conspicuously absent from the diagnosis of the nephritic syndrome.

4. Mixed Nephrotic and Nephritic Syndromes
Because glomerular diseases exist on a continuum, it is possible to have a mixture of nephrotic and nephritic presentations. In these cases, elements of each syndrome exist, and patients usually present with proteinuria and edema in the context of hematuria, renal insufficiency, and hypertension.

5. Chronic Kidney Disease
This condition is discussed in more detail in later chapters. With several types of glomerular diseases, the injury is insidious and slowly progressive, and it remains undetected until the kidney function has deteriorated considerably (the symptoms of chronic kidney disease are discussed in Chapter 12). The patient can have hypertension, edema, and variable

hematuria of varying degrees. In these instances, the presence of dysmorphic (i.e., misshapen or varying in shape with blebs on the surface) red blood cells (RBCs) and casts of several types in the urine sediment under a microscope can often indicate glomerular disease.

2. The Nephrotic Syndrome
In some types of glomerular diseases, massive proteinuria is the predominant finding. When the urinalysis indicates a loss of protein in the urine of more than 3.5 g/day (in adults), the condition is designated as the *nephrotic syndrome*. This is usually in the context of a classic tetrad that includes massive proteinuria, hypoalbuminemia, edema, and hyperlipidemia. When the filtration apparatus of the glomerulus breaks down in the nephrotic syndrome, there is

I. Nephrotic: Proteinuria
  A. Massive proteinuria (>3.5 g/1 g of creatinine)
  B. Hypoalbuminemia
  C. Edema
  D. Hyperlipidemia
II. Nephritic: Inflammation of the glomeruli
  A. Oliguria and hematuria (smoky, cola-colored urine)
  B. Hypertension
  C. Signs of active urine sediment (dysmorphic red blood cells, red blood cell casts)

decreases in kidney function. With these patients, it is also possible to detect either hematuria and/or proteinuria, which would substantiate the suspicion of glomerular damage.

B. Urinalysis in Glomerular Disease

Urinalysis (see Chapter 10) is one of the most critical steps in the diagnosis and classification of renal disease and other urinary abnormalities. Freshly collected urine is centrifuged and examined by light microscopy (of the sediment) and chemical-sensitive dipsticks (of the supernatant). These tests can detect many different factors, but of most relevance to the diagnosis of glomerular pathology are RBCs and protein.

1. Red Blood Cells

RBCs can be detected by dipstick analysis (which detects hemoglobin) or light microscopy (>2–3 RBCs per high-power field is abnormal), and they can sometimes be seen grossly as a reddening or darkening of the urine.

The mere presence of blood in the urine, however, says little about the source of the blood. RBCs can originate from anywhere in the urinary tract, so one cannot automatically assume a glomerular disease. When visualized under the microscope, there are two microscopic indications that hematuria is attributable to a glomerular disorder:
  1. The RBCs are dysmorphic, varying in size, shape, appearance, and hemoglobin content and featuring numerous surface blebs and distortions.
  2. The urine contains RBC casts. These are cigar-shaped masses of mostly glycoproteins that are secreted by the thick ascending limb of the loop of Henle and formed in the renal tubules; they have RBCs embedded in them.

2. Protein

Although low-molecular-weight proteins (e.g., immunoglobulin light chains, small peptides) can freely move across the capillary wall, the filtration of larger macromolecules (e.g., albumin, globulins) is restricted. Among patients with glomerular disease, the

filtration apparatus breaks down and allows abnormal amounts of protein to enter the urine. Although a high amount of urinary protein is often indicative of glomerular injury, this finding is by no means sufficient for a diagnosis.

The presence of protein in the urine can be tested in several ways. The easiest and most convenient test is the urinary dipstick test. This procedure is semi-quantitative and easy to perform, but it tests primarily for albumin, thereby neglecting other protein components and contributors to disease (e.g., immunoglobulins and light chains in multiple myeloma). The more sensitive sulfosalicylic acid turbidity test can be used to test for all proteins; this is particularly useful for 24-hour quantifications, which should not exceed 150 mg per day in a healthy adult (Box 8-4).

Finally, a more sensitive approach is to use antibodies that are directed against albumin. This is most useful in the context of microalbuminuria, where small amounts of albumin are lost through the chronically diseased glomerulus, such as occurs in patients with diabetes mellitus (more information about this topic is provided later in this chapter).

C. Laboratory Studies in Glomerulonephritis

Serologic studies of the blood are an important method of diagnosing glomerular diseases. Many glomerular diseases are mediated by immune mechanisms, and serologic tests are helpful for their diagnosis. In some instances, circulating antibodies or antigens that are either a cause or a consequence of the glomerular insult may be noted in the blood (Table 8-1). It is important to note that the results of these serologic tests are supportive of—but may not be sufficient for—a diagnosis of glomerular disease.

A 10-year-old boy is seen in the clinic for darkened urine. A dipstick urinalysis test comes back positive for heme, but the protein result comes back only as trace. How can these findings be explained? What further work must be done to confirm them?

Red blood cells: The positive dipstick test in combination with the visible darkening of the urine makes a strong argument for hematuria. However, blood in the urine can be attributable to a number of sources, so this result must be confirmed by analyzing the urinary sediment under the microscope and looking for red blood cell casts and/or dysmorphic red blood cells.

Protein: In this instance, the absence of detectable protein by dipstick indicates that, although the glomerular injury has led to the passage of cells from the capillaries into the Bowman's space, the passage of protein molecules across the capillary walls has only been modest.

Table 8-1. Antigens and Antibodies in Glomerular Diseases

Antibody	Associated glomerular disease	Antigen
Antineutrophil cytoplasmic antibodies (ANCA)	Systemic vasculitis	PR3 (C-ANCA) MPO (P-ANCA)
Antinuclear antibody	Systemic lupus erythematosus	Variety of antigens (e.g., DNA, histones)
Anti-glomerular basement membrane	Anti-glomerular basement membrane disease, Goodpasture syndrome	α_3 Type IV collagen
Immunoglobulin A immunoglobulins	Immunoglobulin A nephropathy	Unknown
Immunoglobulin G	Membranous nephropathy	Unknown
Immunoglobulin G	Poststreptococcal glomerulonephritis	NAPlr or zSpeB/SpeB

D. Microscopic Evaluation of Glomeruli in Renal Biopsy

By far the best diagnostic tool for glomerular disease comes from the examination of a tissue biopsy. This is not always practical given the invasiveness of the procedure, but it yields the most information about the condition. The biopsy of the kidney can be useful for justifying therapy with medications that may have significant side effects. Biopsy also provides information regarding patient outcome. Collected tissue is analyzed with various forms of microscopy. The simplest method is with the use of light microscopy. This is most useful for localizing and assessing the extent of damage, although in some instances pathologic examination provides definitive clues (e.g., crescent formations in anti-GBM disease). In addition to hematoxylin and eosin (H & E) staining, special stains such as periodic acid–Schiff (PAS) and periodic acid–methenamine (PAM) can be helpful for elucidating the precise location and nature of the insult.

Samples can also be processed for immunofluorescence microscopy by incubating the sample with fluorescent antibodies that are directed against human immunoglobulins or complement components. This technique is most useful for studying the distribution of immunoglobulins and complement proteins, and it can help to clarify the immunologic mechanism that may be responsible for the glomerular disease.

Finally, diagnoses that remain elusive can be analyzed under the electron microscope to reveal ultrastructural changes that are not otherwise visible by light microscopy. In this case, insults that result in the disruption of the filtration barrier can be directly visualized, including changes in the GBM and alterations in the podocyte foot process.

The combination of all of these techniques is very powerful for diagnosis and monitoring treatment responses, although invasiveness as well as expense must be carefully considered before a renal biopsy is performed.

III. MECHANISMS OF GLOMERULAR INJURY

Mechanisms of tissue injury in glomerulonephritis may be unknown, in which case the disease is called *idiopathic*. Known glomerular disease mechanisms can be classified into two broad categories: immune or nonimmune.

Immune mechanisms present as depositions of antibodies or immune complexes made of antibody-antigen complexes. The glomerulus is especially susceptible to trapping these complexes, which causes severe disruption of the filtration apparatus. In some instances, the immune complexes are located in the subepithelial layers or right outside of the GBM, beneath the podocyte foot processes. In these cases, the mechanism of deposition is thought to involve infiltration of antibodies and binding to antigens on the podocytes (i.e., the *in-situ* formation of immune complexes). The immune complexes in this location are less exposed to the circulatory system and fail to trigger immune responses; they do not show increased glomerular cellularity. Because they injure the podocyte and the filtration barrier, they lead to massive proteinuria and present with the nephrotic syndrome. By contrast, immune complexes deposited in the subendothelial layer are closer to the vascular space and elicit an inflammatory response with increased cellularity in the glomerulus as well as the disruption of the capillary wall, thereby leading to the nephritic syndrome.

In some cases that present with massive proteinuria and the nephrotic syndrome, there is clearly a deficiency

in the glomerular capillary barrier. However, there may be no evidence of cellular proliferation or the deposition of immunoglobulins in the glomeruli, which suggests that immune cells, antibodies, and immune complexes are not involved. Electron microscopic visualization reveals the diffuse effacement (also described erroneously by some as fusion) of the fingerlike foot processes of the podocytes. Although the exact mechanisms are poorly characterized, the podocytes are the site of injury in these instances. These disorders, which are also referred to as *podocytopathies,* may be caused by inherited abnormalities in different proteins that are crucial to maintaining the structure and function of the podocyte, infectious agents such as human immunodeficiency virus (HIV), drugs such as bisphosphonates, or possibly circulating factors from lymphocytes.

Many cases of clinical glomerulonephritis are the result of other disease processes. These diseases include systemic lupus erythematosus, diabetes mellitus, amyloidosis, and multiple myeloma. Vasculitis also has very important implications for the kidney; this condition is discussed at the end of this chapter.

IV. PATHOLOGY OF GLOMERULAR DISEASES

The following section addresses examples of glomerular pathology and correlates histologic findings with clinical presentation; it also suggests mechanisms of injury and treatment options. This is not meant to be a comprehensive list of how to recognize and treat these conditions, but it should serve to expose the reader to a variety of diseases and help him or her recognize how to think about their similarities and differences.

A. Primary Nephrotic Syndrome Glomerular Pathology

1. Minimal Change Nephrotic Syndrome

Previously thought to be lipid nephrosis caused by the cellular accumulation of lipids in the renal tubular cells, this condition tends to affect children and young adults. The patient with the minimal change nephrotic syndrome has proteinuria, edema, hypoalbuminemia, and hyperlipidemia. Hematuria, hypertension, and renal failure are uncommon.

Both light microscopy (Figs. 8-1 and 8-2) and immunofluorescence reveal no significant pathologic changes (hence the term *minimal change*). By contrast, the electron microscope shows effacement of the foot processes of the epithelial podocytes (Fig. 8-3). Minimal change disease is usually very responsive to therapy with antiinflammatory medications (e.g., prednisone). Although the microscopic results are illustrative of the condition, the presentation is well recognized now, so it is uncommon to perform

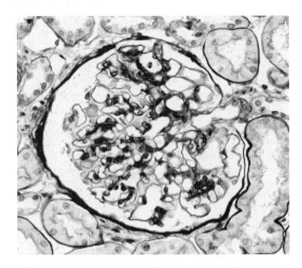

Figure 8-1. Light microscopy of a normal glomerulus. Periodic acid–Schiff stain shows a normal glomerulus with a small amount of mesangial matrix, thin glomerular basement membranes, patent capillary lumens, and two to three cells per mesangial area away from the vascular pole (400×).

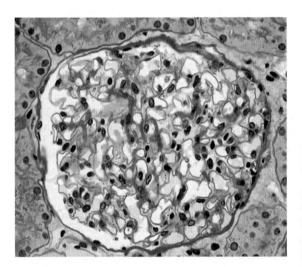

Figure 8-2. Light microscopy of minimal change disease. Periodic acid–Schiff stain shows a normal-appearing glomerulus (400×).

diagnostic biopsies in children with the nephrotic syndrome unless the children's conditions are refractory to treatment with prednisone.

Despite its well-characterized histology and ease of treatment, the pathogenesis of minimal change nephrotic syndrome is not clearly understood. Although circulating toxins have been suspected, the nature of these factors is unclear. What is known is that the pathology is a result of the loss of the net negative charge associated with the foot processes, thereby breaking down the glomerular capillary barrier.

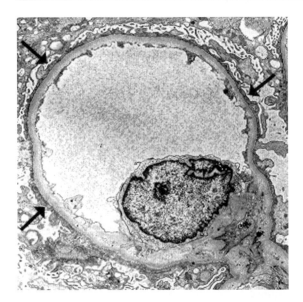

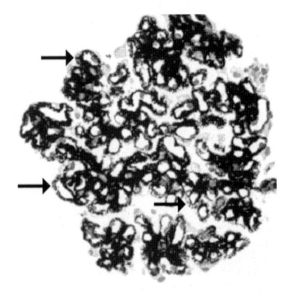

Figure 8-3. Electron microscopy of a glomerulus with minimal change disease. The electron micrograph shows the severe foot process effacement *(arrows)* of visceral epithelial cells without electron-dense deposits. The glomerular basement membrane is of normal thickness. The adjacent mesangium is unremarkable.

Figure 8-4. Light microscopy of membranous nephropathy. Periodic acid–methenamine stain shows glomerular basement membrane thickening and spikes *(arrows)* protruding from the outer aspects of the glomerular basement membranes (600×).

2. Membranous Nephropathy

This condition is a slowly progressive disorder that has been documented in adults of both genders. Similar to minimal change disease, it usually presents as a relatively pure nephrotic syndrome that includes proteinuria, low serum albumin levels, edema, and hyperlipidemia. Increased concentrations of blood urea nitrogen and serum creatinine levels may present later during the course of the disease.

The microscopic findings are again critical for the diagnosis. Although light microscopic findings using hematoxylin and eosin staining may be normal, periodic acid–methenamine staining reveals the marked thickening of the GBM, with spikes that occur as a result of the GBM response to immune complex depositions (Fig. 8-4). Furthermore, immunofluorescence reveals this glomerular deposition to be composed of C3 complement protein and immunoglobulin G (IgG), which form the granular appearance along the glomerular capillary walls (Fig. 8-5). This immune complex deposition is confirmed by electron microscopy in the form of electron-dense deposits along the subepithelial aspect of the GBM (Fig. 8-6).

Although some patients have been noted to have spontaneous remission in the disease, most patients—especially when they have large urinary protein losses—can have progressive kidney failure. Therapy with immunosuppressive medications such as prednisone, cyclophosphamide, or chlorambucil is useful to induce remission. The deposition of immune

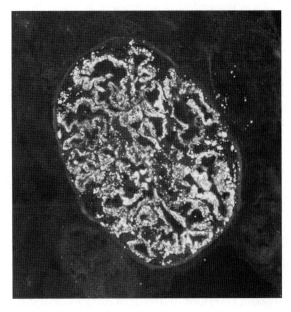

Figure 8-5. Immunofluorescence microscopy of membranous nephropathy. Immunofluorescence stain shows granular immunoglobulin G deposits along the glomerular basement membranes (400×).

complexes (antibody–antigen complexes) along the GBM has been attributed to a number of antigens, including exogenous antigens such as allergens, drugs, or infectious agents and endogenous antigens such as nuclear antigens and cancer antigens. However, in many cases, the antigens are unknown (idiopathic).

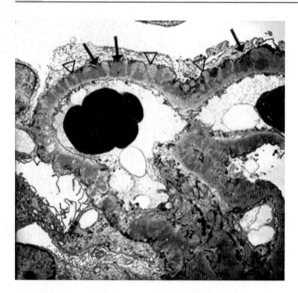

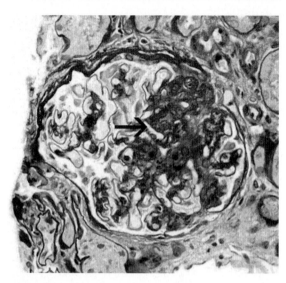

Figure 8-6. Electron microscopy of membranous nephropathy. The electron micrograph demonstrates subepithelial electron-dense deposits *(arrows)*, basement membrane spikes *(arrowheads)*, and foot process effacement.

Figure 8-7. Light microscopy of focal segmental glomerulosclerosis. Periodic acid–Schiff stain shows segmental sclerosis *(arrow)* of the glomerulus involving a portion of the glomerular tuft (400×).

3. Focal Segmental Glomerulosclerosis

Also known as *focal sclerosing glomerulopathy,* focal segmental glomerulosclerosis is simultaneously one of the most identifiable and one of the least understood diseases. Patients with this condition present with symptoms that are reminiscent of minimal change disease. However, the course of the kidney disease is not benign, and progressive kidney failure occurs. The findings on light microscopy reveal the curious hallmark of this condition that sets it apart from other nephrotic diseases: it is a disease that characteristically only affects distinct portions of the glomeruli. Specifically, one can observe sclerotic changes (i.e., the thickening of capillary walls with hyaline deposits) in only some of the glomeruli (focal) and affecting only portions of the glomerular tuft (segmental; Fig. 8-7). However, on electron microscopy, widespread podocyte foot process effacement is seen. The visceral epithelial cell (podocyte) is the site of primary damage in this disease process, which results in proteinuria and the nephrotic syndrome. Familial forms of focal glomerulosclerosis are being identified as being caused by inherited defects in various proteins in the podocytes and the slit diaphragms, which anchor the adjacent foot processes to one another close to the GBM. An example is an inherited defect in the gene that encodes the protein nephrin in the Finnish type of congenital nephrotic syndrome.

The mechanisms of the acquired forms of focal segmental glomerulosclerosis remain mysterious. Immunofluorescence microscopy reveals only minimal glomerular deposits of immunoglobulin M and complement component C3, but there is otherwise a lack of immune complexes. Frequently, focal segmental glomerular sclerosis is the result of other disease processes, including HIV infections, especially in patients of African-American ethnicity. The glomeruli often show collapse of the capillary loops with an increase in the number of surrounding podocytes. This variant of focal glomerulosclerosis is called *collapsing glomerulopathy.* It is thought that HIV infects the podocytes. Focal segmental glomerulosclerosis may also be seen in patients with unilateral renal agenesis, sickle-cell disease, obesity, or vesicoureteral reflux. In these cases, a decrease in renal mass appears to be the culprit. The possibility exists that the reduction of renal mass leads to increased blood flow to the remaining nephrons and results in increased glomerular hydrostatic pressures. In these cases, hyperfiltration is considered to be the cause of glomerular damage and sclerosis.

In some patients with focal segmental glomerulosclerosis, it has been noticed that renal allografts show signs of disease recurrence as early as several weeks after transplantation. This suggests that there may be a circulating factor or toxin that is causing the scattered damage. This hypothesis is supported by anecdotal reports of plasmapheresis reducing the degree of proteinuria. Although circulating factors that affect permeability have been noted in patients with focal segmental glomerulosclerosis, all attempts to characterize these factors have been unsuccessful.

B. Secondary Nephrotic Syndrome Glomerular Pathology

1. Diabetic Nephropathy

Also known as *diabetic glomerulosclerosis,* diabetic nephropathy is one of the most frequent complications in patients with either diabetes mellitus type 1 or type 2. The earliest indication is usually microalbuminuria with progressive increases in the amount of protein excretion, which ultimately leads to the nephrotic syndrome and kidney failure. Both light microscopy and electron microscopy are helpful for diagnosing this disease, primarily identifying changes in the mesangial matrix that include the diffuse expansion of the mesangial matrix and the uniform thickening of the capillary walls (Fig. 8-8). These characteristic regions of increased mesangial matrix are known as Kimmelstiel–Wilson nodules. These are caused by an increased synthesis of the matrix material. Hyaline deposits in both the afferent and efferent arterioles of the glomeruli are characteristic of diabetic nephropathy. GBM thickening is best noted on electron microscopy (Fig. 8-9).

Although immunofluorescence microscopic examination reveals linear staining of IgG and albumin in the glomerular capillary basement membranes (which is thought to be the result of increased capillary permeability to proteins), the glomerular damage is not immune mediated. Rather, the glomerular damage hinges on and has been correlated with uncontrolled glucose levels and the glycosylation of tissue proteins. Glomerular hyperfiltration as well as systemic hypertension are believed to play important roles in the development and progression of diabetic nephropathy. Medications that block the renin–angiotensin system are very effective for decreasing both glomerular hypertension and proteinuria,

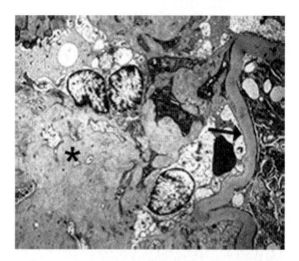

Figure 8-9. Electron microscopy of diabetic nephropathy. The electron micrograph shows marked thickening *(arrow)* of the glomerular basement membranes and widening of the mesangial regions *(asterisk).*

preserving kidney function, and preventing the need for renal replacement therapy, especially when they are started early. Not all patients with diabetes mellitus develop this nephropathy, but those who do can progress to kidney failure.

2. Renal Amyloidosis

Amyloidosis is the name for a number of diseases that result from the tissue deposition of proteinaceous fibrils. Two major types of amyloidosis are recognized by the protein composition of the fibrils. One is AL amyloidosis, in which the fibrils are composed of light chains of immunoglobulins. This is often the type of amyloidosis that is seen in patients with multiple myeloma, which is a malignant process of plasma cells. The other type is AA amyloidosis, which is noted in patients with chronic inflammatory diseases such as rheumatoid arthritis or chronic osteomyelitis or in patients with familial Mediterranean fever. The fibrils in AA amyloidosis are composed of an acute-phase protein that is called *protein AA.* The kidney deposition of amyloid material may be seen in the glomeruli and blood vessels as well as in the interstitium and around the tubules. The deposits are eosinophilic and amorphous, and they stain with special stains, such as Congo red or crystal violet. Congo-red–stained tissue of amyloid deposits, when visualized with polarizing microscopy, gives a unique green birefringence. Electron microscopy also detects the fibrillary deposits (Fig. 8-10). Patients with these conditions have increased proteinuria that is often in the nephrotic range and varying extents of (often progressive) kidney failure.

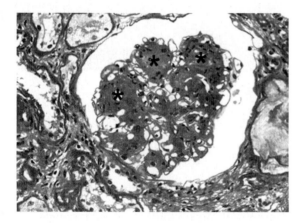

Figure 8-8. Light microscopy of diabetic nephropathy. Periodic acid–Schiff stain demonstrates nodular glomerulosclerosis. There is widening of the glomerular mesangial regions with several rounded, acellular, eccentric mesangial nodules (Kimmelstiel–Wilson nodules; *asterisks*) (400×).

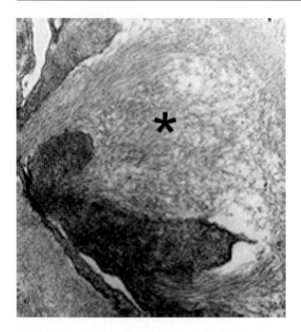

Figure 8-10. Electron microscopy of amyloidosis. The electron micrograph shows randomly arranged, nonbranching amyloid fibrils *(asterisk)* in the subepithelial area of the glomerular basement membrane.

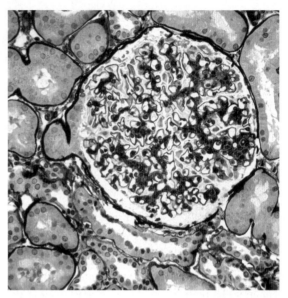

Figure 8-11. Light microscopy of immunoglobulin A nephropathy. Periodic acid–methenamine stain reveals global mesangial matrix expansion and hypercellularity (400×).

C. Primary Nephritic Syndrome Glomerular Pathology

1. Immunoglobulin A Nephropathy

Also known as *Berger disease,* immunoglobulin A (IgA) nephropathy is the most common primary glomerular disease in the world. It also has one of the most dramatic presentations: nearly half of all patients present with episodes of visible hematuria that typically last 1 to 2 days after an infection. This is the prevailing finding, and it is often benign, although the disease can progress to a nephrotic picture with proteinuria during later stages. The finding of hematuria in and of itself is not enough to establish the diagnosis of IgA nephropathy because other conditions (e.g., urinary tract infections) can also result in grossly visible blood in the urine. Therefore, a clear diagnosis requires not only substantiation by renal biopsy but also the elimination of infection as a possible cause.

The examination of renal biopsy tissue by light microscopy reveals increases in mesangial cellularity, although some patients have only focal proliferation of intrinsic glomerular cells (Fig. 8-11). This increase in mesangial cellularity is substantiated by electron microscopy, which also shows electron-dense deposits within the glomeruli. Immunofluorescence, in this case, is particularly diagnostic because it can detect IgA deposition in the glomerular mesangium (Fig. 8-12).

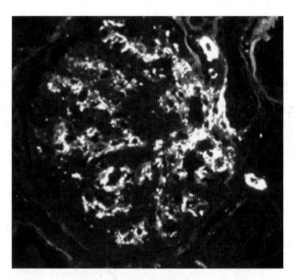

Figure 8-12. Immunofluorescence microscopy of immunoglobulin A nephropathy. Immunofluorescence microscopy shows numerous granular mesangial immunoglobulin A deposits (400×).

The cause of IgA nephropathy remains elusive. Some have reported correlations with bacterial and upper respiratory tract infections, but no single mechanism of disease development is known. Despite the dramatic presentation of this condition, many patients have a benign course. However, the possibility exists that this condition may progress, requiring dialysis or renal transplantation.

2. Anti-glomerular Basement Membrane Disease

Primarily a disease of adults, anti-GBM disease is an uncommon but very serious disease. As is characteristic of nephritic diseases, patients present with hematuria. However, the disease course can rapidly progress to kidney failure, and therefore it is often referred to as *rapidly progressive glomerulonephritis*. A variant of this disease known as *Goodpasture syndrome* additionally involves the lungs and presents with pulmonary hemorrhage and respiratory failure.

Although the exact pathogenetic mechanism is not known, it is evident that anti-GBM disease and Goodpasture syndrome are autoimmune diseases. Circulating antibodies react with an antigen on the α_3-chain of type IV collagen in the GBM (and, in the case of Goodpasture syndrome, an antigen on the pulmonary alveolar basement membrane as well). This prompts the activation of other immune mediators, such as complement proteins and coagulation factors, which leads to tissue damage. Cell-mediated immune mechanisms may also play a role in the inflammatory process. As a consequence of these immune processes, blood appears in the Bowman's space. As the damage continues, the glomeruli become increasingly sclerotic until the disease progresses to kidney failure.

Anti-GBM antibodies in the serum are detected by serologic testing and are diagnostic of the disease. Light microscopy reveals characteristic focal areas of necrosis of the glomerular capillaries and cellular accumulations in the Bowman's space called *crescents* (Fig. 8-13). Crescents are the result of the proliferation of Bowman's capsule cells as well as of accumulations of macrophages. Immunofluorescence microscopy also shows a characteristic linear or ribbon-like pattern of deposition of IgG along the glomerular capillary wall (Fig. 8-14). This pattern emerges as a result of the binding of antibodies to the antigen in the GBM, and it stands in contrast with the immune complex diseases in which the deposition of IgG occurs in a discontinuous pattern, thereby producing a granular appearance on immunofluorescence microscopy. Electron microscopy of the glomerulus does not reveal electron-dense deposits. The disruption of the GBM and the increases in the number of cells in the Bowman's space are also noted on electron microscopy.

The treatment of this condition includes immunosuppressive medications to prevent antibody production in combination with plasmapheresis to remove the circulating antibodies in the serum. However, the response to therapy is only effective when therapy is initiated early during the course of the disease. If left untreated, the patient inevitably progresses to kidney failure. Renal transplantation is effective, but it is advisable to wait until anti-GBM antibodies disappear from circulation because recurrence of the disease in the kidney allograft can develop.

3. Thin Basement Membrane Nephropathy and Alport Syndrome

Thin basement membrane nephropathy is a common inherited autosomal-dominant renal disease with an estimated prevalence of up to 10% in the

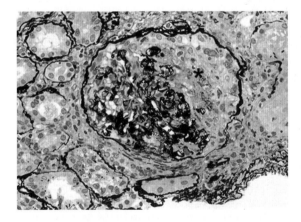

Figure 8-13. Anti-glomerular basement membrane mediated crescentic glomerulonephritis: light microscopy of anti-glomerular basement membrane glomerulonephritis. Periodic acid-methenamine stain shows a cellular crescent *(asterisk)* and compressed capillary loops on the right of the glomerulus. There is periglomerular interstitial inflammation with mononuclear leukocyte infiltration (400×).

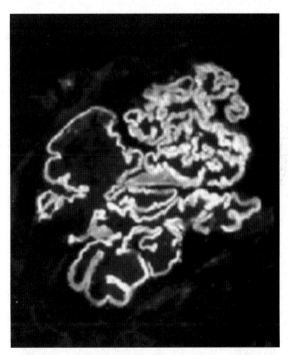

Figure 8-14. Immunofluorescence microscopy of anti-glomerular basement membrane disease. Direct immunofluorescence microscopy demonstrates linear staining for immunoglobulin G along the glomerular basement membranes (400×).

general population. Patients are asymptomatic and present primarily with hematuria that is noted on urinalysis. Blood pressure and kidney function are normal. This disease is usually benign, and it is also known as *benign familial hematuria*. Kidney biopsy shows normal-appearing glomeruli on light microscopy, but diffuse thinning of the GBM is noted on electron microscopy.

By contrast, a more severe form of inherited kidney disease is Alport syndrome. With this condition, patients present with microscopic hematuria, but they can develop a progressive decline in kidney function at an early age, especially in affected men. On electron microscopy, the glomeruli shows extensive changes, with GBM thickening, splitting, and lamination (Fig. 8-15). The kidney disease is usually accompanied by extrarenal findings such as nerve deafness and ocular disorders (most commonly lens dislocations and cataracts).

Alport syndrome and thin basement membrane nephropathy are two disorders that represent the spectrum of a genetically heritable disease in which mutations in the genes for type IV collagen, which is present in the GBM, are responsible. Males are primarily and more severely affected in Alport syndrome because the predominant form is inherited as an X-linked trait. Autosomal variants of Alport syndrome are also known, but they are exceedingly rare. Diagnosis is made on the basis of family history, clinical presentation, and renal biopsy.

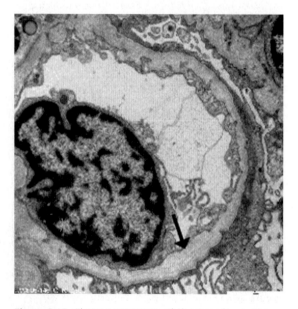

Figure 8-15. Electron microscopy of Alport syndrome. The electron micrograph shows thickening, splitting, and lamination *(arrow)* of the glomerular basement membrane.

D. Secondary Nephritic Syndrome Glomerular Pathology
1. Lupus Nephritis
Systemic lupus erythematosus (SLE) is a multisystem autoimmune disease that affects the heart, the vessels, the skin, and the joints in addition to the kidneys. This disease affects women more frequently than men.

Renal involvement in these patients is as variable in presentation as SLE itself, and it can range from minimal hematuria to the nephrotic syndrome or kidney failure. However, when hematuria is seen in conjunction with the nephrotic syndrome, SLE should be high on the differential diagnosis.

The exact mechanism of renal injury is poorly understood, but it is thought to be a prototypical immune complex disease. Evidence for this hypothesis stems from the detection of DNA and anti-DNA antibody immune complexes in the serum as well as in the glomerular deposits. These immune complexes may be noted in many areas of the glomeruli, including subepithelial, subendothelial, or mesangial locations. It is likely that the immune complexes mediate the disease by the activation of the complement system, because complement proteins are also usually noted in the glomeruli.

The findings on kidney biopsy are variable from patient to patient. As many as six different classes of kidney biopsy changes have been noted in patients with SLE and glomerulonephritis (classes I to VI). In the most severe variety, light microscopic findings are characterized by diffuse proliferation (i.e., increases in endothelial and mesangial cells in more than 50% of the glomeruli) along with glomerular capillary wall thickening as a result of deposits that stain with periodic acid–Schiff stain. The mesangium can show increases in the matrix as well as increased cellularity (Fig. 8-16). The less-severe types show changes in some segments of some glomeruli or changes that are confined to the mesangial regions only. Immunofluorescence microscopy is probably the most diagnostic in that different immunoglobulin classes (e.g., immunoglobulins G, A, and M) as well as complement components (e.g., C3, C4, and C1q) can all be detected in the glomeruli along the capillary walls in a granular pattern (Fig. 8-17). This is a reflection of immune complex deposition in this disease. Nuclear antigens can also be demonstrated in these glomerular deposits, which supports the autoimmune nature of SLE. The electron microscope reveals electron-dense deposits in the subendothelial layers of the capillary walls as well as in the mesangium and the GBM (Fig. 8-18). Although patients with lupus nephritis can develop kidney failure, early treatment with immunosuppressive medications, including prednisone, cyclophosphamide, and mycophenolate mofetil, is often effective for controlling the disease and inducing lasting remission.

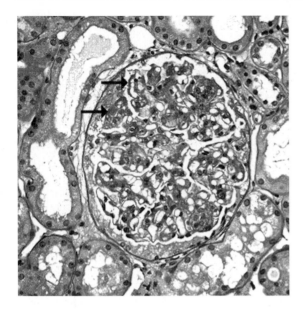

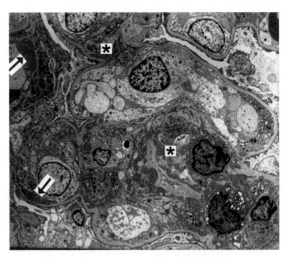

Figure 8-18. Electron microscopy of lupus nephritis. The electron micrograph shows numerous mesangial *(asterisks)* and subendothelial *(arrows)* electron-dense deposits.

Figure 8-16. Light microscopy of lupus nephritis class IV. Periodic acid–Schiff stain shows global endocapillary proliferation, wire-loop deposits, and hyaline thrombi *(arrows)* (400×).

2. Membranoproliferative Glomerulonephritis

Patients with membranoproliferative glomerulonephritis usually present with hematuria and the nephrotic syndrome, so the disease may resemble lupus nephritis. Although the exact cause is not known, membranoproliferative glomerulonephritis has been seen in patients with chronic hepatitis C infections who may also have cryoglobulins (i.e., immunoglobulins that precipitate at room temperature). The kidney biopsy findings can be variable. On light microscopy of the kidney tissue, the glomeruli are usually large and lobular in appearance and have increased cellularity. The capillary walls are often split into a double layer with a "tram-track" appearance as a result of the interposition of the mesangium (Figs. 8-19 and 8-20). Immunofluorescence microscopy may reveal only the C3 component of complement without any immunoglobulin deposits. Electron-dense deposits may be noted in a subendothelial location (Fig. 8-21). In some patients with membranoproliferative glomerulonephritis on electron microscopy, the GBM is replaced with long, extremely dense deposits. This condition is also called the *dense deposit disease*.

3. Poststreptococcal (Postinfectious) Glomerulonephritis

A few weeks after the onset of some (nephritogenic) strains of a group A β-hemolytic streptococcal infection, some patients can suffer from a bout of hematuria. Usually this condition has been reported in epidemics of streptococcal infection, and it has been seen mostly in developing countries. Although many patients develop streptococcal infections, only a few have clinical kidney disease. It is unclear why some

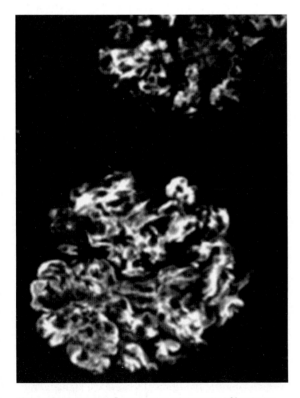

Figure 8-17. Immunofluorescence microscopy of lupus nephritis. Direct immunofluorescence stain shows C1q deposits in the mesangium and along the glomerular basement membranes (400×).

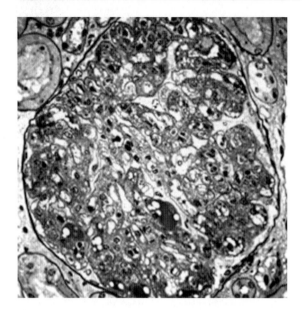

Figure 8-19. Light microscopy of membranoproliferative glomerulonephritis. Periodic acid–Schiff stain shows global endocapillary cellular proliferation and glomerular basement membrane reduplication *(double contours)* (600×).

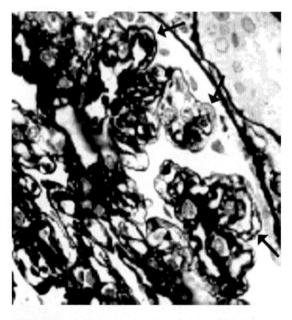

Figure 8-20. Light microscopy of membranoproliferative glomerulonephritis. Periodic acid-methenamine stain shows endocapillary proliferation, increased mesangial matrix, and glomerular basement membrane reduplication *(arrows)* (600×).

people develop this renal complication. Sporadic cases of poststreptococcal glomerulonephritis may also occur. It appears that the glomerular binding of the streptococcal protein nephritis-associated streptococcal plasmin receptor (NAP1r) and the subsequent

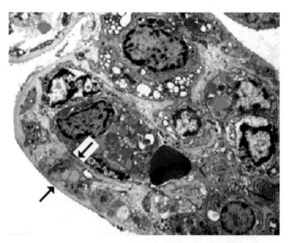

Figure 8-21. Electron microscopy of membranoproliferative glomerulonephritis. Electron micrograph shows glomerular basement membrane reduplication with mesangial interposition *(arrows)*. There is endocapillary proliferation, and the glomerular capillary lumen is narrowed.

inflammatory reaction may be responsible for the glomerular damage. In addition, circulating immune complexes that are composed of a streptococcal serine proteinase in the streptococcal exotoxin (zSpeB/SpeB) and IgG antibodies may be deposited in the glomeruli with subsequent immune damage.

Histologic findings under light microscopy in the patient with poststreptococcal glomerulonephritis include enlarged and swollen glomerular tufts, with a marked proliferation of endothelial cells as well as the infiltration of capillary tufts by neutrophils (Fig. 8-22). Immunofluorescence may show coarse glomerular deposits consisting of IgG or complement components such as C3. Electron microscopy shows fairly characteristic semilunar dome-shaped, electron-dense "humps" in the subepithelial layer (Fig. 8-23). Rarely are the histologic findings necessary for a diagnosis other than to evaluate disease courses that are abnormal. Most patients with poststreptococcal glomerulonephritis have a relatively benign course, despite the persistence of symptoms for many months. In general, the symptoms (e.g., edema, hypertension) are treated until the disease abates.

V. MECHANISMS OF VASCULAR INJURY

A. Systemic Vasculitis

Inflammation of the blood vessels may be present with different clinical syndromes. Because the kidney contains many blood vessels, it is reasonable to anticipate adverse renal consequences in patients with systemic vascular diseases. If large arteries are the sites of the disease process, then the occlusion of the blood vessels leads to infarction of the kidney and other organs. This

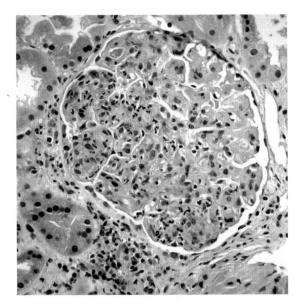

Figure 8-22. Light microscopy of acute postinfectious glomerulonephritis. Hematoxylin and eosin stain shows marked endocapillary hypercellularity with a large number of polymorphonuclear leukocytes and closure of capillaries (400×).

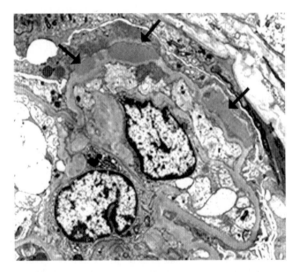

Figure 8-23. Electron microscopy of acute postinfectious glomerulonephritis. The electron micrograph shows hump-like subepithelial electron-dense deposits *(arrows)*.

occurs in the classic form of polyarteritis nodosa. However, inflammation can involve the smaller arteries, the arterioles, the glomerular capillaries, and the venules, and this results in a different clinical picture. This is seen in conditions such as Wegener's granulomatosis, microscopic polyangiitis, and the Churg–Strauss syndrome (Fig. 8-24). Vasculitis may also involve the glomerular capillaries and show focal area necrosis of glomerular tufts and cellular crescents in Bowman's

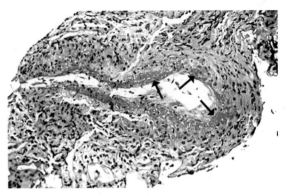

Figure 8-24. Light microscopy of vasculitis and necrotizing glomerulonephritis. Hematoxylin and eosin stain shows arterial fibrinoid necrosis *(arrows)* with fibrin deposition and inflammatory infiltration into the wall (600×).

urinary space (Fig. 8-25). In addition, in Wegener's granulomatosis, accumulations of inflammatory cells (e.g., multinucleated giant cells) are seen in many organs, especially in the upper and lower respiratory tracts. Because immunoglobulin and complement deposits in the glomeruli are insignificant in patients with vasculitis, the term *pauci-immune crescentic glomerulonephritis* is often used to describe this condition.

In patients with vasculitis, antineutrophil cytoplasmic antibody (ANCA) that reacts with proteins in the cytoplasmic granules of neutrophils may be detected

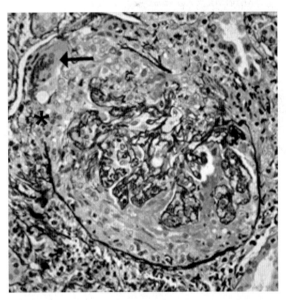

Figure 8-25. Light microscopy of vasculitis and necrotizing glomerulonephritis. Periodic acid–methenamine stain shows a cellular crescent and focal destruction *(asterisk)* of Bowman's capsule and the glomerular basement membrane. There is extensive interstitial inflammation with a multinucleated giant cell *(arrow)* (600×).

in the serum. One type of ANCA binds to a protein-ase 3, and on immunofluorescence microscopy appears as a diffuse granular pattern of immunofluorescence. This type is called *cytoplasmic ANCA* (C-ANCA). Patients with C-ANCA–positive vasculitis often have features that are typical of Wegener's granulomatosis with multiorgan involvement.

Alternatively, in patients with a kidney-only form of vasculitis, P-ANCA, which is directed against myeloperoxidase in the neutrophilic granules, is often noted. When studied by immunofluorescence microscopy, these granules accumulate around the nucleus in a perinuclear distribution; hence, this antibody is known as *P-ANCA*. Low levels of ANCA may be seen in patients with SLE. On occasion, patients with ulcerative colitis and Crohn disease may have P-ANCA positivity as a result of antibodies directed against elastase and other proteins.

Little is known about the generation of ANCAs or the mechanism by which ANCAs mediate kidney injury. It has been noted that target antigens for ANCA appear on the surface of neutrophils when they are stimulated by viral infections and cytokines. ANCAs can then bind to neutrophils, which leads to neutrophilic activation and tissue injury from the release of free radicals and other inflammatory mediators. Given this immune component of the disease, the treatment of patients with vasculitis with drugs such as prednisone, cyclophosphamide, or mycophenolate mofetil has been useful for inducing remission.

B. Thrombotic Microangiopathies

With disorders that are referred to as *thrombotic microangiopathies* (TMAs), vascular injury to the endothelial cell layer of the blood vessel occurs. This injury may be caused by diverse mechanisms such as bacterial toxins, medications, or abnormalities in platelet function. In TMAs, the endothelial cells lose their natural thromboresistance, which results in abnormal platelet activation and fibrin deposition (Fig. 8-26). Thus, it is vascular occlusion rather than inflammation that compromises and damages the vasculature.

Hemolytic uremic syndrome (HUS) is one example of a thrombotic microangiopathy in which primarily the renal microvasculature is affected. The patient presents with a classic clinical triad of thrombocytopenia (depletion of platelets from consumption), microangiopathic hemolytic anemia (anemia with signs of intravascular RBC fragmentation and schistocytes in the peripheral blood smear), and a decline in kidney function. Some forms of HUS are the result of a toxin that is produced by some strains of *Escherichia coli* (particularly strain O157:H7). This is the mechanism involved with the periodic outbreaks of bloody diarrhea that accompany foods that are contaminated with this organism. In many cases, however, HUS presents in the absence of any gastrointestinal illness. Endothelial injury and HUS may be seen in patients with malignancy

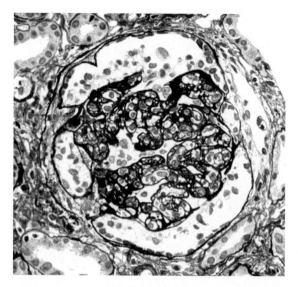

Figure 8-26. Light microscopy of thrombotic microangiopathy. Periodic acid–methenamine stain shows glomerular basement membrane thickening and reduplication with mesangial interposition (600×).

that is treated with agents such as bleomycin or cisplatin. Cyclosporine therapy or kidney failure during pregnancy and after childbirth or bone marrow transplantation can also at times be the result of TMA.

Thrombotic thrombocytopenic purpura (TTP) is another example of a TMA that also causes prominent neurologic dysfunction and fever. Patients with TTP have a decrease in the activity of the von Willebrand factor–cleaving protein (a zinc metalloproteinase called *ADAMTS13*) in the plasma. This could be caused by an inherited defect in the function of the protein, or it may be the result of the presence of an immunoglobulin in the plasma that interferes with the function of this protein. The unusually large von Willebrand factor multimers that develop induce platelet activation, intravascular thrombi, multiorgan damage. Plasmapheresis with the replacement of fresh plasma (which removes the offending immunoglobulin and supplies the defective protein) is often effective in patients with TTP. Antiplatelet agents and immunosuppressive medications are useful on occasion.

VI. SUMMARY

This chapter addressed the approach to pathophysiology of several types of glomerular diseases. By understanding the components of the glomerulus that are subject to damage, this can be correlated with the findings of the physical examination, the laboratory tests, and the histologic appearance. Knowledge of the mechanisms of pathogenesis is limited, but it can help a physician solidify a diagnosis and establish a management strategy.

Clinical Case

A 7-year-old girl is referred to a kidney specialist by her pediatrician for lower extremity and periorbital edema of a few weeks' duration. Her physical examination is normal aside from the edema. Blood chemistries are significant for an albumin level of 2.5 g/dl, a serum creatinine level of 0.6 mg/dl, and a cholesterol level of 270 mg/dl. Urinalysis reveals no blood, but 4+ protein by the dipstick and the microscopy of the sediment shows hyaline casts and several fat globules. A Maltese-cross shape is noted when the urine sediment is viewed under polarized light, and protein excretion is more than 8 g in a 24-hour urine collection.

Is this a nephrotic or a nephritic presentation?

This patient has the four important features of the nephrotic syndrome: generalized edema, 4+ proteinuria, decreased serum albumin level, and elevation in serum cholesterol.

What should the physician expect to see on renal biopsy under light microscopy and under electron microscopy?

Given the patient's age and presentation, this is likely minimal change disease. Both light microscopy and immunofluorescence will reveal no significant pathologic changes (hence the term *minimal change*). The electron microscopic study of the glomeruli will show effacement of the foot processes of the podocytes.

What is the proposed site and mechanism of this disease?

The pathogenesis of minimal change nephrotic syndrome is not clearly known. Although circulating toxins have been suspected, the nature of these factors is unclear. What is known is that the pathology is a result of the loss of the net negative charge associated with the podocyte foot processes, thereby breaking down the glomerular capillary barrier.

Suggested Readings

Hricik DE, Chung-Park M, Sedor JR: Glomerulonephritis. *N Engl J Med* 339:888–899, 1998.

Tryggvason K, Patrakka J, Wartiovaara J: Hereditary proteinuria syndromes and mechanisms of proteinuria. *N Engl J Med* 354:1387–1401, 2006.

PRACTICE QUESTIONS

1. A 27-year-old man presents with a 1-month history of blood in his urine. He reports that this finding occurred spontaneously, and he cannot recall being sick any time during or before the onset of his urinary findings. His physical examination indicates no clinical evidence of edema, and he has no serologic markers or abnormalities; he has normal creatinine and blood urea nitrogen levels as well as normal levels of clotting factors. What finding is most consistent with his condition?

  A. Crescentic proliferation in the glomeruli
  B. A family history of deafness or eye problems
  C. Evidence of schistocytes in the peripheral blood smears
  D. Effacement of the podocytes from the GBM

2. A 17-year-old woman presents with hematuria a few weeks after having a streptococcal infection of her throat. Which of the following findings is not consistent with poststreptococcal glomerulonephritis?

  A. The proliferation of endothelial cells in the glomerulus
  B. The presence of polymorphonuclear leucocytes in the glomeruli
  C. Immunofluorescence staining that reveals a granular pattern of IgG deposition
  D. Diffuse effacement of the foot processes of glomerular podocytes

3. A pathologist at a major hospital receives a tissue specimen from a nephrologist who forgets to write down the name of the patient to which it belongs. Clearly, it is in the pathologist's best interest to call the physician to clarify the mistake. However, feeling very confident of his abilities, the pathologist first decides to try figuring out for himself to whom the specimen belongs simply by correlating his findings with the history and symptoms of the nephrologist's list of patients. He finds that the immunofluorescence staining detects weak linear staining of IgG along the capillary wall, and a periodic acid–Schiff stained sample reveals uniform thickening of the glomerular capillary walls. To confirm his initial suspicion, the pathologist prepares a sample for electron microscopy and finds that there is mesangial expansion into the nodules and hyaline material in the capillary wall. Knowing the diagnosis, the pathologist checks the nephrologist's patient list to compare his results with the clinical findings. Which of the following patients would the pathologist most likely discuss with the nephrologist with regard to the histologic findings?

  A. A 34-year-old man who has microalbuminuria and a HbA1c level of 10%
  B. A 47-year-old man who had a lung biopsy that demonstrated granuloma during the evaluation of hemoptysis
  C. A 55-year-old woman who had a rapid onset of fever, acute kidney failure, and a low platelet count
  D. A 9-year-old boy with periorbital edema and 4+ protein in the urinalysis

Cystic Diseases of the Kidney

Kristin M. Lyerly
Arjang Djamali

OUTLINE
  I. Introduction to Cystic Diseases
 II. Hereditary Polycystic Kidney Disease
     A. Autosomal Dominant Polycystic Kidney Disease
     B. Autosomal Recessive Polycystic Kidney Disease
III. Cystic Diseases of the Renal Medulla
     A. Nephronophthisis–Medullary Cystic Kidney
        Disease Complex
  B. Medullary Sponge Kidney
 IV. Miscellaneous Hereditary Renal Cystic Disorders
     A. Tuberous Sclerosis
     B. von Hippel–Lindau Syndrome

Objectives

- Know the pathogenesis of cystic kidney diseases.
- Recognize the clinical presentation of cystic kidney diseases, especially ADPKD.
- Understand the role of diagnostic imaging in cystic kidney diseases.
- Know the factors involved in disease progression.
- Understand therapeutic principles: dialysis and transplantation.

Clinical Case

A 40-year-old female nurse comes to the emergency department with her husband and two children complaining of a severe, constant headache that began 2 hours before she arrived. According to her husband, the headache was preceded by a brief period of unconsciousness after his wife collapsed while mowing the lawn. Upon awakening, she was confused. There is no prior history of severe headache. Her medical history is significant for two uncomplicated term pregnancies, occasional urinary tract infections, and hypertension. She denies medications and drug allergies. The patient is adopted, and her family history is unknown to her. Her social history is unremarkable, with the exception of two cases of mumps having been diagnosed at her daughter's school within the past month. Her vital signs reveal a blood pressure of 170/95 mm Hg, a pulse rate of 85 beats per minute, and a respiration rate of 16 breaths per minute. On physical examination, the woman is a moderately obese woman who appears to be her stated age. Her lungs are clear. The cardiac examination is remarkable for a systolic click; rate and rhythm are normal. Her abdomen is somewhat difficult to assess as a result of her obesity. Marked hepatomegaly is noted, along with the presence of an indistinct but palpable and firm abdominal mass. The extremities are without edema, and the peripheral pulses are 2+ throughout. The neurological examination is unremarkable, with the exception of mild confusion.

What would be the most appropriate next step in this patient's diagnosis and treatment after the stabilization of her airway, breathing, and circulation and routine blood tests? What is the most likely cause of her headache? Are her children at risk for developing the same condition?

I. INTRODUCTION TO CYSTIC DISEASES

Cystic diseases of the kidney are a mixed group of acquired, hereditary, and developmental disorders with various causes, histopathologies, and clinical presentations. Despite the vast diversity within this group, they all share a common feature: cysts.

In general, a renal cyst is a fluid-filled sac made of tubular epithelium. Cysts may develop anywhere along the tube or the nephron, from Bowman's capsule to the tip of the papilla. They may or may not be visible to the naked eye.

Normal growth and differentiation of the kidney require a balance between cell proliferation and apoptosis. However, these fundamental processes are dysregulated in polycystic kidneys, which results in the formation of cysts with undifferentiated or immature epithelia (Fig. 9-1). The increased burden of apoptosis destroys most of the functional parenchyma and enables the cystic epithelia to proliferate. The basement membrane adjacent to the cyst thickens, and inflammatory cells appear in the interstitium. The cyst may eventually separate from the parent tubule segment as

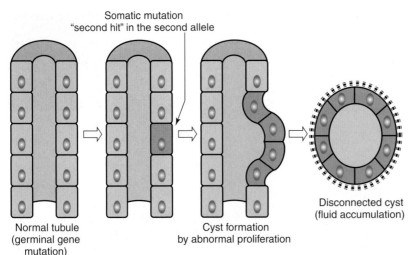

Somatic mutation
"second hit" in the second allele

Normal tubule
(germinal gene
mutation)

Cyst formation
by abnormal proliferation

Disconnected cyst
(fluid accumulation)

Figure 9-1. Pathogenesis of cyst formation in autosomal dominant polycystic kidney disease.

it enlarges, or it may remain attached. Transepithelial fluid secretion results in the accumulation of fluid within the cyst.

Among the acquired forms, simple cysts are generally benign, and they develop in the kidneys as a consequence of dialysis, aging, and drugs. Patients with kidney failure on dialysis are likely to develop cysts that can increase in size; some may become malignant with time.

Hereditary cystic diseases have greater pathologic consequences. This chapter will explore three general categories: hereditary polycystic kidney disease, cystic diseases of the renal medulla, and hereditary renal disorders.

II. HEREDITARY POLYCYSTIC KIDNEY DISEASE

A. Autosomal Dominant Polycystic Kidney Disease

As the name implies, autosomal dominant polycystic kidney disease (ADPKD) is a cystic disease of the kidney with a pattern of autosomal-dominant inheritance.

Multiple large cysts form in the kidney, which affect kidney function. Presentation is highly variable, and progression toward complete kidney failure occurs most often during middle age and later. Cysts can form anywhere in the nephron, and they may be grossly visible both within the kidney and on the surface. The kidneys are bilaterally and uniformly cystic and enlarged (Fig. 9-2).

ADPKD is the most common form of hereditary kidney disease worldwide. There are currently about 500,000 patients with ADPKD in the United States, and there are 4 to 6 million worldwide. It affects all racial groups, and estimates of incidence range from 1 in 500 to 1 in 1000 live births. Approximately 60% to 80% those affected report a family history of ADPKD, whereas 10% to 15% of cases appear to result from spontaneous mutations. Ultimately, ADPKD is the cause of kidney failure in 7% to 10% of patients.

There are two principal types of ADPKD that result from mutations in two different genes. *PKD1* gene mutations, which are found on chromosome 16, are the more common of the two, accounting for 85% of cases. *PKD1* is also the more severe form of ADPKD,

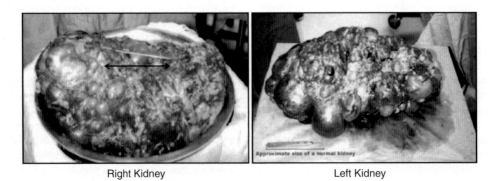

Right Kidney

Left Kidney

Figure 9-2. Nephrectomy samples from a patient with autosomal dominant polycystic kidney disease. *(Courtesy of Yolanda Becker, MD.)*

with a median age of kidney failure of approximately 53 years. *PKD2* gene mutations, which are found on chromosome 4, affect only 15% of patients with ADPKD. In this population, the median age of kidney failure is 69 years (Table 9-1 and Box 9-1). There may be a rare third form of the disease, although the proposed gene (*PKD3*) has not yet been identified.

To date, approximately 200 *PKD1* and more than 50 *PKD2* mutations have been identified. These genetic mutations result in the abnormal, truncated proteins polycystin-1 and polycystin-2, which are transmembrane molecules and components of a novel multifunctional signaling pathway (Fig. 9-3).

Polycystin-1 is a membrane receptor that is involved in cell–cell adhesion (adherens junctions) and cell–matrix contacts (focal adhesions), whereas polycystin-2 typically acts as a transmembrane calcium ion channel. In physiology, complex downstream signaling pathways from polycystins—together with intracellular second messengers and growth factors—regulate the proliferation, differentiation, and morphogenesis of renal tubular epithelial cells. Abnormal polycystin-1 and polycystin-2 proteins are associated both with increased apoptosis and the increased intrinsic capacity for proliferation and survival. Epithelial cells from patients with ADPKD (and autosomal recessive polycystic kidney disease, which is described later in this chapter) are unusually susceptible to the proliferative stimulus of epidermal growth factor. In these cells, the ~~calcium/~~ sodium potassium-ATPase pump is abnormally present in the apical membrane (instead of the basolateral

membrane), and this contributes to fluid secretion into the cyst (Fig. 9-4).

In patients with ADPKD, all renal tubular epithelial cells have germinal gene mutations in the *PKD1* or *PKD2* genes. However, it is believed that a second mutation (this one somatic, called the *second hit*) in the other allele is required for abnormal cell proliferation and cyst formation (see Fig. 9-1). Kidneys become progressively enlarged, potentially up to 15 times larger than normal. They can weigh up to 8 kg and measure up to 40 cm (the normal kidney weight is 400 to 500 mg, and the normal size is 10 to 12 cm). Renal function is compromised as well. An early decrease in renal concentrating ability often results in nocturia, which is one of few early clinical symptoms; the glomerular filtration rate (GFR) is initially conserved. In fact, decreased GFR is a sign of disease progression. Common endocrine complications of ADPKD involve increased renin and erythropoietin production, which often result in hypertension and polycythemia. Manifestations of ADPKD fall into two general categories: renal and extrarenal (Box 9-2).

Renal symptoms include cystic enlargement of the kidneys in virtually everyone with ADPKD. This can result in flank or back pain, early satiety, digestive symptoms, and lower extremity edema as a result of the compression of the inferior vena cava. Hypertension is very common and often results from the activation of the renin–angiotensin–aldosterone system from the stretching of the arteries and the microvasculature by cysts. Urinary tract infections are seen in up to 50% of patients who experience either pyelonephritis or cyst infection. Microscopic and gross hematuria may result from microvascular damage or cyst rupture into the collecting system. Nephrolithiasis or kidney stones (commonly uric acid) are seen in up to 20% of those patients with ADPKD. As mentioned previously, chronic pain is common, and so are acute pain complications related to infections, stones, hemorrhages into the cyst, cyst torsion, and other causes. Ultimately, kidney failure and uremic symptoms occur.

Extrarenal abnormalities are generally the result of cysts as well. Cerebral aneurysms, which are the most serious complication, may rupture, and this may lead to subarachnoid or intracerebral bleeding. The incidence of aneurysms is fairly low, however, at approximately 4% in young adults and up to 10% in older adults. Patients may be electively screened by magnetic resonance imaging (MRI) for aneurysm if there is a family history of aneurysm or cerebral bleeding, if they work high-risk jobs (e.g., piloting airplanes), if they experience new-onset severe headaches, or for patient's peace of mind. Massive hepatic cysts can occur in up to 50% of patients, especially women with histories of multiple pregnancies. Although cysts are caused by the same mechanism as in the kidney, liver dysfunction and portal hypertension rarely occur, regardless of the cyst burden. Cysts

Table 9-1. Genetics of Autosomal Dominant Polycystic Kidney Disease

Gene	PKD1	PKD2
Chromosome	16	4
Percentage of autosomal dominant polycystic kidney disease cases	85%	15%
Protein	Polycystin-1	Polycystin-2
Disease progression	Aggressive	Mild
Mean age to kidney failure	53 years	69 years

Box 9-1. Types of Autosomal Dominant Polycystic Kidney Disease

PKD1: More common, more severe
PKD2: Less common, less severe

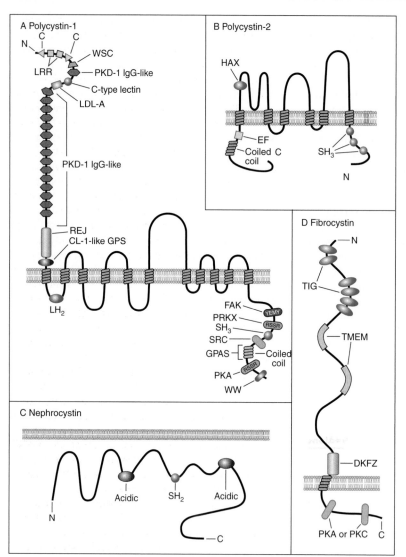

Figure 9-3. The gene for autosomal dominant polycystic kidney disease (*PKD1*) encodes the 462-kD protein polycystin-1 *(A)*. The gene for autosomal dominant polycystic kidney disease (*PKD2*) encodes polycystin-2 *(B)*. The gene for juvenile nephronophthisis (*NPH1*) encodes nephrocystin *(C)*. The gene for autosomal recessive polycystic kidney disease (*PKHD1*) encodes fibrocystin *(D)*. *(Modified from Wilson PD: Polycystic kidney disease. N Engl J Med 350:151–164, 2004.)*

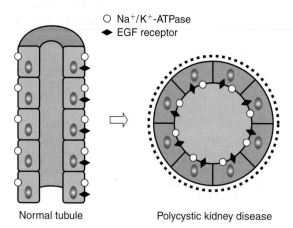

Figure 9-4. The polarization of epidermal growth factor receptor and sodium/potassium-ATPase in the epithelium from a normal kidney and from a patient with polycystic kidney disease.

may also be seen in the pancreas, the spleen, or both. Mitral valve disease is found in up to 25% of ADPKD patients, and abdominal wall and inguinal hernias are seen in up to 45%. Colonic diverticula, drooping upper eyelids, and seminal vesicle cysts are other potential related conditions.

With regard to diagnostic studies, the urinalysis in ADPKD is normal during the early stages. With disease progression, microscopic or gross hematuria and proteinuria (non-nephrotic) can be present. Serum creatinine and blood urea nitrogen levels progressively rise, and, although anemia of chronic kidney disease is common, polycythemia as a result of increased erythropoietin production may be present in some patients.

Imaging is very important for diagnosing ADPKD, with kidney ultrasound being the gold standard for diagnosis (Fig. 9-5). In people who are less than

Box 9-2. Renal and Extrarenal Manifestations of Autosomal Dominant Polycystic Kidney Disease

Renal

Hypertension (+ + +; 80% at >30 years old)

Urinary tract infections (+ + +)

Kidney stones (20–35%)

Decreased urine concentration

Kidney failure (50–75%)

Polycythemia

Hematuria
   Gross
   Microscopic

Mechanical (increased kidney size)
   Pain (60%)
   Acute
   Chronic
   Cyst rupture and bleed

Extrarenal

Central nervous system
   Intracranial saccular aneurysms (3–5%)
   Subarachnoid hemorrhage (often fatal)

Cardiovascular
   Hypertension
   Mitral valve prolapse (25%)
   Left ventricular hypertrophy

Other
   Liver cysts
   Pancreatic cysts

kidney parenchyma and to evaluate the degree of liver involvement. MRI is also available if necessary, with the advantage of very early disease detection (i.e., cysts <0.5 mm in diameter).

Molecular genetic testing may be indicated for the evaluation of at-risk individuals with equivocal imaging results, younger at-risk individuals as living-related kidney donors, and individuals with atypical or de novo renal cystic disease. The role of genetic testing in ADPKD may be greater in the future if effective drugs become available or if the genotype of the patient influences the treatment decision.

Currently, there is no cure for ADPKD. Treatment is directed toward the symptoms of the disease. Blood pressure is carefully monitored in an attempt to maintain levels of less than 130/80 mm Hg. Angiotensin-converting enzyme inhibitors and angiotensin receptor blockers are often the first line of medications employed. Calcium-channel blockers may also be highly effective for the treatment of ADPKD. Diuretics may be used with caution because hypokalemia may worsen cysts. The avoidance of renal trauma, especially contact sports, is recommended. The source of gross hematuria should be determined by imaging studies, and patients may benefit from reduced activity and bed rest. If infection is suspected, pyelonephritis must be differentiated from cyst infection and treated appropriately.

Pain management is a critical component of ADPKD treatment. Chronic pain is managed with appropriate analgesics, with care taken to avoid nephrotoxic nonsteroidal antiinflammatory drugs. Disabling pain can also be treated with percutaneous or intraoperative cyst decompression or, ultimately, nephrectomy. Acute or changing pain requires special attention with regard to the cause of the pain. Typically, acute pain may be the result of urinary tract infection, stones, or cyst rupture.

For patients reaching kidney failure, there are two options: dialysis and transplantation. Dialysis is often used as a bridge until an appropriate donor kidney becomes available. Although the cystic disease will

30 years old with a family history of ADPKD, the presence of just two renal cysts (either unilateral or bilateral) makes the diagnosis likely. In the 30- to 59-year-old age group, at least two cysts in each kidney are required. Among patients 60 years old and older, at least four cysts in each kidney are necessary to suspect the diagnosis. The absence of cysts in patients who are less than 20 years old likely excludes carrier status.

If kidney ultrasound is equivocal, a computed tomography (CT) scan may be useful to assess the

Figure 9-5. The diagnosis of autosomal dominant polycystic kidney disease (ADKPD).

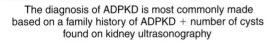

The diagnosis of ADPKD is most commonly made based on a family history of ADPKD + number of cysts found on kidney ultrasonography

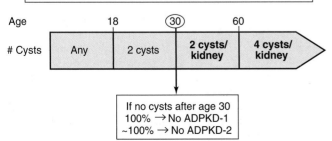

not recur in the transplanted kidney, transplant does not treat the extrarenal manifestations of ADPKD.

In any case, genetic counseling should be made available to those affected by ADPKD regarding the transmission of this disease of autosomal-dominant inheritance.

Prognosis varies with the type of disease present and the degree to which the symptoms are managed. The presence of *PKD1* (as compared with *PKD2*), male sex, hypertension, and recurrent insults (i.e., urinary tract infections, nephrotoxic drugs) all contribute to a faster rate of disease progression toward kidney failure (Fig. 9-6). Therefore, it is recommended to promptly manage modifiable risk factors as previously described.

B. Autosomal Recessive Polycystic Kidney Disease

Autosomal recessive polycystic kidney disease (ARPKD) is a cystic disease of the kidney that typically presents during infancy (Box 9-3). As its name indicates, genetic transmission is autosomal recessive, with variable degrees of expression. ARPKD is characterized by fusiform dilation of the renal collecting ducts; the remainder of the nephron is not affected. In addition to the kidney manifestations, hepatic cysts are also common, with varying degrees of periportal fibrosis and lung abnormalities such as impaired development and pulmonary hypoplasia.

The incidence of ARPKD in the general public is estimated to be between 1 in 10,000 and 1 in 20,000 live births per year. The diagnosis of ARPKD carries with it a very poor prognosis for some because 9% to 24% of those affected will die during the first month of life. Those who survive that first month, however, will likely live to be teens or older with current treatment options.

ARPKD can be attributed to a genetic mutation in a very large gene called *polycystic kidney and hepatic disease 1* (*PKHD1*), which is located on chromosome 6. This gene codes for a protein called *fibrocystin*, which is also known as *polyductin*.

Fibrocystin is a 447-kd transmembrane protein with extracellular protein interaction sites and intracellular phosphorylation sites. *PKHD1* mutations result in an

abnormal C-terminus of fibrocystin, which affects the intracellular signaling sites. Not much is known about the role of this protein in health and disease. However, it is presumed that cyst formation mechanisms are comparable in ARPKD and ADPKD. One remarkable difference, however, is that in ADPKD, large cysts arise in every tubule segment and rapidly close off from the nephron of origin. However, in ARPKD, small cysts are derived from collecting tubules and remain connected to the nephron of origin (Fig. 9-7).

Because of the variable expression in ARPKD, clinical manifestations range widely, even among siblings. Severe cases are often discovered with antenatal ultrasound. These patients are likely to succumb to complications of the disease within the first month of life. Signs and symptoms of less-severe presentations include progressively worsening renal failure and liver findings that include fibrosis, dilation, and hyperplasia of the bile ducts, which eventually lead to portal hypertension.

The diagnosis of ARPKD is usually made with ultrasound. Antenatal ultrasound may incidentally detect large kidneys, or it may be indicated with situations such as polyhydramnios (too much amniotic fluid) or oligohydramnios (insufficient amniotic fluid). Ultrasound is also useful for evaluating newborns and children with renal insufficiency, abdominal mass, or portal hypertension. Enlarged cystic kidneys are the typical finding. CT and MRI are more sensitive diagnostic options if further investigation is warranted.

The mainstay of treatment for ARPKD is supportive. Hypertension is controlled with angiotensin-converting enzyme inhibitors, calcium-channel blockers, β-blockers, and judicious diuretic use. A

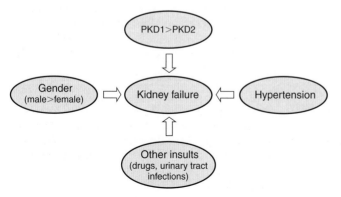

Figure 9-6. Factors that accelerate the disease progression rate in autosomal dominant polycystic kidney disease.

Normal Nephron

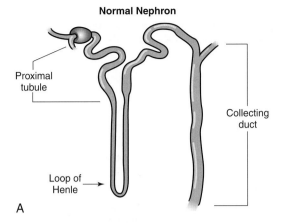

Proximal tubule

Collecting duct

Loop of Henle

A

Cyst Formation in Autosomal Dominant Polycystic Kidney Disease

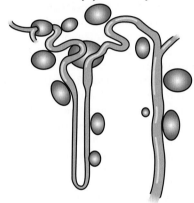

B

Cyst Formation in Autosomal Recessive Polycystic Kidney Disease

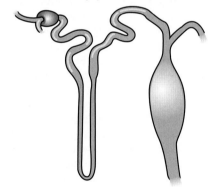

C

Figure 9-7. Cyst formation in cystic kidney disease. *(Modified from Wilson PD: Polycystic kidney disease.* N Engl J Med *350: 151–164, 2004.)*

high index of suspicion is maintained for urinary tract infection and vesicoureteral reflux, both of which must be treated promptly. Renal osteodystrophy screening is achieved with routine parathyroid hormone measurements and treated with calcium and vitamin D supplementation as well as

phosphate binders. Routine blood counts are obtained to monitor anemia, which is subsequently improved with erythropoietin. Growth hormone is administered to counteract the stunting effects of uremia. Eventually, the need for dialysis and transplantation will arise.

III. CYSTIC DISEASES OF THE RENAL MEDULLA

A. Nephronophthisis–Medullary Cystic Kidney Disease Complex

Nephronophthisis–medullary cystic kidney disease (NPH–MCKD) complex is a collection of similar diseases that share the following characteristics:
1. They are inherited.
2. They progress to kidney failure.
3. Large amounts of urine are produced as a result of a decreased ability to concentrate urine.
4. Bilateral renal cysts are found in the medulla or the corticomedullary junction.

The things that differentiate these two diseases are the specific gene with which each is associated, the pattern of inheritance, the age of onset (Fig. 9-8), and the associated features. NPH and MCKD will be discussed as two similar but distinct disorders.

1. Nephronophthisis
The term *NPH* refers to a group of autosomal-recessive inherited renal disorders that are characterized by the four previously listed criteria. NPH typically presents during childhood, and it is often associated with extrarenal involvement. It is the most common genetic cause of kidney failure in European children and adolescents (>15%), although it is seen less frequently among the U.S. population. Three common genetic mutations are known:
1. NPH1: Associated with juvenile NPH
   a. Associated with up to 85% of NPH cases
   b. Encodes for a protein called *nephrocystin-1* that has an important function in cell–matrix interactions
2. NPH2: Associated with infantile NPH
   a. Encodes for the protein *inversin*
   b. Age at onset of kidney failure is typically less than 30 months and always less than 5 years
3. NPH3: Associated with adolescent NPH
   a. Specific protein has yet to be revealed
   b. Median age at kidney failure is approximately 19 years

In individuals with NPH, both kidneys are small, and renal cysts are restricted to the medulla or the corticomedullary junction. Typical clinical manifestations include salt wasting, growth retardation, anemia, polyuria, and progressive kidney failure. Kidney failure and death occur during late childhood (mean age, 13 years) without treatment, which is limited to dialysis or transplantation.

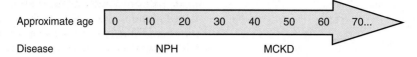

Figure 9-8. Age at diagnosis in cases of nephronophthisis (NPH) and medullary cystic kidney disease (MCKD).

2. Medullary Cystic Kidney Disease

MCKD is a group of autosomal-dominant inherited renal disorders that are characterized by the four criteria listed previously. MCKD typically presents during early adulthood. It is a rare condition, with approximately 50 new cases reported in the U.S. every year. There are two types: MCKD1 type 1 and MCKD2 type 2.

The two variants are clinically indistinguishable, although type 2 may be more severe. Manifestations are often subtle and nonspecific (the most common presenting sign is elevated serum creatinine), which results in frequent misdiagnosis. Similarly, polyuria and polydipsia, which are symptoms of progressive renal insufficiency, hypertension, hyperuricemia, and gout, are also known to occur in patients with MCKD. Diagnosis may be made by family history, clinical suspicion, ultrasound (this may reveal shrunken kidneys with cysts), renal biopsy (this may show medullary cysts with tubulointerstitial nephritis but no tubular basement membrane thickening), and genetic testing (available for patients with type 2 disease). Kidney failure typically occurs between the ages of 20 and 60 years. Treatment is supportive until kidney transplantation is required.

B. Medullary Sponge Kidney

A somewhat common and generally benign disease, medullary sponge kidney (MSK) is characterized by the cystic dilation of the terminal collecting ducts in the pericalyceal region of the renal pyramids. Cysts range in size from microscopic to large, and they are typically diffuse and bilateral. Despite the name, the kidney does not resemble a sponge either microscopically or macroscopically.

It is estimated that 1 in 5000 people have MSK, and it is more frequently seen in women. The average age of diagnosis is 27 years. The disease is not currently thought to be genetically transmitted, although some families seem to show autosomal-dominant inheritance patterns.

Most patients are asymptomatic, and progression to kidney failure is quite rare. The condition is often discovered incidentally as a result of imaging for other reasons, including kidney stones, hematuria, and urinary tract infections. These three conditions are common complications of MSK.

Diagnosis most often is based on excretory urography; other diagnostic studies may include intravenous pyelography, ultrasound, and CT scanning. Treatment is symptomatic and based on complications. With proper care, the prognosis for MSK is generally excellent.

IV. MISCELLANEOUS HEREDITARY RENAL CYSTIC DISORDERS

A. Tuberous Sclerosis

Tuberous sclerosis (TS) is a neurocutaneous disease in which "tubers" or hamartomas are deposited throughout the body, most often in the skin (adenoma sebaceum), the brain, the kidneys, and other organs. It affects 1 in 5000 to 1 in 10,000 live births, and it is inherited in an autosomal-dominant manner, although the majority of cases are attributed to new mutations. The pathophysiology of TS involves defects in the production of either the protein *hamartin* or the protein *tuberin*, each of which regulates different aspects of cellular differentiation and proliferation.

Clinical presentation may vary but typically will include seizures, mental retardation, and adenoma sebaceum. Diagnosis most often occurs in children who are less than 7 years old.

Diagnostic criteria, which include major and minor features, have been established to aid in the identification of TS. Definitive diagnosis involves the identification of either two major features or one major and two minor features (Box 9-4).

Renal manifestations of TS may include the following:

1. Angiomyolipomas, which are composed of thick-walled blood vessels, smooth muscle, and adipose tissue, are seen in approximately 80% of those affected with TS. Incidentally, up to 90% of angiomyolipomas found in the general population are sporadic and unrelated to TS. They are most often seen bilaterally and in large quantities. Angiomyolipomas most often become symptomatic as they enlarge to greater than 4 cm in size, when they cause complications such as pain (abdominal or flank), bleeding into a lesion, and hematuria.
2. Benign cysts are less commonly found, and they are seen in approximately half of TS patients. These cysts may be unilateral or bilateral, and they rarely cause symptoms.

Angiomyolipomas and benign cysts present at an average age of 9 years, and their size and number

Major features
1. Facial angiofibromas or forehead plaque
2. Nontraumatic ungual or periungual fibroma
3. Hypomelanotic macules (>3)
4. Shagreen patch (connective tissue nevus)
5. Multiple retinal nodular hamartomas
6. Cortical tuber
7. Subependymal nodule
8. Subependymal giant cell astrocytoma
9. Cardiac rhabdomyoma (single or multiple)
10. Lymphangiomyomatosis
11. Renal angiomyolipoma

Minor features
1. Multiple randomly distributed pits in the dental enamel
2. Hamartomatous rectal polyps
3. Bone cysts
4. Cerebral white-matter migration lines
5. Gingival fibromas
6. Nonrenal hamartoma
7. Retinal achromic patch
8. "Confetti" skin lesions
9. Multiple renal cysts

Definite tuberous sclerosis complex: Either two major features or one major feature and two minor features
Probable tuberous sclerosis complex: One major feature and one minor feature
Possible tuberous sclerosis complex: Either one major feature or two or more minor features

Data from Gomez MR, Sampson JR, Whittemore VH: Tuberous Sclerosis Complex, 3rd ed. New York, Oxford University Press, 1999.

tend to increase over time. Renin-dependent hypertension, chronic kidney disease, and renal cell carcinoma are other potential but rare renal complications.

The treatment of TS involves a multidisciplinary care team to address the various manifestations that are present within each individual. With specific regard to renal disease, blood pressure and renal function should be monitored annually. Renal ultrasonography or CT scanning is performed at diagnosis and then routinely thereafter as indicated by the initial study. Logically, the symptomatic treatment of complications and, if possible, the surgical resection of concerning tumors are other important therapeutic interventions.

TS is a progressive disease with variable expression patterns, the severity of which help to predict prognosis. An estimated 25% of children with TS die before the age of 10 years, and another 50% fail to reach the age of 25 years. The most common causes of death are central nervous system tumors and kidney failure.

B. von Hippel–Lindau Syndrome

von Hippel–Lindau (VHL) syndrome is an uncommon disorder that is characterized by the presence of various visceral cysts and benign tumors, many of which undergo malignant transformation. Common manifestations of VHL include hemangioblastomas of the central nervous system and retina, pheochromocytomas, and cysts of the kidney, liver, and pancreas. Because the clinical presentation varies widely from patient to patient, the discovery of any of these findings or a suspicious family history warrants a thorough investigation into the possibility of VHL.

VHL is inherited as an autosomal-dominant trait, and the gene for it is located on the short arm of chromosome 3. Approximately 1 in 36,000 individuals are born with the germ-line mutation, although initial signs and symptoms are not typically recognized until a mean age of 26 years. The pathophysiology of VHL likely follows the two-hit model, like ADPKD, in which an individual is born with one nonfunctioning allele. The loss of the complementary allele later in life results in a malfunctioning tumor-suppressor gene, unregulated growth, and eventually, the sequelae of VHL.

Forty percent of those affected with VHL will eventually present with clear-cell renal carcinoma, which is responsible for most deaths from VHL. Renal cysts are considered premalignant; therefore, diligent screening and surveillance are imperative. Diagnostic studies include CT, MRI, and ultrasound to detect primary tumors and genetic testing to confirm the existence of VHL.

Other than routine surveillance, treatment is primarily surgical. Renal-sparing surgical techniques, such as partial nephrectomy and radiofrequency ablation, have been shown to be as effective as total nephrectomy with fewer undesirable consequences, including the need for dialysis. Although outcomes have improved with such therapeutic advances, VHL is still a devastating disease that involves an average life expectancy of 49 years.

Clinical Case

A 40-year-old female nurse comes to the emergency department with her husband and two children complaining of a severe, constant headache that began 2 hours before she arrived. According to her husband, the headache was preceded by a brief period of unconsciousness after his wife collapsed while mowing the lawn. Upon awakening, she was confused. There is no prior history of severe headache. Her medical history is significant for two uncomplicated term pregnancies, occasional urinary tract infections, and hypertension. She denies medications and drug allergies. The patient is adopted, and her family history is unknown to her. Her social history is unremarkable, with the exception of two cases of

mumps having been diagnosed at her daughter's school within the past month. Her vital signs reveal a blood pressure of 170/95 mm Hg, a pulse rate of 85 beats per minute, a respiration rate of 16 breaths per minute. On physical examination, the woman is a moderately obese woman who appears to be her stated age. Her lungs are clear. The cardiac examination is remarkable for a systolic click; rate and rhythm are normal. Her abdomen is somewhat difficult to assess as a result of her obesity. Marked hepatomegaly is noted, along with the presence of an indistinct but palpable and firm abdominal mass. The extremities are without edema, and the peripheral pulses are 2+ throughout. The neurological examination is unremarkable, with the exception of mild confusion.

What would be the most appropriate next step in this patient's diagnosis and treatment after the stabilization of her airway, breathing, and circulation and routine blood tests?

Explore the presenting or the most pressing problem first, which is the headache. CT scanning of the brain would be the most appropriate way to look for an acute process such as bleeding or swelling. An ultrasound of the liver and kidneys is probably required in the future, but this patient's immediate condition does not warrant this test. CT scanning of the abdomen and pelvis is helpful for evaluating abdominal masses, but again, this is not her most important complaint. Electrocardiography would be helpful if the physician was considering a cardiac cause of the problem, which is possible but not at the top of the list. Finally, lumbar puncture would be indicated if meningitis was a high possibility for the differential diagnosis. However, at this time it is not.

What is the most likely cause of her headache?

This patient has a laundry list of the signs and symptoms of ADPKD, including occasional urinary tract infections, hypertension, systolic click (as a result of

mitral valve prolapse), hepatomegaly, and palpable abdominal mass. If her family history was known, it would likely reveal evidence of renal disorders. However, the extrarenal symptom of ADPKD that is perhaps the most interesting to test writers is cerebral aneurysm with the potential for intracranial bleeding. Meningitis would certainly cause a headache, but the probability is remote given the acute presentation and the likelihood of having contracted the disease from such a remote exposure. Similarly, migraine would not likely present in such an abrupt manner with a loss of consciousness. Elevated blood pressure can certainly cause a headache; however, unless the elevated pressure results in intracranial bleeding (i.e., stroke), one would not suspect the collapse followed by a period of unconsciousness that was experienced by this patient.

The patient recovers well and the result of the CT scan of the brain is normal. What symptoms does the patient have an increased risk of experiencing?

This patient is likely to experience all of the symptoms of ADPKD, which include needing dialysis or a kidney transplant during the next 10 to 20 years, having recurrent episodes of hematuria, having chronic back pain, and developing kidney stones.

Suggested Readings

Hildebrandt F: Nephronophthisis–medullary cystic kidney disease. In Avner ED, Harmon WE (eds): *Pediatric Nephrology*, 5th ed. Baltimore, Lippincott Williams & Wilkins, 2004, p 665.

Wilson PD: Polycystic kidney disease. *N Engl J Med* 350: 151–164, 2004.

Yendt ER: Medullary sponge kidney. In Schrier RW, Gottschalk CW (eds): *Diseases of the Kidney*, 5th ed. Boston, Little, Brown, 1993, pp 525–532.

PRACTICE QUESTIONS

1. Both of the children of the patient in this chapter's clinical case appear to be healthy. With the use of ultrasound imaging for confirmation, at what age could these children be told with near certainty that they will not inherit their mother's condition?

    A. 10 years
    B. 15 years
    C. 30 years
    D. 40 years

2. A 25-year-old man presents to your office with a chief complaint of hematuria. Upon further questioning, you discover that he is also concerned about progressively worsening hearing loss. Which of the following conditions is at the top of your differential diagnosis?

    A. Thin basement membrane nephropathy
    B. VHL syndrome
    C. Alport syndrome
    D. ADPKD

Urinalysis and an Approach to Kidney Diseases

10

A. Vishnu Moorthy
Frederick J. Boehm III

OUTLINE

I. Introduction
II. Dipstick Urine Testing
   A. Hematuria
   B. Proteinuria
   C. Other Dipstick Abnormalities
III. Microscopic Analysis of the Urine Sediment
   A. Red Blood Cells in the Urine Sediment
   B. Other Cells in the Urine Sediment
   C. Casts in the Urine Sediment
   D. Crystals in the Urine Sediment

IV. Quantification of Urinary Protein
V. Microalbuminuria
VI. Syndromes in Nephrology
   A. Proteinuria and the Nephrotic Syndrome
   B. Hematuria with Kidney Failure: The Nephritic Syndrome
   C. Other Kidney Disorders with Abnormalities in the Urine Sediment
   D. Urinary Abnormalities in the Asymptomatic Patient

Objectives

- Know the methods to analyze urine: dipstick testing for protein, blood, and other substances and microscopic evaluation of urine sediment.
- Know the significance of finding protein in the urine by the dipstick.
- Know the significance of a positive blood test by the dipstick.
- Know what microalbuminuria is and understand its significance in a patient with diabetes mellitus.
- Know the various cells, casts, and crystals that can be seen on microscopy of the urine sediment and their clinical significances.
- Be able to correlate urinary abnormalities with some common kidney diseases.

Clinical Case

A 62-year-old African-American man with a 10-year history of diabetes mellitus type 2 visits the primary care clinic where a second-year medical student is working with her preceptor. The patient tells the student that he has no new concerns and that he is visiting the doctor for a routine health assessment and diabetes check. When reviewing the patient's chart, the student sees that the patient's most recent visit was approximately 1 year ago. His current medication regimen includes only glipizide (for lowering blood sugar levels). A random finger-prick blood glucose level is 203 mg/dl, and the hemoglobin A1c level is 7.7 mg/dl. The patient has a negative dipstick test for protein in the urine. The student also decides to check the urine for microalbuminuria, and this value is found to be 210 mg albumin/1 g creatinine. All previous urine albumin-to-creatinine ratios were less than 20 mg protein/1 g creatinine.

Why is there albumin in the patient's urine? How does the albuminuria relate to his diabetes?

I. INTRODUCTION

Urinalysis is a simple and useful test for diagnosing diseases of the kidney. Every patient with suspected kidney disease should have an analysis of his or her urine. Urinalysis is of great diagnostic value for several types of kidney disease, and it is often described as a "liquid kidney biopsy." Urine abnormalities (e.g., bloody urine) may be visible to the naked eye. At other times, the urine may appear normal, but abnormalities may be detected by chemical testing of the urine.

II. DIPSTICK URINE TESTING

A specialized strip of plastic with paper tabs impregnated with different reagents is used to detect the presence of various substances in the urine. The two most important abnormal substances in the urine are blood (hematuria) and protein (proteinuria).

A. Hematuria

Hematuria may arise from disease in any part of the urinary tract. Urologic causes include diseases of the urethra, prostate, bladder, ureter, or renal pelvis, such

as cancer, infections, or kidney stones. Kidney paren-chymal causes include various types of glomerular diseases.

An examination of the urinary sediment is useful for differentiating between these two groups of diseases that cause hematuria.

Increasing amounts of blood in the urine cause color changes in the dipstick. The color changes are the result of the heme pigment, and therefore this test may be positive if the urine contains free hemoglobin (which is noted in patients with intravascular hemolysis and hemoglobinuria) or myoglobin (which is seen in patients with muscle damage).

B. Proteinuria

In the normal, healthy state, the glomerular capillary wall is an effective barrier to the filtration of proteins. Small amounts of low-molecular-weight proteins (e.g., immunoglobulin light chains) cross the glomerular capillary wall and are reabsorbed by tubular epithelial cells. They are subsequently metabolized by the tubular epithelial cells. In glomerular disease, damage to the glomerular capillary wall and the podocyte leads to the appearance of protein in the urine. Dipstick testing for proteinuria is a qualitative test. The resulting color change is read as negative or trace (noted in healthy subjects) or 1+ to 4+, with these values indicating increasing amounts of proteinuria. The dipstick test for urinary protein is specific for albumin, and it may not detect proteins other than albumin, such as immunoglobulin light chains. Light chains may be noted in the urine of patients with plasma cell disorders (e.g., multiple myeloma). Other procedures, such as the precipitation of protein with sulfosalicylic acid or urine protein electrophoresis, may be necessary for detecting urinary proteins other than albumin.

C. Other Dipstick Abnormalities

Urinary glucose, which is also called *glycosuria*, may be seen in patients with diabetes mellitus and hyperglycemia or in renal glycosuria, where the blood glucose levels are normal but glucose appears in the urine as a result of a defect in proximal tubular reabsorption of glucose, as is seen in patients with Fanconi syndrome. Other substances noted in the urine by dipstick include ketones (acetoacetic acid, which is noted in patients with diabetic ketoacidosis), bilirubin and urobilinogen (in patients with liver disease), leukocyte esterase (when the urine may contain leukocytes, as in urinary tract infection), and nitrite (produced by bacteria from nitrate and suggestive of urinary tract infection). The dipstick can also measure urine pH and specific gravity (Table 10-1).

Table 10-1. Significance of Dipstick Analysis

Finding on dipstick analysis	Significance
Blood	Urologic or nephrologic lesions
Albumin	Glomerular disease
Glucose	Diabetes mellitus or renal glycosuria
Ketones	Diabetic ketoacidosis
Bilirubin and urobilinogen	Liver disease
Leukocyte esterase	Urinary tract infection
Nitrite	Urinary tract infection

III. MICROSCOPIC ANALYSIS OF THE URINE SEDIMENT

Examination of the unstained sediment of a fresh sample of urine (within 60 minutes of voiding) spun in a centrifuge at 3000 rpm for 5 minutes can detect several types of cellular elements in various diseases of the urinary system. A phase-contrast microscope, if available, will be useful for the study of the urine sediment.

A. Red Blood Cells in the Urine Sediment

It is within the normal range to identify up to two to three red blood cells (RBCs) per high-power field. The presence of RBCs in the urine sediment confirms that the positive dipstick is indeed caused by blood and not by hemoglobinuria or myoglobinuria. In many glomerular diseases, the glomerular capillary wall is disrupted and thus permits RBCs to pass into the tubules. The RBCs are then excreted in the final urine either as gross hematuria or as clear urine with RBCs that are seen only in the urine sediment; this finding is known as *microscopic hematuria*. In these disorders, the RBCs in the urine sediment are abnormal in shape and often have small, bubble-like projections that result from defects in the cell membrane. These cells are described as *dysmorphic erythrocytes*. RBC casts and dysmorphic erythrocytes in the urine sediment are indicative of glomerular disease. If blood in the urine arises in the renal pelvis or bladder as a result of infection, neoplasm of the urinary tract (often noted in patients >50 years old), or renal calculi, then the RBCs in the urine sediment are regular-appearing biconcave discs and are described as *monomorphic* or *isomorphic RBCs*.

B. Other Cells in the Urine Sediment

Other cellular elements noted on urine microscopy can include white blood cells (WBCs) in patients with urinary tract infection. WBCs are larger than RBCs and have large, multilobed nuclei and granular cytoplasm. Eosinophils in the urine sediment can be identified with the use of special stains (e.g., Hansel's stain), and they may be noted in allergic tubulointerstitial disease with acute kidney injury, such as what is seen after exposure to antibiotics. Epithelial cells may also be noted in the urine sediment. In women, it is common to find varying numbers of large squamous epithelial cells from the vagina. Renal tubular epithelial cells may be seen in the urine sediment of patients with ~~both interstitial and glomerular diseases~~ acute tubular necrosis. Fat globules (epithelial cells full of lipid) may be noted in patients with the nephrotic syndrome. The fat globules appear like a Maltese cross when the urine sediment is studied under polarized light. Malignant cells may be detected in the urine sediment with the use of special stains in patients with cancer at any site of the urinary tract (Table 10-2).

C. Casts in the Urine Sediment

At times, urine sediment can contain cigar-shaped structures called *casts*. These are often translucent, and they have a ground-glass appearance. They are formed in tubules, and they are composed of a glycoprotein (Tamm–Horsfall protein) that is secreted by the epithelial cells of the loop of Henle; these are called *hyaline casts*. A few hyaline casts may be seen at times in healthy people with normal concentrated urine, but they are also seen in large numbers in patients with numerous kidney diseases. The hyaline matrix of the cast can be embedded with RBCs if the glomeruli are diseased and allowing for the passage of RBCs into the tubules. RBC casts indicate a glomerular origin of hematuria and are diagnostic of glomerulonephritis. Casts can contain tubular epithelial cells (epithelial cell casts) in various glomerular

and interstitial diseases. Granular casts caused by the precipitation of protein or disrupted cells in the hyaline matrix are nonspecific and may be seen in various forms of chronic kidney diseases. Waxy casts are broad casts with an opaque waxy appearance; they may be seen in the urine sediment of patients with chronic kidney disease. In patients with acute kidney injury (also called *acute tubular necrosis*) and kidney failure, tubular epithelial cell casts, which often appear as muddy brown casts, may be seen in the urine sediment (Fig. 10-1 and Table 10-3).

D. Crystals in the Urine Sediment

Various types of crystals may be seen in the urine sediment (Fig. 10-2 and Table 10-4). These include calcium oxalate crystals, which are shaped like envelopes (seen in patients with kidney stones composed of calcium oxalate); coffin-lid–shaped crystals that contain magnesium ammonium phosphate (also called *triple phosphate* in patients with urea-splitting bacterial [*Proteus* species] urinary infection); rhomboid or needle-shaped urate crystals (when there is increased urinary excretion of urate); hexagonal cystine crystals (seem in patients with increased urinary cystine as a result of tubular transport defect and cystine stones); and fan-shaped or starburst-appearing crystals of indinavir (in patients with human immunodeficiency virus [HIV] or acquired immunodeficiency syndrome [AIDS] who are treated with this medication).

IV. QUANTIFICATION OF URINARY PROTEIN

The dipstick proteinuria is a qualitative test for urinary protein, the amount of protein in a 24-hour collection of urine is a quantitative measure of proteinuria. Reagents such as sulfosalicylic acid are used to precipitate the urine protein that can then be measured. Normally in an adult, 24-hour urinary protein excretion is less than 150 mg of total protein, and albumin accounts for up to 30 mg per day of urinary protein. Tamm–Horsfall mucoprotein secreted by the loop of Henle is another component of urinary protein. In patients with diseases of the glomeruli, the capillary walls become more permeable and allow the excretion of larger amounts of protein. Anyone who excretes more than 3.5 g of protein in a 24-hour urine collection is said to have nephrotic range proteinuria. This is one component of the nephrotic syndrome.

Twenty-four–hour urine collections are not used with the same frequency as they were in the past because they are cumbersome, inconvenient, and possibly inaccurate as a result of collection errors. However, they continue to be used to measure proteinuria in women who are affected by preeclampsia (Box 10-1).

Table 10-2. Significance of Urine Sediment Findings

Finding in urine sediment	Significance
Dysmorphic erythrocytes	Glomerular disease
Monomorphic erythrocytes	Urologic disease
White blood cells	Urinary tract infection
Eosinophils	Allergic tubulointerstitial disease
Renal tubular epithelial cells	Renal interstitial or glomerular disease *(acute tubular necrosis)*
Malignant cells	Urinary tract neoplasm

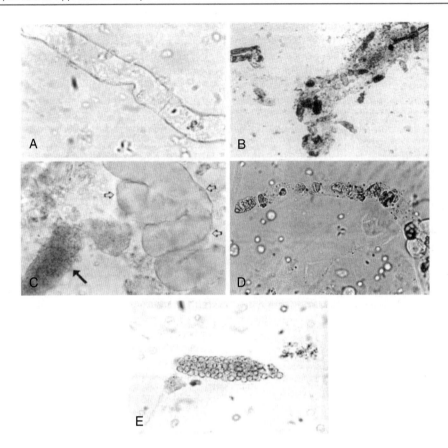

Figure 10-1. Casts in the urine sediment. *A,* Hyaline cast. *B,* Muddy brown granular cast in acute kidney injury. *C,* Granular cast *(closed arrow)* and waxy cast *(open arrows). D,* Epithelial cell cast. *E,* Red blood cell cast. *(From Greenberg A:* Primer on Kidney Diseases, *4th ed. Philadelphia, Saunders, 2005.)*

Table 10-3. Significance of Casts in the Urine

Type of cast	Clinical significance
Hyaline casts	In normal concentrated urine and other kidney diseases
Red blood cell casts	Glomerulonephritis or vasculitis of the kidney
Renal epithelial cell casts or muddy brown casts	Acute kidney injury
Granular casts	Numerous glomerular diseases
White blood cell casts	Tubulointerstitial disease or acute pyelonephritis
Fatty casts	Nephrotic syndrome
Waxy casts	Chronic kidney disease
Broad casts	Chronic kidney disease

In practice, the concentration of creatinine and protein can be measured in a random urine sample and expressed as the protein-to-creatinine ratio. A protein-to-creatinine ratio of less than 0.15 g of protein per 1 g of creatinine is normal and a ratio of more than 3.5 is in the nephrotic range. Lesser amounts of urinary protein excretion (<3.5 g per 1 g of creatinine) may be seen in a variety of kidney diseases. The urine protein-to-creatinine ratio is based on the observation that an average adult excretes approximately 1 g of creatinine in the urine over the course of 24 hours. Of course, muscular adults can excrete more creatinine, whereas older individuals with less muscle mass will produce and excrete less creatinine (Fig. 10-3 and Box 10-2).

V. MICROALBUMINURIA

Small amounts of albumin in the urine may remain undetected by the routine dipstick urinalysis. In these instances, special methods such as enzyme-linked immunosorbent assay with antibodies to albumin can detect minimal amounts of urinary

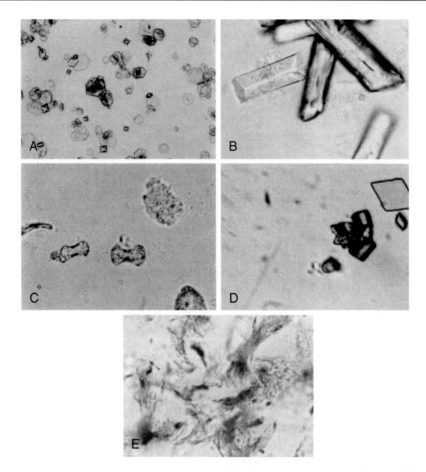

Figure 10-2. Crystals in the urine sediment. *A,* Hexagonal cystine and envelope-shaped oxalate. *B,* Coffin-lid–shaped triple phosphate. *C,* Dumbbell-shaped oxalate. *D,* Rhomboid urate. *E,* Needle-shaped urate. *(From Greenberg A: Primer on Kidney Diseases, 4th ed. Philadelphia, Saunders, 2005.)*

Table 10-4. Significance of Urine Crystals

Urine crystal	Shape	Pathologic significance
Calcium oxalate	Envelope	Calcium oxalate stones
Magnesium ammonium phosphate (triple phosphate)	Coffin lid	Urea-splitting bacterial urinary infection
Urate	Rhomboid or needle	Gout or uric acid stones
Cystine	Hexagon	Tubular transport defect or cystine stones
Indinavir	Fan or starburst	Treatment with indinavir

albumin excretion. Healthy subjects excrete less than 30 mg of albumin in their urine per 1 g of creatinine. Urinary albumin excretion between 30 and 300 mg per 1 g of creatinine is called *microalbuminuria.* Larger amounts of urinary albumin are easily detected on dipstick testing. In patients with diabetes mellitus, persistent microalbuminuria implies the glomerular disease, diabetic nephropathy. If the dipstick is negative for proteinuria in a patient with diabetes mellitus, then microalbuminuria

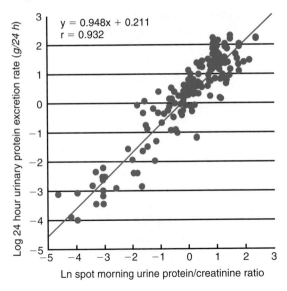

Figure 10-3. Correlation between spot morning urine protein-to-creatinine ratio (natural logarithm [Ln]) and 24-hour protein-uria (decimal logarithm [Log]) in 177 patients without diabetes with chronic proteinuric nephropathy. *(Data from Ginsberg JM, Chang BS, Matarese RA, Garella S: Use of single voided urine samples to estimate quantitative proteinuria.* N Engl J Med *309:1543–1546, 1983.)*

Box 10-2. Important Urine Protein-to-Creatinine Ratios

Normal: <0.15 g protein per 1 g creatinine
Suggestive of glomerular disease: >1.0 g protein per 1 g creatinine
Nephrotic syndrome: >3.5 g protein per 1 g creatinine

---

should be tested to detect early diabetic nephropathy. It is recommended that patients with type 2 diabetes mellitus have microalbuminuria checked at the time of the initial diagnosis and annually thereafter to detect diabetic nephropathy. In patients with diabetes mellitus type 1, microalbuminuria testing is advised 10 years after the initial diagnosis of diabetes.

VI. SYNDROMES IN NEPHROLOGY

The urinalysis is the first step in the evaluation of a patient with kidney disease. One simple way to classify the various types of glomerular diseases is by observing the changes in the urine.

A. Proteinuria and the Nephrotic Syndrome

Patients with large amounts of proteinuria (2+ or 3+ on dipstick or >1 g of protein per 1 g of creatinine) are likely to have a glomerular disease as a cause of the proteinuria. The features of the nephrotic syndrome include urinary protein excretion exceeding 3.5 g per 1 g of creatinine, decreased serum albumin levels with generalized dependent edema, and hyperlipidemia. Lipiduria with fat globules and fatty casts (with a Maltese-cross appearance under polarized light) may be present. Primary kidney diseases that cause the nephrotic syndrome include minimal change disease, membranous nephropathy, and focal segmental glomerulosclerosis. Systemic diseases that can be accompanied by the nephrotic syndrome include diabetic nephropathy, amyloidosis, and systemic lupus erythematosus.

B. Hematuria with Kidney Failure: The Nephritic Syndrome

In patients with various types of glomerular diseases, kidney failure with oliguria and hematuria may be seen with an illness of short duration. The urine sediment in these patients is often described as "active," with numerous RBCs and RBC casts. Diseases associated with this clinical picture include idiopathic crescentic glomerulonephritis (also called *rapidly progressive glomerulonephritis*) as a result of antiglomerular-basement-membrane antibodies and vasculitides, including Wegener's granulomatosis. Patients with crescentic glomerulonephritis may have pulmonary symptoms such as hemoptysis or respiratory failure as a result of anti-glomerular-basement-membrane antibodies reacting with the alveolar basement membrane; this is Goodpasture syndrome. Immune-complex–mediated glomerular diseases (e.g., systemic lupus erythematosus, cryoglobulinemia in association with hepatitis C infection) can present with acute kidney failure with hematuria.

The term *nephritic syndrome* is at times used to describe the clinical condition that is characterized by dark, smoky-colored urine, hypertension, and acute kidney failure with decreasing urine output. Poststreptococcal glomerulonephritis is a common cause of the nephritic syndrome in many parts of the world.

Hematuria and kidney failure can also be seen in patients with endothelial damage in conditions described as *thrombotic microangiopathy*. Infections with certain strains of *Shigella* or *Escherichia coli*, human immunodeficiency virus (HIV)/acquired immunodeficiency syndrome (AIDS), malignant hypertension, progressive systemic sclerosis (scleroderma), bone marrow transplantation, or medication toxicity (e.g., from oral contraceptives, vincristine, or cyclosporine) can lead to thrombotic microangiopathy. These patients have a decrease in the platelet count of the blood, because platelets are consumed during the thrombotic process. Fragmented RBCs (schistocytes) may be noted in the peripheral blood smear. The term *hemolytic uremic syndrome* is often used when describing this condition. Sometimes the patient has a systemic illness with fever and neurologic dysfunction along with thrombotic

microangiopathy. This clinical disorder is called *thrombotic thrombocytopenic purpura.*

C. Other Kidney Disorders with Abnormalities in the Urine Sediment

Although WBCs in the sediment are noted in urinary tract infections, the presence of WBC casts is suggestive of acute pyelonephritis. Microscopic or gross hematuria, often with colicky abdominal pain, is seen in patients with urinary calculi. The urine sediment in these patients can also contain crystals: calcium oxalate, uric acid, or cystine, depending on the type of the calculus. In patients with acute kidney injury, muddy brown granular casts are often seen in the urine sediment. Urinary eosinophils can be identified in the urine sediment by special stains in patients with acute kidney failure as a result of drug-induced interstitial nephritis.

D. Urinary Abnormalities in the Asymptomatic Patient

Microscopic hematuria is not uncommon in patients with urinary tract infection, with diseases of the prostate, or after catheterization of the bladder. Gross or microscopic hematuria may be noted in patients with urinary tract malignancies. Every effort must be used to exclude a urogenital malignancy in patients with unexplained hematuria who are more than 50 years old. Urologic procedures such as cystoscopy or ultrasonography of the kidney may be useful.

The hematuria is likely the result of glomerular disease if urine sediment contains RBC casts or if the RBCs in the sediment are dysmorphic. Glomerular diseases such as immunoglobulin A (IgA) nephropathy, Alport syndrome, and thin basement membrane nephropathy are characterized by microscopic hematuria in patients with minimal symptoms. In these diseases, a modest amount of proteinuria is often noted. The patient with IgA nephropathy may present with repeated episodes of gross hematuria that are often associated with infections, usually of the respiratory tract. At times, hematuria may be transient or remain unexplained.

Microalbuminuria is the earliest abnormality in the patient with diabetes mellitus and diabetic nephropathy. As glomerular changes that result from diabetic nephropathy progress, greater amounts of protein are excreted in the urine. The nephrotic syndrome and kidney failure are noted in patients with advanced diabetic nephropathy.

Clinical Case

A 62-year-old African-American man with a 10-year history of diabetes mellitus type 2 visits the primary care clinic where a second-year medical student is working with her preceptor. The patient tells the student that he has no new concerns and that he is visiting the doctor for a routine health assessment and diabetes check. When reviewing the patient's chart, the student sees that the patient's most recent visit was approximately 1 year ago. His current medication regimen includes only glipizide (for lowering blood sugar levels). A random finger-prick blood glucose level is 203 mg/dl, and the hemoglobin A1c level is 7.7 mg/dl. The patient has a negative dipstick test for protein in the urine. The student also decides to check the urine for microalbuminuria, and this value is found to be 210 mg albumin/1 g creatinine. All previous urine albumin-to-creatinine ratios were less than 20 mg protein/1 g creatinine.

Why is there albumin in the patient's urine? How does the albuminuria relate to his diabetes?

With an elevated hemoglobin A1c level and an elevated random finger-prick blood glucose level, the patient has demonstrated poor blood glucose control and is at great risk for diabetic complications. One complication of diabetes is diabetic nephropathy. The earliest manifestation of diabetic nephropathy is the excretion of increasing amounts of albumin in the urine. A simple and sensitive test to detect microalbuminuria in a patient with diabetes mellitus is by the measurement of the albumin-to-creatinine ratio in a random sample of urine. In healthy individuals, urinary albumin excretion is less than 30 mg per 1 g of creatinine. Urinary excretion of albumin in amounts from 30 to 300 mg per 1 g of creatinine is considered microalbuminuria. In the patient with diabetes, persistent microalbuminuria is predictive of worsening kidney function in the future.

Suggested Readings

Cohen RA, Brown RS: Microscopic hematuria. *New Eng J Med* 348:2330–2338, 2003.

Glassock RJ: Hematuria and proteinuria. In Greenberg A (ed): *Primer on Kidney Diseases.* Philadelphia, National Kidney Foundation and Elsevier/Saunders, 2005, pp 36–46.

PRACTICE QUESTIONS

1. A 22-year-old man is seen in his physician's office with a weeklong history of swelling all over the body and a 10-lb weight gain. Urine testing shows 4+ protein and is negative for blood. This patient is likely to have a disorder of any of the following structures except for which one?

A. The podocyte
B. The glomerular basement membrane
C. The slit diaphragm
D. The proximal convoluted tubule

2. A 72-year-old man is seen in his physician's office with back pain of several months' duration and a recent history of fracture of his femur. He is noted to be anemic and to have an elevated serum creatinine level. His urine is normal on dipstick testing. All of the following would be recommended except for which one?

A. Testing of the urine for protein with sulfosalicylic acid
B. Testing for microalbuminuria

C. Urine protein electrophoresis
D. Urine immunofixation for light chains of immunoglobulins

3. A 24-year-old woman is hospitalized for a 3-week illness that is characterized by skin rash, fever, joint pains, and dark, cola-colored urine. Of the following abnormalities in the urine sediment, which one suggests that the patient is likely to have an illness with glomerular involvement?

A. WBCs
B. RBC casts
C. Uric acid crystals
D. Eosinophils

Acute Kidney Injury

Paul S. Kellerman
Tracy C. Blichfeldt

OUTLINE

I. Incidence and Definitions
II. Categories of Acute Kidney Injury
   A. Prerenal Disease
   B. Postrenal Disease
   C. Intrinsic Kidney Disease
III. Ischemic Acute Tubular Necrosis
   A. Pathophysiology of Tubular Injury and Death
   B. Tubular Necrosis and Decreased Glomerular Filtration Rate
   C. Clinical Phases of Ischemic Acute Tubular Necrosis

IV. Toxic Acute Tubular Necrosis
V. Acute Interstitial Nephritis
VI. Glomerulonephritis As a Cause of Acute Kidney Failure
VII. Diagnosis of Acute Kidney Injury
   A. Clinical History
   B. Physical Examination
   C. Laboratory and Radiologic Testing
VIII. Treatment of Acute Kidney Injury
IX. Mortality and Recovery from Acute Kidney Injury

Objectives

- Understand the definition of *acute kidney injury* and *oliguria*.
- Describe the three main categories of acute kidney injury and the primary causes within each category.
- Describe the effects of acute tubular necrosis on nephron sites, and understand why the glomerular filtration rate decreases with acute tubular necrosis.
- Distinguish between the ischemic and toxic causes of acute tubular necrosis and their clinical courses.
- Describe the clinical presentation of acute interstitial nephritis and acute glomerulonephritis.
- Describe how to find reversible causes of acute kidney injury using the history, the physical examination, and diagnostic studies.
- Describe the indications for dialysis intervention.

Clinical Case

A 50-year-old man presents to the emergency department with nausea, vomiting, and abdominal pain. He has a 20-year history of insulin-dependent diabetes mellitus, and he has been unable to keep food or water down for the last 2 days. His wife has been sick with influenza and at home during the last week. The patient's history also includes hypertension and diabetic retinopathy, but there is no history of nephropathy. Medications include enalapril (an angiotensin-converting enzyme inhibitor), hydrochlorothiazide (a diuretic), and ibuprofen (3 tablets twice a day) for the last 2 weeks to treat a painful big toe. The patient's wife states that he has not urinated since the previous day.

The physical examination reveals a sick man with occasional retching. He is afebrile. His supine blood pressure is 110/76 mm Hg, and his supine pulse is 94 beats per minute; his sitting blood pressure is 90/60 mm Hg, and his sitting pulse is 115 beats per minute. His lungs are clear, and his cardiac examination reveals only tachycardia. His abdomen demonstrates diffuse tenderness but no rebound, and his extremities have no edema.

Laboratory blood testing reveals the following values in the patient's blood (serum): white blood cell count, 15,000/ml; sodium, 145 mmol/L; potassium, 3.7 mmol/L; bicarbonate, 22 mmol/L, blood urea nitrogen, 70 mg/dl; creatinine, 3.4 mg/dl; and glucose 485 mg/dl. Testing of his urine reveals a sodium level of 54 mmol/L and a creatinine level of 37 mg/dl. Urinalysis shows 1+ protein. Urine microscopy shows renal tubular cells and muddy brown casts. Over the next 8 hours, the patient has 75 ml of urine output.

Of the three categories of acute kidney injury, which is the most likely? What is this patient's extracellular fluid volume status? What factors contributed to this patient's volume status? What is the fractional excretion of sodium? Is there evidence of kidney damage? What treatment should be prescribed?

I. INCIDENCE AND DEFINITIONS

The kidney receives 25% of cardiac output. It is one of two major excretory organs, with the other one being the liver. As such, the kidney is subject to insults from any reduction in perfusion as well as from toxins. Approximately 7% of hospitalized patients will experience acute kidney injury (AKI). Given the volume of patient admissions per year in the United States, this is a significant number of patients.

AKI is defined as a decline in the glomerular filtration rate (GFR) that occurs during a period of less than 2 weeks. The decline in GFR is measured by an increase in serum creatinine. The actual increase that defines AKI is not currently agreed on, although it may be an increase in serum creatinine by 0.5 mg/dl or 1.0 mg/dl or by 25% or 50%. This is in contradistinction with chronic kidney disease, in which the decline in GFR occurs over months to years. AKI may be oliguric or nonoliguric. *Oliguria* ("little urine") is defined as less than 500 ml of urine per day or less than 20 ml per hour. *Anuria* ("no urine") is defined as less than 100 ml of urine per day.

Anuria often indicates a blockage of urine flow, and it is less common than other forms of AKI. Oliguria is diagnosed by examining the obligatory amount of cellular waste products that needs to be excreted from an average-sized individual. This approximates 600 milliosmoles per day. The maximal concentrating ability of the kidney is 1200 milliosmoles/L. Thus, the minimal volume to excrete the obligatory waste each day is 600 milliosmoles to 1200 milliosmoles/L, which equals 0.5 L or 500 ml.

Uremia is defined as the clinical signs and symptoms of kidney failure. This results in a lack of secretory as well as excretory function in the kidney. *Azotemia* is defined as increased urea (blood urea nitrogen) in the blood. This is a laboratory abnormality, although it is often used by clinicians synonymously with kidney failure.

II. CATEGORIES OF ACUTE KIDNEY INJURY

AKI is conceptualized into three major categories on the basis of whether the insult is intrinsic to the kidney itself or before or after the kidney.

A. Prerenal Disease

Prerenal disease is diagnosed as a result of decreased kidney perfusion. This accounts for 60% of all AKI. The kidney is an autoregulatory organ that maintains the constancy of blood flow via changes in vasoregulation over a wide range of blood pressures. When the blood pressure falls beneath a threshold level, the kidney is unable to maintain blood flow, and GFR declines. It is important to note that the kidneys are actually not yet injured, just unable to maintain the

blood flow and the GFR. Because kidney injury has not yet occurred, prerenal AKI is reversible if it is recognized.

Decreased kidney perfusion may be related to hypovolemia or, more precisely, to decreased extracellular fluid volume and decreased sodium content. This is manifested by low blood pressure, which results in decreased kidney blood flow. Common examples of hypovolemia include bleeding, gastrointestinal losses (i.e., vomiting and diarrhea), and skin losses with severe burns. Although congestive heart failure has a high intravascular volume, when severe enough, there is decreased cardiac output with a failure to perfuse the kidneys and, consequently, a prerenal state. In patients with sepsis, peripheral vasodilation shunts blood away from the central organs, thereby decreasing perfusion to the kidneys. Other causes of prerenal disease include medications such as nonsteroidal antiinflammatory drugs and immunosuppressive agents such as cyclosporine.

B. Postrenal Disease

Postrenal disease indicates an obstruction to urine flow after the urine has left the tubules. It accounts for approximately 10% of AKI. Obstruction can occur primarily at three anatomic sites (Fig. 11-1).

Ureteral obstruction can occur anywhere, but it typically takes place at the ureteropelvic junction (where the ureter meets the renal calyces) or at the ureterovesical junction (where the ureters implant into the bladder). AKI occurs only if both ureters are obstructed, barring preexisting injury to one of the ureters. Unilateral obstruction (e.g., the type that arises from nephrolithiasis) rarely causes AKI, except when there is a solitary functioning kidney.

Bladder obstruction occurs structurally with bladder tumors and functionally with medications that block acetylcholine (anticholinergics), which is the neurotransmitter that is responsible for normal bladder contraction. Finally, the urethra can be a site of obstruction. This can be the result of strictures or of external compression. Among men, the most common cause of obstructive nephropathy is benign or malignant prostate disease. Among women, the most likely causes of AKI as a result of obstruction are pelvic malignancies and radiation for malignancies.

C. Intrinsic Kidney Disease

Intrinsic kidney disease accounts for 30% of all AKI. This type of kidney injury can be stratified by the compartment in which the injury arises (Fig. 11-2).

Glomerulonephritis causes inflammation in glomeruli. This is an uncommon form of AKI among adults, but it is more common among children. The space between the tubules and the glomeruli is

- Bilateral Ureteral
  Obstruction
  – Extraureteral (cervical CA,
    uterine CA, retroperitoneal fibrosis)
  – Intraureteral (stones,
    clots, papillary necrosis)

- Bladder Obstruction
  – Structural (bladder CA)
  – Functional (anticholinergics, diabetes)

- Urethral Obstruction
  (prostatic hypertrophy, prostate CA)

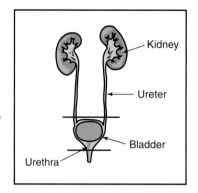

Figure 11-1. Some common causes of urinary obstruction causing postrenal azotemia. *CA*, carcinoma.

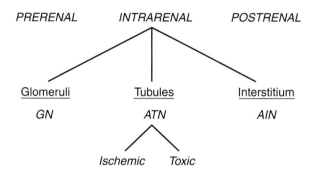

Figure 11-2. Diseases that cause intrinsic acute kidney injury. *AIN*, acute interstitial nephritis; *ATN*, acute tubular necrosis; *GN*, glomerulonephritis.

called the *interstitium*, which, if inflamed, leads to acute interstitial nephritis. Tubules can be injured, which causes acute tubular necrosis (ATN). This accounts for 90% of intrinsic AKI in adults. The primary cause of ATN is decreased kidney perfusion, which is called *ischemic ATN*. If it is severe enough, prerenal disease can eventually result in ATN, which is indicative of true tubular damage. Tubules can also be damaged by toxins such as radiocontrast agents, aminoglycoside antibiotics, platinum-containing chemotherapeutic agents, various antifungal agents, pigments such as myoglobin (a substance that is released during muscle breakdown), and other medications.

III. ISCHEMIC ACUTE TUBULAR NECROSIS

A. Pathophysiology of Tubular Injury and Death
In patients with ischemic ATN, there are two stages of tubular injury that affect different parts of the nephron (Fig. 11-3).

1. Initiation Phase
The initiation phase occurs in the proximal tubule. Proximal tubule cells are energy-dependent, and reabsorb approximately 70% of the glomerular filtrate. They have a large surface area for reabsorption in their brush border, with numerous mitochondria for energy generation to supply the active transport

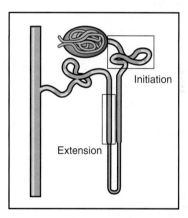

Figure 11-3. Nephron sites of injury in acute kidney injury: "the one–two punch." Initiation occurs in the proximal tubule. Extension occurs in the medullary thick ascending limb of the loop of Henle.

of sodium along with other reabsorbed solutes. The apical brush border membrane is different from the basolateral domain in lipid and protein composition. These differences are maintained by the presence of tight junctions, which are complexes of specific proteins in the basolateral domain. Cells also attach to each other through adhesion molecules and to the basement membrane via transmembrane proteins (integrins) that localize

to the basolateral domain (Fig. 11-4). Specific proteins anchor to one domain as compared with the other via the actin cytoskeleton and associated proteins. For example, sodium/potassium-ATPase is found almost exclusively in the basolateral membrane domain (see Fig. 11-4).

During ischemia, the decrease in perfusion to the kidney results in a lack of the delivery of oxygen and nutrients such as glucose to kidney tubular cells. Adenosine triphosphate (ATP) depletion occurs, thereby disrupting multiple ATP-dependent cellular processes, including intracellular calcium flux, cytoskeletal structure, protein anchoring, and the maintenance of tight junctions, all of which normally maintain cell polarity (Fig. 11-5A). There is a loss of cell polarity that makes cells unable to transport normally (Fig. 11-5B).

Cells may lose their ability to attach to other cells and to the basement membrane (see Fig. 11-5B). Some are simply injured, but many of these cells slough into the urine, often when they are still alive. They can be visualized by urine microscopy. Some cells die during this process through frank necrosis or through programmed cell death (apoptosis).

Blood flow to the kidney may be restored after ischemia (reperfusion). However, the resumption of oxygen delivery can be detrimental after ischemia because of the formation of highly toxic oxygen radicals (Fig. 11-6). After an ischemic insult, ATP degrades to hypoxanthine, and there is an increased formation of xanthine oxidase, which catalyzes hypoxanthine to xanthine as a result of a change in the oxidation-reduction balance of cells. Xanthine

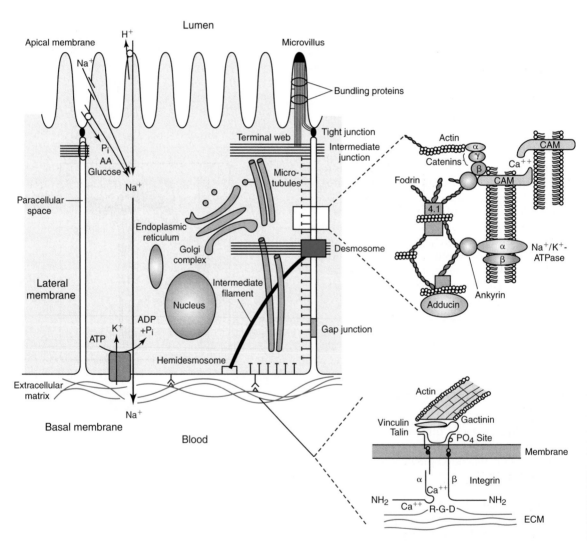

Figure 11-4. Structure of the tubular epithelial cell. The apical and basolateral membrane domains are separated by the tight junction. Cells attach to each other via cellular adhesion molecules and to the extracellular matrix via integrins, all of which interact with the actin cytoskeleton. *(From Fish EM, Molitoris BA: Alterations in epithelial polarity and the pathogenesis of disease states. N Engl J Med 330:1580–1588, 1994.)*

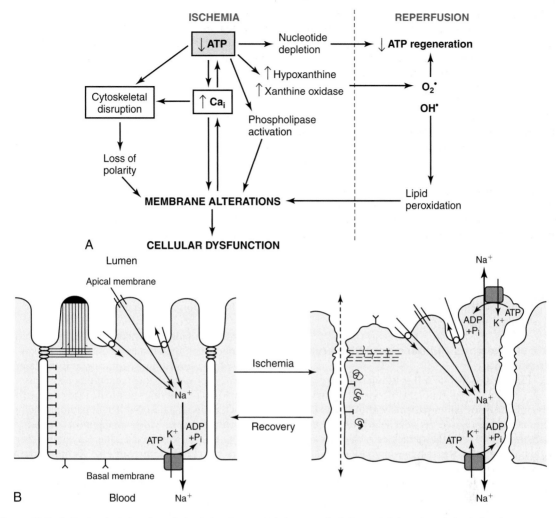

A, Biochemical alterations during ischemic acute tubular necrosis.

B, Structural alterations during ischemic acute tubular necrosis.

Figure 11-5. *A,* Biochemical alterations during ischemic acute tubular necrosis. *B,* Structural alterations during ischemic acute tubular necrosis. *(B, From Fish EM, Molitoris BA: Alterations in epithelial polarity and the pathogenesis of disease states. N Engl J Med 330:1580–1588, 1994.)*

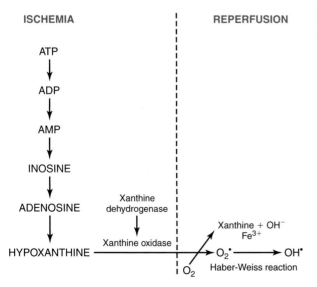

Figure 11-6. Ischemic reperfusion of the kidney and oxygen radical formation.

oxidase, when exposed to oxygen during reperfusion, generates oxygen radicals such as peroxide and hydroxyl radicals. These can damage surrounding cells. Ischemic–reperfusion injury is thought to occur in many tissues in addition to the kidneys, including the brain and the heart.

2. Extension Phase

The kidneys would recover quickly from ischemic AKI were it not for an extension phase that prevents recovery. The distal tubule cells of the thick ascending limb of the loop of Henle function in a relatively hypoxic environment. Although they do not show structural injury during experimental AKI, they experience multiple biochemical changes. During the extension phase, there is endothelial cell activation and impaired vasodilation, with cytokine release to recruit inflammatory mononuclear cells. This leads to leukostasis, platelet activation, and clot formation in small medullary vessels, thereby resulting in further ischemia. Only after the inflammation and vascular stasis ameliorate does AKI eventually recover (Fig. 11-7).

B. Tubular Necrosis and Decreased Glomerular Filtration Rate

The hallmark of ischemic AKI is tubular necrosis, primarily of the proximal tubule. However, although glomeruli look normal in patients with AKI, the GFR is significantly decreased. As cells detach from their basement membranes, they attach to each other and obstruct the tubules, thereby causing back pressure on filtration and decreasing GFR. In addition, there is side-to-side detachment of proximal tubule cells from each other that allows for the back leaking of filtrate between cells.

C. Clinical Phases of Ischemic Acute Tubular Necrosis

There are three clinical phases of AKI that are associated with ischemic ATN (Fig. 11-8). Initially, there is kidney failure, which involves a rising serum creatinine as the kidney fails to excrete creatinine. This can last for days to weeks. Eventually, the serum creatinine plateaus and the urine output increases in volume. This is called the *diuretic phase*. Although the GFR may still be low, this phase is a harbinger of recovery. Last is the recovery phase, when the serum creatinine rapidly falls and the GFR is restored. Because the kidney does not recover its concentrating ability until the serum creatinine is near normal, it is important to maintain adequate kidney perfusion by providing intravenous salt and water to replace urinary losses and to maintain a normovolemic state.

IV. TOXIC ACUTE TUBULAR NECROSIS

The kidney is normally prepared to handle toxins without injury because it is a major excretory organ. However, if the kidney is underperfused, as it is in hypovolemic states, then it may be injured by a toxin. If there are fewer functioning nephrons, as is the case in chronic kidney disease, these remaining nephrons may be injured as a result of greater toxic loads per nephron. Each toxin may have a different pathophysiology. Radiocontrast agents, which are the most common toxins, cause AKI more often if a patient is volume depleted or has chronic kidney disease. Radiocontrast agents cause severe arterial vasoconstriction in the kidney and decrease GFR. They also cause proximal tubule injury similar to the oxygen-free radical damage induced by ischemic ATN. Myoglobin released from

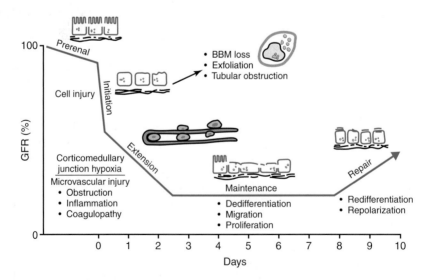

Figure 11-7. Pathophysiologic phases of ischemic acute tubular necrosis and recovery. *BBM,* Basement membrane; *GFR,* glomerular filtration rate. *(From Sutton TA, Fisher CJ, Molitoris BA: Microvascular endothelial injury and dysfunction during ischemic acute renal failure. Kidney Int 62:1539–1549, 2002.)*

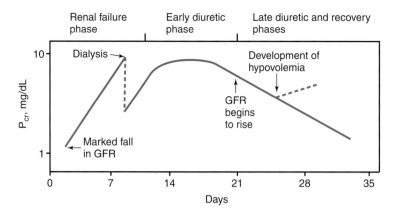

Figure 11-8. Clinical phases of acute tubular necrosis. *GFR,* Glomerular filtration rate; *P_{Cr},* plasma creatinine level.

muscles in patients with rhabdomyolysis is toxic to the proximal tubule cells and causes AKI. Myoglobin can also cause tubular obstruction as a result of cast formation. Aminoglycosides attach to tubular cell apical membrane phospholipids, and they are endocytosed into proximal tubule cells and then isolated in lysosomes. After many days of drug exposure, the lysosomes are overwhelmed and then rupture, thereby resulting in cell injury and death. Newer compounds, including antiretroviral agents and bisphosphonates, can cause AKI either from direct tubular toxicity or tubular obstruction. Overall, toxic ATN is less clinically severe than ischemic ATN, and it is associated with a faster recovery (Box 11-1).

V. ACUTE INTERSTITIAL NEPHRITIS

AKI was originally described as occurring with the antistaphylococcal drug methicillin. On a kidney biopsy one finds infiltration of white blood cells (WBCs; primarily neutrophils and eosinophils) into the interstitium of the kidney (Fig. 11-9). This often is seen in patients who are treated with medications, particularly β-lactam antibiotics (Box 11-2). These patients typically take a β-lactam antibiotic for a week or two, and they often have a rash or

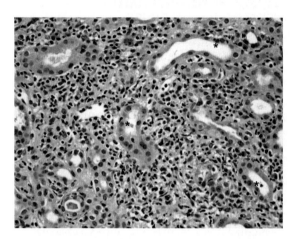

Figure 11-9. Pathology of acute interstitial nephritis demonstrating the infiltration of white blood cells, including eosinophils, surrounding the renal tubules *(asterisk)* in the interstitium. (Hematoxylin and eosin stain, 400×.)

Box 11-1. Acute Tubular Necrosis: Toxins

Radiocontrast agents: Oliguric, within 24 hours of dye, fractional excretion of sodium; risk factors: hypovolemia, chronic kidney disease, diabetes mellitus with chronic kidney disease

Aminoglycosides: Classic nonoliguric, 5 to 7 days of antibiotics

Pigments: Immobility (alcohol, drugs); seizures; trauma; diagnostic triad of acute kidney injury, serum level of creatinine phosphokinase of greater than 1000 U/L, dipstick heme without red blood cells

Cisplatinum: Treatment of squamous cell carcinoma; risk factors: aminoglycosides, chronic kidney disease, hypovolemia

Amphotericin B: Severe hypokalemia, hypomagnesemia; risk factors: chronic kidney disease, hypovolemia, higher dose

Other agents: Antiretrovirals, bisphosphonates, intravenous globulin

---

Box 11-2. Drugs Associated with Acute Interstitial Nephritis

Antibiotics
  Penicillins
  Cephalosporins
  Others (rifampin, sulfonamides)
Nonsteroidal antiinflammatory drugs
Others
  Analgesics
  Diuretics (furosemide)
  Anticonvulsants (phenytoin)
  Miscellaneous (cimetidine, allopurinol)

eosinophilia with a rising serum creatinine level. Urinalysis in these patients shows mild proteinuria, often with WBCs and sometimes with WBC casts, which are diagnostic. The patients may have eosinophils in their urine or on kidney biopsy (Fig. 11-10), and kidney function often returns toward normal simply by stopping the inciting medication, although corticosteroids may enhance recovery. In contrast with a true allergy, reexposure to the medication at a later date usually does not cause the same problem.

There is another type of interstitial nephritis that is seen more often in the outpatient setting. Non-steroidal antiinflammatory drugs, particularly when used in elderly patients for many months, cause a minimal change nephropathy with acute interstitial nephritis. These patients often do not have a rash, eosinophilia, or WBCs in their urine, but they have kidney dysfunction and nephrotic-range proteinuria.

VI. GLOMERULONEPHRITIS AS A CAUSE OF ACUTE KIDNEY INJURY

In children, 50% of intrinsic AKI is the result of glomerulonephritis (GN). Adults may also develop GN and present with AKI. These patients are often said to present with *rapidly progressive GN*. The renal biopsy may show glomerular inflammation with capillary wall necrosis and an accumulation of cells in the Bowman's space. These cells may form crescents, which leads to the term *crescentic GN*. Patients may also have circulating antibodies against the glomerular basement membrane antigens; some of these antibodies can react with the alveolar basement membrane and cause pulmonary symptoms such as hemoptysis. This condition is called *Goodpasture syndrome*. Some patients with a systemic vasculitis can also have AKI; this is seen in patients with diseases such as Wegener's granulomatosis or microscopic polyangiitis. Urinalysis in these patients shows hematuria with dysmorphic red blood cells (RBCs) and RBC casts.

VII. DIAGNOSIS OF ACUTE KIDNEY INJURY

It is critical to identify reversible causes, such as prerenal and postrenal disease, before they cause tubular damage. After ATN is established, there is no specific treatment except supportive therapy until the kidneys recover.

A. Clinical History
Because prerenal disease means decreased kidney blood flow and the three major categories are volume depletion, cardiac failure, and the shunting of blood as a result of peripheral vascular dilation, the history should focus on the patient's volume status (i.e., the extracellular fluid volume). Hypovolemia can result from excess diuretic use, bleeding, or excess fluid loss from gastrointestinal or cutaneous sources. In addition, cardiovascular dysfunction and other causes of hypotension (e.g., sepsis) cause decreased kidney perfusion (Box 11-3).

Postrenal disease means urinary tract obstruction. Thus, a good history is imperative to identify any history of pelvic malignancy or pelvic irradiation in women. In men, symptoms of hesitancy, urgency in micturition, and nocturia suggest prostatism. Also, it is important to recognize that many medications can slow bladder function, such as antihistamines and psychiatric medications.

Intrinsic kidney disease is usually the result of ATN. Thus, a history of hypotension or toxin exposure is important.

B. Physical Examination
For prerenal disease, signs of hypovolemia may be manifested by tenting of the skin when it is pinched gently or the presence of dry mucous membranes. Along with a lack of tears when crying, these are very reliable examination findings in children. However, in adults (particularly the elderly), these are less trustworthy. For adults, the best sign of volume depletion is orthostatic blood pressure and pulse. If taking the blood pressure with the patient in a supine position and standing up or sitting up with the

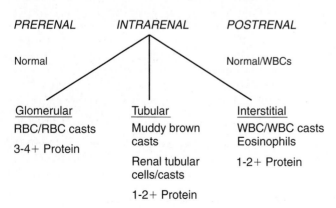

PRERENAL   INTRARENAL   POSTRENAL

Normal   Normal/WBCs

Glomerular   Tubular   Interstitial
RBC/RBC casts   Muddy brown   WBC/WBC casts
                       casts   Eosinophils
3-4+ Protein   1-2+ Protein
                       Renal tubular
                       cells/casts

                       1-2+ Protein

Figure 11-10. Urinalysis for the diagnosis of acute kidney injury. *RBC*, Red blood cell; *WBC*, white blood cell.

Mechanisms of Prerenal Disease

1. Hypovolemia
2. Heart failure
3. Peripheral vasodilation

legs down causes the blood pressure to go down or the pulse to rise, then the patient is said to be orthostatic. A rise in pulse of 20 beats per minute, a decrease in systolic blood pressure of 20 mm Hg, or a decrease in diastolic pressure of 10 mm Hg is considered significant for hypovolemia. There is an important caveat, however: if a drop in blood pressure without an increase in pulse is seen, this may be the result of autonomic dysfunction. This condition is often seen in patients with diabetes, in whom the normal vasoconstriction does not occur with standing as a result of the diabetic involvement of the nerves supplying the blood vessels. The physician must also look for signs of cardiac failure (e.g., rales), peripheral edema, an S3 heart sound, increased jugular venous pressure, and any signs of infection.

For postrenal disease, the presence of abdominal dullness above the pubic bone suggests a distended bladder with outflow obstruction. A mass found on pelvic or rectal examination in a woman or an enlarged prostate in a man is suggestive of possible urinary tract obstruction.

For ATN, the physical examination may show nothing specific.

C. Laboratory and Radiologic Testing

The urinalysis is often very helpful for separating prerenal and postrenal kidney disease from intrinsic kidney disease (see Fig. 11-10). With prerenal disease, because the kidney is not yet injured, the urinalysis is bland (no protein or blood on the dipstick, and no cells or casts). With postrenal disease, the urinalysis again typically shows no protein or blood on the dipstick, and the microscopic examination is also benign, or it may show pyuria. With intrinsic kidney disease, the urinalysis may be very revealing. GN shows large degrees of proteinuria (often 3+ to 4+ on the dipstick), and microscopic examination may demonstrate RBCs, granular casts, and diagnostic RBC casts. ATN manifests lower levels of proteinuria (1+ to 2+), and it may show tubular epithelial cells, tubular cell casts, or muddy brown casts. Tubular cells, tubular cell casts, and muddy brown casts are diagnostic for ATN. Acute interstitial nephritis also displays 1+ to 2+ proteinuria, and urine microscopy often demonstrates WBCs and diagnostic WBC casts.

Obstruction must be ruled out at two levels: at the level of the urethra and bladder and also in the ureters. The passage of a catheter into the bladder or an ultrasonic bladder scan can measure the postvoid residual, which is the amount of urine that is left in the bladder after voiding. A normal postvoid residual is less than 50 ml in young adults and less than 100 ml in the elderly. If a catheter is placed and a large amount of urine is released, the diagnosis is made, and therapy has been initiated as well. Ureteral obstruction must be bilateral, and it is best ruled out with a kidney ultrasound. After obstruction is ruled out, the differential diagnosis is often between prerenal disease and ATN. In addition to the urinalysis, urinary tests can help differentiate these two entities because they ask the following basic question: are the tubules concentrating normally in the face of decreased kidney blood flow?

Multiple urinary substances can be measured (Table 11-1), such as creatinine, osmolality, and sodium, to determine whether tubular epithelial cells are reabsorbing and functional. The most accurate tests are the renal failure index and the fractional excretion of sodium (FE_{Na}), which compare the urinary reabsorption of sodium relative to the creatinine level in oliguric patients:

$$\text{Renal failure index} = \frac{U_{Na}}{U_{Cr}/P_{Cr}}$$

$$FE_{Na}\ (\%) = \frac{U_{Na}/P_{Na}}{U_{Cr}/P_{Cr}} \times 100*$$

This is easily measured by ordering a random urine test for sodium and creatinine levels along with serum sodium and creatinine levels. If the FE_{Na} is less than 1, it is indicative of prerenal disease.

The goal for diagnosis in AKI is to identify reversible causes. There is no single test that is truly diagnostic, although there is the suggestion that certain molecules (e.g., kidney injury molecule 1) may ultimately lead to greater diagnostic precision. Until then, the clinician must use the history, the physical examination, urinalysis, ultrasound, and urinary studies to identify the cause of AKI.

Table 11-1. Laboratory Evaluation of Acute Kidney Injury: Tests of Kidney Function

Test	Prerenal	ATN Intrarenal
Blood urea nitrogen/creatinine (plasma mg/dl)	>40:1	<40:1
Urine sodium (mmol/L)	<20	>40
Urine/plasma creatinine (mg/dl)	>40	<20
Urine/plasma osmolality (mOsm/kg)	>1.5	<1
Renal failure index	<1	>2
Fractional excretion of sodium	<1%	>2%

*U_{Na}, Urine sodium (mmol/L); U_{Cr}, urine creatinine (mg/dl); P_{Na}, plasma sodium (mmol/L); P_{Cr}, plasma creatinine (mg/dl).

VIII. TREATMENT OF ACUTE KIDNEY INJURY

Treatment will be dictated by the cause of AKI. With prerenal insults, the correction of the volume status is often warranted (e.g., fluid administration if the patient is hypovolemic or the use of a diuretic if the patient is experiencing heart failure). If there is urinary tract obstruction, urologic intervention is necessary to reestablish urine flow.

After ATN is established, treatment is supportive. This means maintaining good kidney perfusion, avoiding nephrotoxins (e.g., radiocontrast dye), restricting various solutes (e.g., potassium, phosphorus), and providing nutritional support.

Dialysis is initiated if the kidneys can no longer adequately excrete salt, water, potassium, acid, and uremic toxins. Life-threatening hyperkalemia, severe acidosis, severe pulmonary edema, and profound uremic symptoms (e.g., encephalopathy, pericarditis) are primary indications for emergently initiating dialysis (Box 11-4). A lack of urine output is not an indication per se. Dialysis can either be performed rapidly and intermittently or slowly and continuously. The process of dialysis is discussed in Chapter 13.

Current dialytic therapies for AKI substitute normal kidney function by replacing the filtration function of the glomerulus. However, they do not replace metabolic, immunologic, or endocrine functions. A number of new but still experimental treatments for AKI include new molecules and devices attempt to support these other functions and to maintain volume and electrolyte status.

IX. MORTALITY AND RECOVERY FROM ACUTE KIDNEY INJURY

Historically, once AKI became established (ATN), the disease had a very high mortality rate. During the last decade, however, this seems to have been abating somewhat. It is now being found that, although many patients recover from AKI, a significant proportion of these individuals have an increased risk for chronic kidney disease in the future. AKI usually

arises in conjunction with injury or failure in other organ systems. Indeed, AKI is often part of multisystem organ failure in the intensive care setting. In the unusual event of isolated AKI, the mortality rate is only 5% to 10%. If one other organ system is involved (e.g., respiratory failure on a ventilator), then the mortality rate climbs to just over 50%. If a second organ system is involved (e.g., altered mental status), the mortality remains greater than 75%. Thus, it is critical to identify AKI that is reversible before it becomes ATN (Box 11-5).

Patients with AKI die primarily from infections. They are immunocompromised, and various risk factors (e.g., multiple venous and genitourinary catheters) place them at very high risk for infection and sepsis. These patients also are predisposed to bleeding as a result of uremic platelet dysfunction (Box 11-6). Electrolyte disturbances can give rise to cardiac events and dysrhythmias.

Clinical Case

A 50-year-old man presents to the emergency department with nausea, vomiting, and abdominal pain. He has a 20-year history of insulin-dependent diabetes mellitus, and he has been unable to keep food or water down for the last 2 days. His wife has been sick with influenza and at home during the last week. The patient's history also includes hypertension and diabetic retinopathy, but there is no history of nephropathy. Medications include enalapril (an angiotensin-converting enzyme inhibitor), hydrochlorothiazide (a diuretic), and

---

Box 11-4. Dialysis Indications for Acute Renal Failure

Hard indications
1. Hyperkalemia
2. Symptomatic uremia (pericarditis, encephalopathy)
3. Unresponsive acidosis
4. Sodium and fluid overload (congestive heart failure, pulmonary edema)

Soft indications
1. Bleeding as a result of uremic platelet dysfunction
2. Blood urea nitrogen level of more than 100 mg/dl

Box 11-5. Acute Kidney Injury: The Early Years

Acute kidney injury (AKI) was first recognized by Bywaters and Beall in London during World War II in severe crush injury victims. It was originally described as the acute loss of kidney function in these victims. At that time, the mortality rate was nearly 100% because acute hemodialysis had not yet been developed. During the Korean War, acute hemodialysis was first used for the treatment of military casualties. This decreased the mortality rate to approximately 50%. Since that time, the mortality rate from AKI has remained essentially static, but the demographics of the patients developing AKI have been changed; they often have other comorbid conditions, and they are older. The incidence of AKI has also decreased over time. During World War II, 35% of severely wounded casualties developed AKI, whereas by the time of the Vietnam War, only 0.17% of casualties developed AKI. The credit for this dramatic decrease in incidence of AKI is the result of rapid fluid resuscitation on the battlefield and the evacuation of patients to hospitals by helicopter. This suggested that early intervention may prevent AKI caused by acute tubular necrosis, which has proven to be true.

Box 11-6. Acute Kidney Injury in Young Children: Hemolytic Uremic Syndrome

The most common cause of acute kidney injury in infants and young children is hemolytic uremic syndrome (HUS). HUS can be caused by infection as well as by some medications (e.g., calcineurin inhibitors). It is most commonly associated with some strains of *Escherichia coli* 0157:H7 infections.

   Classic HUS presents as thrombotic microangiopathy with thrombocytopenia, acute hemolytic anemia, and acute kidney injury. An indicator that HUS is caused by *E. coli* 0157:H7 is a presentation of gastroenteritis with bloody diarrhea. *E. coli* 0157:H7 expresses Shigella-like toxin and a lipopolysaccharide that allows it to adhere to intestinal epithelial cells, thereby changing their permeability to water and electrolytes. The Shigella-like toxin also reaches the kidney via the circulatory system, where it damages glomerular endothelial cells and leads to platelet aggregation, microangiopathic glomerular capillary thrombosis, and related tissue injury. The treatment of *E. coli*-associated HUS is supportive, and it may include dialysis when indicated. Antibiotics are typically not used because they can increase the release of more toxin that will further damage organs. The prognosis for childhood HUS is variable: 5% of patients die during the acute phase, 58% recover fully, 11% develop chronic kidney disease, and 17% have hypertension. The best predictor of prognosis is the duration of oliguria or anuria.

ibuprofen (3 tablets twice a day) for the last 2 weeks to treat a painful big toe. The patient's wife states that he has not urinated since the previous day.

   The physical examination reveals a sick man with occasional retching. He is afebrile. His supine blood pressure is 110/76 mm Hg, and his supine pulse is 94 beats per minute; his sitting blood pressure is 90/60 mm Hg, and his sitting pulse is 115 beats per minute. His lungs are clear, and his cardiac examination reveals only tachycardia. His abdomen demonstrates diffuse tenderness but no rebound, and his extremities have no edema.

   Laboratory blood testing reveals the following values in the patient's blood (serum): WBC count, 15,000/ml; sodium, 145 mmol/L; potassium, 3.7 mmol/L; bicarbonate, 22 mmol/L, blood urea nitrogen, 70 mg/dl; creatinine, 3.4 mg/dl; and glucose 485 mg/dl. Testing of his urine reveals a sodium level of 54 mmol/L and a creatinine level of 37 mg/dl. Urinalysis shows 1+ protein. Urine microscopy shows renal tubular cells and muddy brown casts. Over the next 8 hours, the patient has 75 ml of urine output.

Of the three categories of AKI, which is the most likely?

Intrinsic kidney disease as a result of ATN is the most likely cause in this case, as evidenced by an FENa of more than 3% and urinalysis showing muddy brown and renal tubular cell casts. There still could be some component of prerenal disease given that the patient has orthostatic hypotension, which is indicative of hypovolemia. However, if this was purely prerenal disease, the urinalysis would be benign, and the FENa would be less than 1%. Postrenal disease is unlikely, because there is little evidence for obstruction, and the urinalysis is diagnostic for acute tubular injury.

What is this patient's extracellular fluid volume status?

It is decreased. He has no edema, and he is orthostatic, as evidenced by the increase in the pulse and the drop in blood pressure on sitting. Thus, his extracellular fluid volume is low.

What factors have contributed to this patient's volume status?

Poor oral intake, nausea, vomiting, diuretic use (early on), and possibly sepsis all contributed to this patient's hypovolemia.

What is the fractional excretion of sodium?

In this case, it is 3%. This is consistent with ATN.

Is there evidence of kidney damage?

Kidney damage is demonstrated by the urinalysis showing renal tubular cells, muddy brown casts, and proteinuria. The elevation in the serum creatinine level suggests kidney injury.

What treatment should be prescribed?

The hypovolemia should be corrected by giving the patient salt and water (normal saline). Because this patient has primarily ATN and not prerenal disease, the AKI may not respond in terms of increased urine output. If there is no increase in urine output, then the patient may require dialysis.

Suggested Readings

Abuelo G: Normotensive ischemic acute renal failure. *N Engl J Med* 357:797–805, 2007.
Bonventre JV, Weinberg JM: Recent advances in the pathophysiology of ischemic acute renal failure. *J Am Soc Nephrol* 14:2199–2210, 2003.

PRACTICE QUESTIONS

1. A 36-year-old man is admitted for an increased serum creatinine level. He has been taking intravenous antibiotics at home for the past 2 weeks for osteomyelitis caused by *Staphylococcus aureus*. He reports no change in his urine output. On physical examination, his blood pressure was 124/76 mm Hg and his pulse was 82 beats per minute while he was supine and 126/74 mm Hg and 86 beats per minute while he was standing. He has a diffuse fine red maculopapular rash on his trunk and limbs. The remainder of the examination is normal. His serum creatinine level is 2.4 mg/dl today, and it was 1.0 mg/dl a week ago. His other blood laboratory findings include the following: WBC count, 11,000/ml; sodium, 142 mmol/L; potassium, 4.2 mmol/L; and blood urea nitrogen, 34 mg/dl. His urine showed a sodium level of 54 mmol/L and a creatinine level of 39 mg/dl. The urinalysis with dipstick testing showed 1+ protein; the microscopic analysis showed 5 to 10 WBCs/HPF (high-powered field) and an occasional WBC cast. Kidney ultrasound showed no hydronephrosis. What is the most likely diagnosis for this patient?

A. AKI as a result of acute interstitial nephritis
B. Chronic kidney disease as a result of diabetes
C. AKI as a result of ATN
D. AKI as a result of prostate disease

2. A 79-year-old white man comes to the urgent care department with the complaint of not being able to urinate that day. He recently saw his primary care physician for an upper respiratory infection, and he began taking diphenhydramine (an antihistamine) for the relief of nasal congestion. He reports a history that is significant for benign prostatic hypertrophy and hypertension. A Foley catheter was placed, with the return of 1200 ml of urine. Urinalysis was within normal limits. His blood urea nitrogen level was 21 mg/dl, and his creatinine level was 1.5 mg/dl (baseline creatinine level, 1.0 mg/dl). What is the most likely cause of this patient's AKI?

A. Prerenal as a result of hypovolemia
B. Intrarenal as a result of ATN
C. Intrarenal as a result of acute interstitial nephritis
D. Postrenal as a result of obstruction

Chronic Kidney Disease

12

Ryan Kipp
Paul S. Kellerman

OUTLINE
  I. Definition and Incidence of Chronic Kidney Disease
  II. Calculating the Glomerular Filtration Rate
  III. Pathophysiology of Progression
    A. The Special Case of Glomerular Hypertension
    B. Slowing the Progression of Chronic Kidney Disease
  IV. Signs and Symptoms of Kidney Failure
    A. Altered Excretory Function in Chronic Kidney Disease
  B. Bone Disease Associated with Chronic Kidney Disease
  C. Hematologic Consequences
  D. Cardiovascular Consequences
  E. Neurologic Consequences
  F. Other Organ Systems Affected by Uremia
  V. Treatment for Problems Associated with Progressive Chronic Kidney Disease
  VI. Conclusions

Objectives

- Describe the stages of chronic kidney disease.
- Understand the use and limitations of the methods that calculate the glomerular filtration rate.
- Understand the factors that contribute to the progression of chronic kidney disease.
- Describe the therapies that slow the progression of chronic kidney disease.
- Describe the clinical and laboratory abnormalities that are associated with chronic kidney disease.
- List the indications for initiating renal replacement therapy (either dialysis or transplantation).

Clinical Case

A 56-year-old man who has had diabetes mellitus for 27 years has had progressively declining kidney function. His most recent estimated glomerular filtration rate was 22 ml/min/1.73 m². His medications include lisinopril, an ACE inhibitor, and insulin. The physical examination shows a blood pressure of 150/95 mm Hg. His chest is clear to auscultation, but his extremities show 2+ pedal edema. Laboratory tests show a hemoglobin level of 8.5 g/dl, a serum bicarbonate level of 16 mmol/L, a potassium level of 5.9 mmol/L, a phosphorus level of 5.9 mg/dl, and an intact parathyroid hormone level of 558 pg/ml.

What stage of chronic kidney disease does this patient have? What metabolic abnormalities of the condition does he manifest? What could be done to correct these abnormalities?

I. DEFINITION AND INCIDENCE OF CHRONIC KIDNEY DISEASE

Chronic kidney disease (CKD) arises when one or both of the following conditions are present:

1. When there is evidence of kidney damage lasting for at least 3 months, as defined by structural or functional abnormalities of the kidney with or without a decreased glomerular filtration rate (GFR), as demonstrated either by pathologic abnormalities or by markers of kidney damage, including urine or blood abnormalities or abnormalities noted on imaging
2. When the GFR is less than 60 ml/min/1.73 m² for at least 3 months with or without kidney damage

Currently, in the United States, nearly 22% of the adult population has CKD, thereby making it a highly prevalent disease process.

CKD is categorized by the level of the GFR and the presence or absence of proteinuria (Fig. 12-1). Stage 1 includes patients with no decrease in GFR but with kidney abnormalities. Stage 2 includes patients with mild CKD with an estimated GFR (eGFR) of 60 to 89 ml/min/1.73 m² and kidney abnormalities. Stage 3 includes patients with an eGFR of 30 to 59 ml/min/1.73 m², and Stage 4 patients have an eGFR of 15 to 29 ml/min/1.73 m². Stage 5 is kidney failure; this includes patients with an eGFR of less than 15 ml/min/1.73 m². In the United States, more than 6 million people have stage 3, 4, or 5 CKD, with more than 400,000 individuals

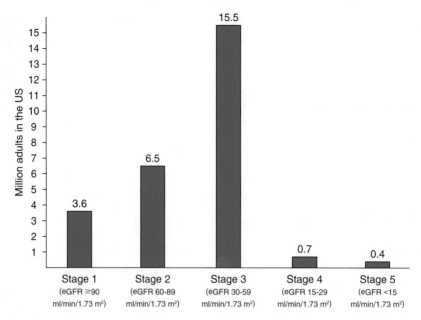

Figure 12-1. Prevalence of chronic kidney disease (CKD) in the adults in the United States. *eGFR*, Estimated glomerular filtration rate.

receiving dialysis or transplantation in 2004. The number of patients with kidney failure in the United States is projected to exceed 600,000 by 2010. After a patient begins dialysis, there is a 1- year mortality rate of approximately 20% and a nearly 75% mortality rate at 5 years. There are now effective methods for slowing the progression of CKD. Recognizing and appropriately treating CKD is imperative to prevent or postpone patients from requiring dialysis or transplantation and to help limit their mortality risk.

II. CALCULATING THE GLOMERULAR FILTRATION RATE

The calculation of GFR is critical for staging CKD. To assess the GFR, an endogenous serum marker is needed to measure clearance by the kidneys. To accurately represent clearance at the glomerulus, this endogenous substance needs to be freely filtered through the glomerular filtration membrane and to not be secreted or reabsorbed from the kidney tubules. The clearance of creatinine, which is naturally formed in the body from the breakdown of creatine (a component of muscle), is the most common substance used to calculate GFR. It is easily measured in serum and urine, it is freely filtered across the glomerulus, and it is not reabsorbed in the tubules. However, there is tubular secretion of creatinine. The most common assays for creatinine err to approximately the same degree, predominantly negating the effect of creatinine secretion by the kidney's tubule cells as long as the GFR is more than 40 ml/min. From urine and serum values, creatinine clearance can be directly calculated; from

serum values alone, GFR can be estimated. Other agents such as inulin, which is freely filtered and not secreted or reabsorbed, are more accurate and thus are used to study GFR. In addition, iothalamate is also used to assess GFR. Unfortunately, these agents require an intravenous infusion because they are not endogenous; thus, they are not as easily obtainable in the standard clinical setting.

All equations using creatinine depend on the inverse relationship between kidney function and serum creatinine: as kidney function declines in patients with CKD, the daily excretion of creatinine is reduced, and this leads to a higher serum level. Creatinine clearance, which is a close surrogate for GFR, can be calculated from a timed urine collection with the use of the following formula:

$$\text{Creatinine clearance (ml/min)} = \frac{U_{Cr}\ (\text{mg}/\text{dl}) \times \text{volume (ml)}}{P_{Cr}\ (\text{mg}/\text{dl}) \times \text{time (min)}}$$

The Cockcroft-Gault equation can also estimate creatinine clearance. Aging contributes to changes in GFR; on average, individuals lose 1 ml/min/year after the age of 30 years. Second, serum creatinine is dependent on muscle mass, so the ideal body weight is used to calculate the creatinine clearance or the GFR rather than the true body weight, particularly for obese patients. Third, there are sex differences in muscle mass, which are represented by the correction factor for females in the Cockcroft-Gault equation:

$$\text{Creatinine clearance (ml/min)} = \frac{(140 - \text{age in years})(\text{weight in kg})}{72 \times \text{Serum Cr (mg/dl)}} \times 0.85$$

One can also use the Modification of Diet in Renal Disease (MDRD) equation to estimate GFR:

$$\text{GFR (ml/min/1.73 m}^2) = 186 \times$$
$$(\text{Serum creatinine})^{-1.154} \times (\text{Age})^{-0.203} \times$$
$$(0.742 \text{ if female}) \times (1.210 \text{ if African American})$$

The MDRD equation takes into account age, sex, and race or ethnicity, with a correction for African American patients. The MDRD equation is more accurate for estimating GFR than the other methods when the GFR is less than 60 ml/min/1.73 m². Calculators are readily found at several sites online (e.g., www.kidney.org).

III. PATHOPHYSIOLOGY OF PROGRESSION

Historically, the idea that CKD would progress led to several critical and foundational hypotheses about the condition. In most diseases that lead to CKD, the end result appeared to be that nephrons maintained a well-defined pattern of function. This is characterized by adaptation. As the number of functioning nephrons declines, the work per remaining functioning nephrons will increase to accommodate the needs of the organism. Over time in patients with progressive CKD, the remaining nephrons will increase the fractional excretions of sodium, water, and phosphorus while increasing the tubular secretion of potassium and the hydrogen ion secretion per nephron. All of this is also influenced by the attempt to increase the GFR per single nephron.

These physiologic changes have potentially deleterious effects in the kidney itself that can enhance progression. The increased GFR per nephron can accelerate glomerular injury. The increase in tubular function can hasten tubular injury via various mechanisms that lead to tubular epithelial cell fibrosis. The increase in the fractional excretion of sodium may change an individual's ability to maintain volume status over time and in fact may augment sodium reabsorption at a different threshold, theoretically hastening progression. Changes in tubular secretion of cations (e.g., hydrogen, ammonium) can augment tubulointerstitial disease. Finally, altered calcium-phosphate

---

Box 12-1. History of Chronic Kidney Disease

As recent as the mid 20th century, chronic kidney failure and uremia were called *Bright disease* in tribute to English physician Richard Bright, who first described symptoms of kidney disease in 1836. Emily Dickinson, President Chester Arthur, and presidential wives Alice Lee Roosevelt (Theodore) and Ellen Wilson (Woodrow) died of Bright disease. Famed chemist Linus Pauling was treated for Bright disease by Dr. Addis.

---

metabolism and excretion can affect bone health in the setting of CKD.

Many of these changes by themselves can stimulate endogenous inflammatory and fibrogenic signaling pathways, thus setting into motion the gradual loss of functional kidney cells. In addition, it has been suggested that albuminuria can potentially induce tubular cell inflammation. Albuminuria occurs when the glomerular selectivity barrier is disrupted through injury, disease, or genetic abnormalities. This can be a consequence of direct podocyte injury or injury to the surrounding cells in the glomerulus. Albuminuria has been well validated as a marker of kidney disease and also of cardiovascular disease. Treatments that reduce albuminuria (e.g., angiotensin-converting enzyme [ACE] inhibitors) limit progression of CKD. However, the direct mechanism by which albuminuria effects changes in the kidney parenchyma has been somewhat difficult to establish. Cell-based studies suggest that albumin may be reabsorbed into tubular epithelial cells and that it may initiate inflammation by activating nuclear factor κB, thereby initiating a cascade of events that can eventually lead to fibrosis and even the possibility of tubular cell transformation into myofibroblast-like cells. This would further reduce the number of functional kidney cells and exacerbate the propagation of collagen and fibrosis in the surrounding interstitial milieu.

A. The Special Case of Glomerular Hypertension

Glomerular hypertension is a major factor that contributes to CKD progression. GFR is dependent on glomerular capillary pressure (P_{GC}). In a healthy kidney, a normal P_{GC} helps to maintain a normal GFR. In a diseased kidney, higher P_{GC} may be needed to maintain GFR, but it will simultaneously contribute to further damage. Experimental studies in which animals experienced a reduction in kidney mass (5/6 nephrectomy model) demonstrated that glomerular hypertension leads to the damage of the remaining nephrons. The remaining nephrons are "hyperfiltering," which results in glomerular hypertension.

Glomerular capillary pressure is dependent on systemic blood pressure as well as local factors that are responsible for vasoregulation at the level of the efferent and afferent arteries. Vasodilation of the afferent artery or constriction of the efferent artery increases P_{GC}, whereas constriction of the afferent artery or dilation of the efferent artery decreases P_{GC}. Angiotensin II, which is produced from the cleavage of angiotensin I by ACE, works as a potent vasoconstrictor by raising systemic blood pressure and constricting the efferent artery, thereby raising P_{GC}. Angiotensin II also increases sodium reabsorption in the proximal tubule and stimulates aldosterone production, thus further increasing sodium reabsorption and raising the systemic and glomerular blood pressures. Finally,

angiotensin II, through blood-pressure-independent effects, can directly lead to scarring and fibrosis in kidney tissue, in part through the activation of transforming growth factor-β (Fig. 12-2).

Glomerular hypertension contributes to glomerular injury through a number of potential mechanisms, including direct endothelial damage, effects on tubuloglomerular feedback, and shear stress on adjacent mesangial cells that produce cytokines and other inflammatory molecules. These include transforming growth factor-β and platelet-derived growth factor, which produce fibrosis and increased extracellular matrix formation.

Elevated P_{GC} is also an effect of increased protein delivery into the nephron. This can then increase glucagon, insulin-like growth factor I, and kinin release, all of which increase kidney blood flow, P_{GC}, and GFR. A high-protein diet also increases the amount of amino acids filtered, which increases sodium transport out of the proximal tubule via sodium-amino-acid cotransport, which decreases the amount of sodium that is detected by the macula densa. This activates tubuloglomerular feedback and results in increased GFR and glomerular hypertension.

Other factors that are associated with the exacerbation of CKD progression include tubulointerstitial fibrosis, hyperglycemia, hyperlipidemia, phosphate retention, increased aldosterone, altered prostanoid metabolism, metabolic acidosis, ammonium, anemia, retained uremic toxins, iron toxicity, corticosteroids, decreased nitric oxide, and increased fibrotic gene expression.

B. Slowing the Progression of Chronic Kidney Disease

The progression of CKD can be slowed by controlling these contributing factors. Both animal and human studies over the last several decades have demonstrated that controlling hypertension slows progression, regardless of the cause. The goal blood pressure for patients with CKD is less than 130/80 mm Hg;

achieving this often requires the use of two to three medications.

The blockade of angiotensin II substantially slows progression as well. Medications known as ACE inhibitors or angiotensin receptor blockers (ARBs) lower systemic blood pressure as well as P_{GC}. ACE inhibitors and ARBs also reduce urinary protein excretion. Their ability to slow the progression of both diabetic- and nondiabetic-related kidney disease can be attributed in part to effects that are independent of blood pressure. Not only have ACE inhibitors and ARBs become the cornerstone of therapy for CKD, they are now being used in combination for synergistic effects on the reduction of proteinuria as well.

Dietary protein restriction has also been demonstrated to slow the progression of CKD, particularly in patients with diabetes. In these patients, the rate of CKD progression was delayed by more than 75% in patients who were placed on protein restriction as compared with patients without protein restriction. Multiple smaller studies in nondiabetics showed similar results; however, a large, randomized trial in nondiabetic kidney disease demonstrated no significant benefit from dietary protein restriction (the MDRD study). For individuals with diabetes, protein restriction to 0.6 gm/kg of the ideal body weight if the urinary protein excretion is less than 3 g per day or to 0.8 gm/kg of the ideal body weight if urinary protein excretion is more than 3 g per day is nutritionally safe.

The control of the blood glucose level in individuals with diabetes can slow the development of microalbuminuria as well as the progression from microalbuminuria to overt proteinuria. Strict glucose control with glycosylated hemoglobin levels of less than 7% is also recommended for diabetic patients with CKD.

IV. SIGNS AND SYMPTOMS OF KIDNEY FAILURE

Uremia is a term that describes the clinical manifestations of kidney failure. These result from the retention of toxins that are normally excreted by the kidney and/or the lack of hormones that are normally produced by the kidney. Symptoms usually do not manifest themselves until the GFR is less than 10 to 15 ml/min/1.73 m², although some clinical problems (e.g., anemia, secondary hyperparathyroidism) can be present as early as stage 3 CKD.

The identity of the toxins that cause uremia remains elusive. Urea has been ruled out as the cause of most of the symptoms. For many years, the middle molecule hypothesis suggested that compounds with a molecular weight of 1 to 10 kDa were possible uremic factors. This hypothesis was based on the observation that patients who were receiving peritoneal dialysis, which is a modality that efficiently removes molecules weighing 1 to 10 kDa, had fewer uremic symptoms for the degree of azotemia than similar

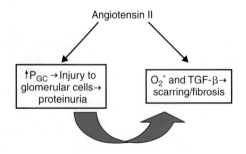

Angiotensin II

$\uparrow P_{GC} \rightarrow$ Injury to glomerular cells $\rightarrow$ proteinuria

$O_2^\cdot$ and TGF-β $\rightarrow$ scarring/fibrosis

Figure 12-2. Angiotensin II causes progressive kidney damage by causing glomerular hypertension and increasing proteinuria as well as by inducing fibrogenic cytokines, such as transforming growth factor-β (TGF-β) and reactive oxygen species ($O_2^\cdot$). P_{GC}, glomerular capillary pressure.

patients on hemodialysis. However, other studies showed that, when the molecules extracted by peritoneal dialysis weighing 1 to 10 kDa were injected into healthy rats, the animals exhibited uremic symptoms similar to those seen in humans. These molecules decrease chemotaxis and lymphocyte proliferation, lower oxidative metabolism, and impair intracellular bacterial killing. The various systems affected by CKD are shown in Box 12-2.

A. Altered Excretory Function in Chronic Kidney Disease

One of the kidney's primary functions is to regulate electrolytes within the extracellular fluid. As kidney function declines, the ability of the kidney to maintain a normal electrolyte environment within the body also fails. The kidney may fail to excrete sodium, free water, potassium, acid, and phosphorus.

Sodium is one of the primary electrolytes handled by the kidney. The ability of the kidney to respond to variations in dietary sodium and to alter its reabsorption and excretion of sodium is impaired in chronic kidney disease (Fig. 12-3). This lack of flexibility as a result of a reduced nephron mass leads to hypertension and, at times, to edema with excess sodium intake as well as to hypotension and intravascular volume depletion with low sodium intake.

Similarly, the inability to alter the amount of water reabsorbed or excreted as a result of kidney failure potentially leads to hyponatremia when excess water is ingested and to hypernatremia when a patient's free water intake is insufficient.

As CKD progresses, hyperkalemia may develop. This usually does not occur from CKD alone until the GFR decreases to less than 10 ml/min/1.73 m^2 because there is significant single-nephron adaptation to increase potassium excretion as the functional nephron number declines.

Hyperkalemia is usually attributable to multiple causes, including increased intake (oral or intravenous potassium supplements, foods high in potassium) and decreased excretion as a result of drugs such as potassium-sparing diuretics, ACE inhibitors, or ARBs (Box 12-3). In addition, a shift of potassium from

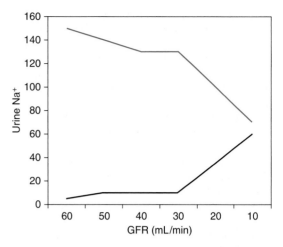

Figure 12-3. As kidney function declines, the kidneys are less able to maintain sodium (Na$^+$) homeostasis. At low levels of glomerular filtration rate (GFR), the kidneys are not able to excrete the excess of sodium ingested, and patients are more prone to developing volume excess *(green line)*. The kidneys are also not able to retain sodium when there is decreased sodium intake, thereby making the patient more susceptible to volume depletion *(black line)*.

Box 12-3. Drugs and Conditions That Increase Serum Potassium in Chronic Kidney Disease

- Potassium supplements
- Potassium-sparing diuretics
- Angiotensin-converting enzyme inhibitors
- Angiotensin receptor blockers
- Uncontrolled diabetes (lack of insulin)
- Acidosis
- Adrenergic blockade (β-blockers)

Box 12-2. Organ Systems Affected by Chronic Kidney Disease

- Electrolytes/volume status
- Cardiovascular
- Endocrine
- Immunologic
- Gastrointestinal
- Hematologic
- Neurologic
- Skin

intracellular to extracellular domains may occur as a result of acidosis as well as from clinical situations, such as β-blocker use or the presence of uncontrolled diabetes, which alter functional Na$^+$/K$^+$-ATPase activity and reduces the entry of potassium into the cells from the extracellular fluid.

Hydrogen ion handling is also impaired in CKD, and it worsens in the presence of kidney failure. The acidosis of CKD may be associated with either a high anion gap or the absence of an elevated anion gap. As kidney function declines, the ability of the proximal tubule cells to form ammonia from glutamine for the excretion of hydrogen also declines. Ammonia acts as a "sink" for hydrogen ions that are excreted in the distal tubule (Fig. 12-4).

Decreased levels of ammonia in the distal tubule lead to the decreased formation of ammonium ions and reduced hydrogen ion binding in the cortical collecting duct. This allows free hydrogen ions to diffuse back into the plasma, causing a nonanion gap acidosis.

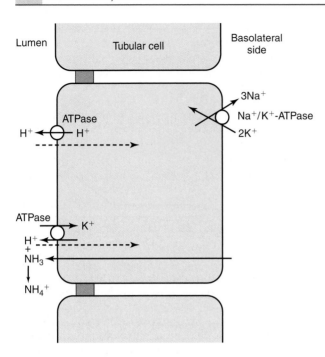

Figure 12-4. Renal tubular acidosis in chronic kidney disease. The loss of proximal tubule function results in decreased ammonia production available to the cortical collecting duct to combine with hydrogen ion in the tubular lumen to form ammonium ion. Thus, unbound hydrogen ion in the tubular lumen is reabsorbed back into the blood. H^+, Hydrogen; K^+, potassium; Na^+, sodium; NH_3, ammonia; NH_4, ammonium.

As kidney failure evolves, the retention of negatively charged uremic toxins leads to an anion gap acidosis. Acidosis has many consequences on the musculoskeletal system. It stimulates the catabolism of branched-chain amino acids, it contributes to insulin resistance, and it leads to osteopenia as a result of calcium carbonate in bone acting as a buffer for the acidosis.

As kidney function declines, there is also decreased phosphorus excretion with resultant increases in serum phosphorus, along with decreases in 1,25-dihydroxycholecalciferol (vitamin D_3; Fig. 12-5). 25-Hydroxycholecalciferol undergoes 1-α-hydroxylation in the kidney, which leads to active vitamin D_3 (1,25-dihydroxycholecalciferol or dihydroxyvitamin D_3). In patients with CKD, there is decreased intestinal calcium absorption, which lowers the serum calcium level. The serum calcium level may decline as the result of a lack of the production of dihydroxyvitamin D_3 and ongoing combination with phosphorus with the deposition of calcium phosphate in tissues, which is called *metastatic calcification*. This calcification may significantly contribute to vascular calcification in the heart and the periphery in patients with CKD. The relative hypocalcemia associated with CKD stimulates parathyroid hormone (PTH) secretion, which results in metabolic bone disease and secondary hyperparathyroidism (Fig. 12-6).

B. Bone Disease Associated with Chronic Kidney Disease

CKD is often accompanied by a loss of bone mass. There are several types of bone disease that are associated with CKD, including osteitis fibrosa (an adynamic and low-turnover bone disease) and acidosis-induced osteopenia. Each has a different cause, but all result in similar clinical manifestations.

Osteitis fibrosa cystica is the pathologic manifestation of renal osteodystrophy and secondary hyperparathyroidism (see Fig. 12-6). Histologically, in osteitis fibrosa, there is increased osteoblast and osteoclast activity, with large amounts of unmineralized and abnormally formed bone matrix. This results from a high rate of bone turnover associated with elevated PTH that is known as *secondary hyperparathyroidism*. The excess PTH secretion stimulates increased bone reabsorption.

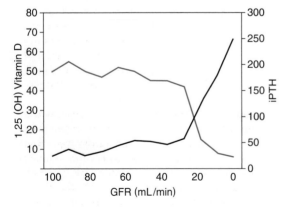

Figure 12-5. In patients with chronic kidney disease, as the glomerular filtration rate (GFR) declines, the serum level of intact parathyroid hormone (iPTH) increases, and the serum level of 1,25-dihydroxyvitamin D3 declines.

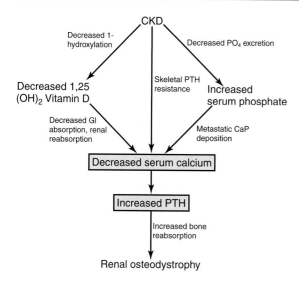

Figure 12-6. Pathophysiology of renal osteodystrophy. *CaP,* Calcium phosphate; *CKD,* chronic kidney disease; *GI,* gastrointestinal; *PO₄,* phosphate; *PTH,* parathyroid hormone.

Hyperphosphatemia is an independent stimulator of PTH secretion and as well as of osteoclasts.

The term *adynamic bone disease* refers to a decreased rate of matrix production and bone mineralization that is related to decreased PTH secretion (relative to osteitis fibrosa) and decreased bone formation. The very low levels of PTH seen in this disorder can be caused by overtreatment with 1,25-dihydroxycholecalciferol or simply in association with certain other disease states (e.g., diabetes mellitus). Histologically, there are increased osteoid seams with decreased osteoblast and osteoclast activity. Adynamic bone disease can be distinguished from high-turnover bone disease either by bone biopsy or by PTH level. The treatment of metabolic bone disease involves a balance of suppressing renal osteodystrophy without causing low-turnover bone disease. When diagnosing bone disease in patients with CKD, it is important to obtain a serum level of intact PTH.

Acidosis also contributes to bone disease in patients with CKD. Calcium carbonate from bone is leached out to act as a buffer for excess hydrogen ions, thereby reducing bone calcium content. Acidosis also stimulates osteoclast activity and decreases osteoblast activity, thereby further reducing bone mass.

There are other gradations of bone disease in CKD that represent an admixture of the two forms of disease that have already been discussed. These include mixed renal osteodystrophy and even osteomalacia with failure to calcify the cartilaginous bone matrix. Regardless of the form, the symptoms of metabolic bone disease are similar. Individuals may have bone pain and an increased risk of fractures. Spontaneous tendon ruptures, pruritus from calcium deposits in the skin, ocular calcification, and calcification of the joints also frequently accompany renal osteodystrophy. Vascular calcification theoretically contributes to mortality risk through impaired myocardial function, coronary artery disease, peripheral vascular disease, and comorbid complications.

All forms of renal bone disease cause osteopenia and osteomalacia to some extent. Classic findings in renal osteodystrophy are the reabsorption of distal phalangeal cortical bone and terminal tufts on hand radiographs. Frequently, pseudofractures (also called *Looser zones*) are observed. These are characterized by increased bands of radiolucency perpendicular to the long axis of the bone. Stress fractures and bone deformations are also commonly identified.

The treatment of renal osteodystrophy includes the suppression of PTH through dietary phosphorus restriction and therapy with 1,25-dihydroxycholecalciferol. Phosphate binders are given at mealtimes to bind phosphorus and prevent absorption. Vitamin D and calcimimetic agents (compounds that block the G-protein–coupled calcium-sensing receptor) can be administered because both suppress parathyroid gland activity. On occasion, parathyroid adenomas become autonomous and do not respond to these measures; patients should then undergo parathyroidectomy. To prevent acidosis-induced osteopenia, sodium bicarbonate is given to patients with CKD to maintain serum bicarbonate levels of more than 20 mmol/L. This is particularly important in children with CKD because the acidosis can prevent growth.

C. Hematologic Consequences

CKD has detrimental affects on all hematologic cell lines, resulting in anemia, increased bleeding risk, and increased rates of infection. The kidney, as the primary site of erythropoietin production, regulates red blood cell (RBC) production. As CKD progresses, erythropoietin production in the kidney declines. Anemia can be seen in patients as early as stage 3 CKD, and it is normocytic and normochromic, with a low reticulocyte count for the degree of anemia. It is primarily the result of decreased RBC production and decreased RBC lifespan, especially as CKD progresses. The half-life of RBCs improves in dialyzed patients, which confirms that the uremic environment accounts for the short RBC half-life.

Erythropoietin was first introduced into clinical trials during the mid 1980s, and since the early 1990s, it has become a cornerstone of anemia management in CKD at all stages when anemia occurs. Recombinant human erythropoietin or other erythropoietic stimulating agents (e.g., darbepoetin alfa) are effective for maintaining steady hemoglobin levels, and they involve less risk of viral infections than repeated transfusions. Therapy with recombinant human erythropoietin is usually instituted in stage 4 and 5 CKD patients to maintain hemoglobin levels between 10 and

12 g/dl. Concurrent iron therapy (either oral or intravenous) is needed to provide an ongoing iron source for RBC production.

Platelet–vessel and platelet–platelet interactions are also impaired in CKD, which leads to impaired hemostasis. Various molecules in the uremic state interfere with von Willebrand-factor–binding proteins that are necessary for platelet adhesion to the vascular walls. This functional platelet disorder is usually seen very late in CKD. It can cause increased bleeding complications such as gastrointestinal bleeding, subdural hematomas, and even hemorrhagic pericarditis and cardiac tamponade. Desmopressin (synthetic antidiuretic hormone, also called *DDAVP*) corrects the defect in von Willebrand-factor–binding proteins, and it is the primary modality used for the treatment of emergent bleeding complications.

Impaired immunologic function results in infection in individuals with kidney failure. Infection is the second most common cause of death among individuals on dialysis, after cardiovascular complications. Uremia has detrimental effects on granulocyte and monocyte function, which increases patient susceptibility to infections. Decreased chemotaxis, phagocytosis, and the generation of reactive oxygen species by granulocytes as well as abnormal T-cell cytokine responses cause patients with kidney failure to be very susceptible to both bacterial and viral infections. The abnormality in immune response is best demonstrated by the need for four rather than three hepatitis B immunizations to attain immunity rates of more than 90% in this population; these patients are also predisposed to *Staphylococcus aureus* colonization of the skin.

D. Cardiovascular Consequences

Cardiovascular complications are the leading cause of death for patients with CKD, accounting for 40% to 45% of all deaths of dialysis and transplant patients. A patient on hemodialysis has a 10% chance per year of having a myocardial infarction or a 10- to 100-fold increased risk of having a myocardial infarction as compared with a matched patient without CKD. By the time patients present for dialysis, 35% will have CHF, and only 15% will have a normal echocardiogram.

Uremia itself may have unique effects on the heart, although it is difficult to separate out the effects of other concurrent risks, like hypertension and diabetes. Uremic cardiomyopathy, which results in CHF with both systolic and diastolic dysfunction, has an echo-cardiographically defined course, with left ventricular thickening over time followed by left ventricular dilatation. Other causes or contributors to cardiomyopathy include anemia, increased effective circulating volume, fluid overload, and hypertension.

Seventy-five percent of patients who start dialysis have left ventricular hypertrophy. Hypertrophy becomes maladaptive as the muscle mass increases

and demands energy beyond what the blood vessels can supply. The energy deficiency results in apoptosis and myocardial fibrosis, with rearrangement of the muscle fibers. This further reduces cardiac systolic contraction and inhibits diastolic relaxation. The fibrosis also causes conduction abnormalities and slower calcium reuptake, thereby resulting in increased ventricular stiffness and diastolic dysfunction. As the systolic failure progresses, there is decreased perfusion of the kidneys, fluid retention, and increased circulating volume. The heart undergoes concentric hypertrophy, which leads to a left ventricle with increased left ventricle pressures and decreased cardiac output, thereby resulting in increased myocardial energy demand. Thus, CKD is associated with an increased risk of left ventricular hypertrophy, myocardial infarction, arrhythmias, congestive heart failure, and overall increased mortality (Fig. 12-7).

Atherosclerotic ischemic heart disease is the most common cardiac complication among patients with CKD and, ultimately, kidney failure. The degree of atherosclerosis is an independent predictor of mortality, and, as such, it needs to be aggressively treated. Patients with CKD in general are at very high risk for atherosclerotic vascular disease as a result of increased inflammation, dyslipidemia, and hyperphosphatemia.

Approximately 30% to 50% of patients with kidney failure have inflammation, which is demonstrated by increased C-reactive protein (CRP), increased interleukin-6, and decreased albumin levels. CRP contributes to atherosclerosis by binding to injured cells, promoting complement activation and low-density lipoprotein aggregation, and monocyte activation. The cause of inflammation in this patient population is probably multifactorial and includes unrecognized infections; ongoing systemic illnesses (or, in the case of dialysis patients, the back filtration of endotoxins or other inflammatory mediators from dialysate water during dialysis); and the bioincompatibility of the

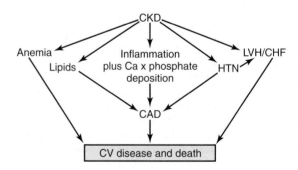

Figure 12-7. Mechanisms for increased risk of cardiovascular (CV) disease in patients with chronic kidney disease (CKD). *CAD*, Coronary artery disease; *CHF*, congestive heart failure; *HTN*, hypertension; *LVH*, left ventricular hypertrophy.

hemodialysis membranes. Inflammation, as measured by CRP levels, is associated with an increased risk of a cardiovascular event and increased mortality while on dialysis.

Dyslipidemia occurs more frequently with decreasing GFR. Although decreases in high-density lipoprotein and increases in cholesterol, low-density lipoprotein, and triglycerides are commonly seen, the classic pattern in kidney failure is a type IV hyperlipidemia, predominantly with hypertriglyceridemia. Fifty percent of patients on hemodialysis and 70% of patients on peritoneal dialysis develop dyslipidemia.

Hyperphosphatemia is also strongly associated with cardiovascular disease in patients with CKD and kidney failure, primarily with the deposition of calcium phosphate in atherosclerotic plaque, increased plaque size, decreased luminal area, and increased plaque instability. The increased inflammation, dyslipidemia, and hyperphosphatemia all result in patients with CKD being highly susceptible to atherosclerosis and cardiovascular events.

Hypertension is present in 70% to 80% of patients with CKD. Hypertension is dependent on both volume overload and vasopressors, but as kidney function declines, volume overload becomes an increasingly important factor. Pressor-dependent hypertension early in CKD is caused by increased peripheral resistance that often results in increased left ventricular afterload and the exacerbation of heart failure. Unfortunately, more than half of all patients with CKD have an average blood pressure of more than 140/90 mm Hg.

Proteinuria has recently been defined as an independent risk factor for cardiovascular disease in patients with and without CKD. Studies have shown that the degree of proteinuria correlates with the progression of CKD and heart disease, as well as mortality. Because patients with CKD often have proteinuria as well as multiple other risk factors that contribute to an increased risk of cardiovascular disease, the reduction of proteinuria by angiotensin blockade is especially important.

The adequate treatment of the cardiovascular manifestations of CKD often relies on aggressive pharmacotherapy and interventions in addition to lifestyle changes. The goal for the treatment of hypertension in CKD is a blood pressure level of less than 130/80 mm Hg. Blood pressure treatment usually incorporates vasodilators, diuretics, and ACE inhibitors. For heart failure, patients may receive loop diuretics, ACE inhibitors, β-blockers, and calcium-channel blockers. As patients progress to kidney failure, volume overload may become an indication for the initiation of dialysis. For ischemic heart disease, ACE inhibitors, β-blockers, and aspirin are currently the drugs of choice. Statins and diet control are often used to control dyslipidemia, recognizing that statins by themselves may have

disparate effects among dialysis patients; they lower cholesterol effectively but in limited clinical studies, have had little impact on mortality. Proteinuria is often treated with ACE inhibitors and ARBs. Anemia is treated with erythropoietic stimulating agents and hyperphosphatemia with dietary phosphate restriction and phosphate binders. Kidney failure patients can do exceedingly well with coronary revascularization, but data regarding their outcomes are limited because CKD has often been a contraindication for cardiovascular study enrollment.

E. Neurologic Consequences

Without treatment, patients with kidney failure may develop uremic encephalopathy with confusion, tremors, and even delirium and coma. The severity as well as the rapidity of kidney failure correlates with the degree of uremic encephalopathy. The pathophysiology of uremic encephalopathy is unknown, but, along with the uremic state, secondary hyperparathyroidism and elevated levels of ammonia may contribute to neurologic changes. Deposits of calcium have also been found in the gray matter of patients with uremic encephalopathy, thereby further supporting secondary hyperparathyroidism as a contributor to uremic encephalopathy. Electroencephalogram changes of uremic encephalopathy may also resolve with parathyroidectomy. The encephalopathy can also resolve with daily dialysis. The neurologic symptoms that develop are always nonfocal. If there are focal defects, another process (e.g., stroke) should be considered.

Another neurologic complication that often develops in late CKD is peripheral neuropathy. Complications include restless leg syndrome, which is found in 15% to 40% of patients on dialysis, and sensory neuropathy (burning foot syndrome). Sensory neuropathy from uremia is difficult to distinguish from diabetic neuropathy. The motor neuropathies are generally late in onset, and they are less common than sensory neuropathies.

F. Other Organ Systems Affected by Uremia

Other organ systems that are affected include the respiratory system, the gastrointestinal system, the skin, and sexual function. Patients with kidney failure have a greater tendency to manifest sleep apnea in the context of various sleep disturbances. In addition, they may experience nausea and vomiting as well as anorexia.

Patients with CKD often have significant pruritus. This is usually the result of calcium-phosphate deposition. Porphyria cutanea tarda results in bullous lesions in sun-exposed areas, commonly in patients with CKD. Recently, a new syndrome called *nephrogenic systemic fibrosis*, which involves the thickening of the skin over the hands and limbs, has been described, and it may be related to exposure to the

gadolinium contrast agents used in radiologic procedures.

Sexual dysfunction and infertility are often seen in patients with CKD. Studies have shown that sexual dysfunction as a result of physical impairment is more common among women and that it increases with decreasing GFR. Infertility as a result of the disruption of the hypothalamic-pituitary axis as well as the impaired cyclic release of gonadotropin-releasing hormone and luteinizing hormone leads to the reduced release of testosterone and sperm production in males as well as impaired ovulation in females. Although there have been exceptions, it is rare for women with kidney failure to carry pregnancies to term. Even women with mild to moderate CKD have an increased risk for miscarriage, small-for-gestational-age infants, and preeclampsia. Impotence is also common among men with kidney failure.

V. TREATMENT FOR PROBLEMS ASSOCIATED WITH PROGRESSIVE CHRONIC KIDNEY DISEASE

Box 12-4 summarizes CKD-associated problems and their accompanying treatments.

Kidney or *renal replacement therapy* is appropriately named because it is used when the kidneys can no longer perform the functions that are vital to life. Indications for chronic dialysis are given in Box 12-5.

VI. CONCLUSIONS

Currently there are effective methods for slowing the progression of CKD, including strict blood pressure control, the blockade of angiotensin, protein restriction, and glucose control. Nevertheless, many patients will still have progressive CKD. For these patients, it is important that physicians recognize,

---

Box 12-4. Treatment of Chronic Kidney Disease: Maintenance of Metabolic Balance

- *Acidosis:* Oral sodium bicarbonate
- *Secondary hyperparathyroidism:* Oral 1,25-dihydroxyvitamin D, phosphate binders, low phosphorus diet
- *Anemia:* Erythropoietic stimulating agents and oral or intravenous iron
- *Fluid overload:* Diuretics, sodium restriction
- *Hypertension:* Antihypertensives, sodium restriction
- *Hyperkalemia:* Removal of medications causing hyperkalemia, potassium restriction
- *Infectious risk:* Vaccinations against hepatitis B, *Streptococcus pneumoniae*, influenza
- *Hyperlipidemia:* Lipid lowering medications
- *Bleeding risk:* Desmopressin for surgical procedures

Box 12-5. Indications for Starting Chronic Dialysis

- Symptomatic uremia: anorexia, nausea, vomiting, encephalopathy, pericarditis, severe fatigue
- Fluid overload not responsive to diuretics
- Hyperkalemia not controlled with diet or loop diuretics
- Glomerular filtration rate of less than 10 ml/min/1.73 m^2 or of less than 15 ml/min/1.73 m^2 in patients with diabetes

---

understand, and properly treat the associated problems to reduce the morbidity and mortality of CKD.

Clinical Cases

A 56-year-old man who has had diabetes mellitus for 27 years has had progressively declining kidney function. His most recent eGFR was 22 ml/min/1.73 m^2. His medications include lisinopril, an ACE inhibitor, and insulin. The physical examination shows a blood pressure of 150/95 mm Hg. His chest is clear to auscultation, but his extremities show 2+ pedal edema. Laboratory tests show a hemoglobin level of 8.5 g/dl, a serum bicarbonate level of 16 mmol/L, a potassium level of 5.9 mmol/L, a phosphorus level of 5.9 mg/dl, and an intact PTH level of 558 pg/ml.

What stage of CKD does this patient have?

This patient has stage 4 CKD, with a GFR of 15 to 29 ml/min/1.73 m^2.

What metabolic abnormalities of the condition does he manifest?

This patient exhibits several metabolic disturbances of CKD. He has azotemia with the retention of nitrogenous waste products as shown by an elevated blood urea nitrogen level. He has the impaired ability to excrete ingested sodium, which has led to hypertension and pedal edema. He has excessive body stores of potassium as noted by hyperkalemia. He has metabolic acidosis with the depressed serum bicarbonate level. Anemia is likely to be a consequence of the deficiency of erythropoietin production by the kidney. The decreased renal excretion of ingested phosphorous has led to an increase in the serum phosphorous level, and the depressed serum calcium level has caused secondary hyperparathyroidism as noted by a significant increase in serum level of parathyroid hormone.

What could be done to correct these abnormalities?

This patient would benefit from the dietary restriction of protein, sodium, and potassium. Diuretics and antihypertensive agents to normalize his blood pressure will be necessary. ACE inhibitors and/or ARBs are the preferred agents for patients with CKD as a result of diabetic nephropathy and proteinuria. Oral phosphate binders taken with food to prevent the absorption of

dietary phosphorous, erythropoietin to stimulate RBC, and 1,25-dihydroxyvitamin D to suppress the elevated intact PTH level are the other therapeutic agents that will be necessary.

Suggested Readings

Vassalotti JA, Stevens LA, Levey AS: Testing for chronic kidney disease: A position statement from the National Kidney Foundation. *Am J Kidney Dis* 50:169–180, 2007.

Gillespie BS, Inrig JK, Szczech L: Anemia management in chronic kidney disease. *Hemodialysis Int* 11:15–20, 2007.

Toto RD: Treatment of hypertension in chronic kidney disease. *Semin Nephrol* 25:435–439, 2006.

PRACTICE QUESTIONS

1. A 63-year-old African-American woman with type 2 diabetes mellitus and hypertension for 17 years is seen in the clinic for worsening pedal edema. Her history reveals that she underwent laser surgery for diabetic retinopathy. Her medications include metoprolol (50 mg twice daily), hydrochlorothiazide (25 mg daily), and insulin. On physical examination her blood pressure is 148/88 mm Hg, and her pulse rate is 85 beats per minute. She has 2+ pedal edema. Laboratory tests show a serum creatinine level of 0.7 mg/dl and a blood urea nitrogen level of 32 mg/dl. The glycosylated hemoglobin level is 7.5%. Urine testing shows 4+ protein by dipstick. Which of the following statements is true?

   A. This patient does not have CKD.
   B. This patient has stage 1 CKD.
   C. This patient has stage 2 CKD.
   D. This patient has stage 3 CKD.

2. Which of the following factors is not likely to increase the progression of CKD for the patient in the previous question?

   A. Female gender
   B. 4+ proteinuria
   C. Blood pressure of 144/88 mm Hg
   D. Glycosylated hemoglobin level of 7.5%

3. In a patient with CKD, certain pathophysiologic mechanisms have a role in kidney injury and in the progressive decline in kidney function. Which of the following factors may be less likely to be a cause?

   A. Increased tubular fibrosis mediated by ammonia synthesis
   B. Tubular transcription factors (e.g., nuclear factor κB) increased by proteinuria
   C. Decreased glomerular hydrostatic pressure
   D. Angiotensin II–mediated production of fibrosing cytokines

Replacement Therapy for Kidney Failure: Dialysis

13

Joshua David Lindsey
Paul S. Kellerman

OUTLINE

I. History of Dialysis
II. Principles of Dialysis
  A. Diffusion
  B. Ultrafiltration
  C. Convection
III. Types of Dialysis
  A. Hemodialysis
  B. Peritoneal Dialysis

IV. Complications of Dialysis
  A. Hemodialysis
  B. Peritoneal Dialysis
V. Mortality on Dialysis
VI. Conclusions

Objectives

- Understand the concepts of diffusion, convection, and ultrafiltration and their application to hemodialysis and peritoneal dialysis.
- Describe the major complications of dialysis.
- Understand the reasons for starting chronic dialysis.
- Understand the reasons for dialysis mortality.

Clinical Case

A 56-year-old man with stage 5 chronic kidney disease had a peritoneal catheter placed to initiate dialysis. After 6 weeks of peritoneal dialysis, his blood pressure is 170/100 mm Hg, and he has 2+ edema; however, his nausea has resolved, and his appetite is better. He currently does four exchanges of 2 L every 6 hours. He is using two peritoneal dialysis fluid bags of 1.5% glucose and two of 2.5% glucose daily. His serum albumin level is 3.4 g/dl.

What can you do to improve this patient's edema? Why is his serum albumin level low? Are there other treatment options for the patient if he does not improve?

I. HISTORY OF DIALYSIS

The first attempts to replace kidney function through mechanical means occurred during the early part of the twentieth century. Abel, Rowntree, and Turner developed insights into this process through research focusing on diffusion devices. Haas and others expanded on that work by attempting to apply it to humans. However, it was in the midst of World War II that Dr. Willem Kolff performed the first true hemodialysis procedure in 1944.

Kolff's artificial kidney consisted of a large rotating drum wrapped with cellophane tubing (sausage casing). Blood was drawn from the patient into a large pail, anticoagulated, and then elevated above the drum, with gravity drawing the blood through the tubing. While the blood was drawn through the tubing, the drum would rotate, and the blood would temporarily pass through dialysate solution (Fig. 13-1). The blood would then drain to another bucket below the drum and be infused back into the patient. By the conclusion of the following decade, during the Korean conflict, the US Army Surgical Research Team would make great strides in the understanding of the physiology of dialysis, and a gradual evolution of dialysis technology would occur. With the creation of Teflon-containing tubes by Scribner and colleagues in Seattle, which could link arteries and veins for vascular access, hemodialysis moved from an acute treatment to one that could be repeated and considered for use for a much longer duration.

The principle at work in the original dialysis machine, which involved solute transferring down a concentration gradient from an area of high concentration (blood) to an area of low concentration (dialysate) across a semipermeable membrane, is still in use today. The difference is that modern dialysis machines use higher rates of blood removal with rapid blood flow from the patient as well as dialysate flow. In addition, hollow-fiber artificial kidneys dramatically improve dialysis efficiency and safety (Box 13-1).

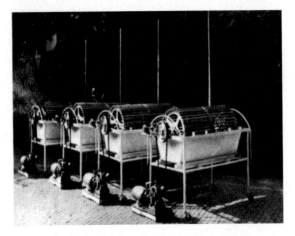

Figure 13-1. A rotating drum dialyzer. *(From Kolff WJ, Berk HT, ter Welle M, et al: The artificial kidney: A dialyser with a great area.* J Am Soc Nephrol 8[12]:1959–1965, 1997.)

II. PRINCIPLES OF DIALYSIS

Dialysis is based on the dynamic laws of solute transport. *Solute* is simply the particles that are dissolved in the solvent. The solute in dialysis is the collected

waste products of body metabolism that are normally excreted on a daily basis by the kidneys. In patients with kidney failure, the function of the kidneys is severely impaired, and waste accumulates in the blood, thereby leading to uremic symptoms.

A. Diffusion

Diffusion is the process by which a concentration gradient provides the energy for solute transfer. Solute particles flow down their concentration gradient until they reach equilibrium across a semipermeable membrane. Equilibrium can be prevented by the continuous removal of solute from one side of the membrane (Fig. 13-2A).

A *semipermeable membrane* is a physical membrane of some type that allows for the passage of some—but not all—particles across it. Particles may not be able to move across the membrane as a result of size, electrical charge, or other physical characteristics. In the case of dialysis, metabolic waste products are the particles, and the semipermeable membrane can be either an artificial filter (as in hemodialysis) or the peritoneum (as in peritoneal dialysis). On one side of the membrane is the blood from the patient, and on the other side of the membrane is the dialysate.

DIFFUSION

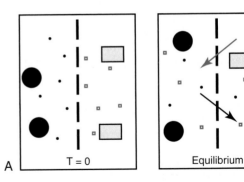

A   T = 0   Equilibrium

DIALYSIS – Solute Diffusion
Constant gradient is maintained, never reaches equilibrium due to dialysate flow

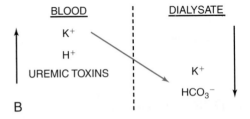

B

Figure 13-2. *A,* The principle of diffusion. Solute moves down a concentration gradient from an area of high concentration to an area of lesser concentration across a semipermeable membrane. Over time, if there is no removal of solute, a state of equilibrium is reached. The continuous removal of solute can prevent a state of equilibrium. *B,* How dialysate works to support the principle of diffusion in actuality.

Diffusion is the principal method of solute removal by hemodialysis and peritoneal dialysis.

The *dialysate* is an artificial solution that is created to favor the withdrawal of various solutes from the blood. For example, patients with kidney failure may become hyperkalemic. The dialysate for these patients has a low concentration of potassium to favor potassium removal from the bloodstream.

The continuous flow of dialysate prevents equilibrium from occurring and provides for the continuous removal of waste products (Fig. 13-2*B*).

B. Ultrafiltration

Ultrafiltration is the process by which an external pressure gradient moves fluid across a semipermeable membrane from one compartment to another (Fig. 13-3*A*).

The process is different from diffusion in that there is a *pressure* gradient that moves fluid as opposed to a *concentration* gradient to move solute, as is seen in diffusion. In hemodialysis, a transmembrane pressure gradient is created artificially, and fluid is forced from the blood to the dialysate (Fig. 13-3*B*).

In hemodialysis, the fluid pressure is maintained by the dialysis machine. Ultrafiltration is used to remove excess extracellular fluid from patients with expanded extracellular fluid volume. Patients with kidney failure may make little to no urine. Therefore, all sodium and water that are taken in by the mouth and not excreted by means of feces, sweat, and insensible losses remain as extracellular body fluid. This fluid needs to be removed, and this is accomplished by ultrafiltration. The goal with the ultrafiltration portion of dialysis is to remove adequate amounts of fluid during each session to allow for an appropriate amount of extracellular volume (including plasma volume) so that the patient has a stable blood pressure without evidence of edema.

C. Convection

Convection is solute transport that occurs as a byproduct of ultrafiltration. The water that is moved by the transmembrane pressure of ultrafiltration drags solute particles in mass transfer across the membrane (Fig. 13-4).

Convection is important in the setting of acute kidney injury, where patients may be treated with intermittent hemodialysis or slower continuous dialysis, which is also called *continuous renal replacement therapy* (CRRT). There are several modes of CRRT, but they all basically use slow continuous dialysis with a very "leaky" membrane, which results in large fluid losses with convective losses of solute. CRRT can clear solutes through convection alone or in combination with diffusion using a dialysate as well.

In summary, diffusion, ultrafiltration, and convection are the forces that lead to solute and fluid transfer across a membrane during any dialysis procedure. Managing these principles is the means by which

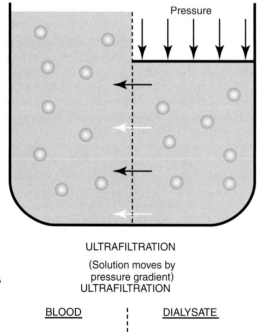

ULTRAFILTRATION
(Solution moves by pressure gradient)
ULTRAFILTRATION

A

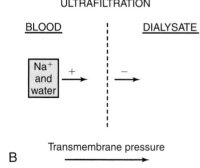

B

Transmembrane pressure

Figure 13-3. *A*, Ultrafiltration. An external pressure is applied to fluid on one side of the semipermeable membrane to move it to the other side using the pressure gradient as the physical force. *B*, How ultrafiltration works as part of a dialysis treatment. Either a positive pressure is applied from the blood side to push fluid across or a negative pressure is applied from the dialysate side to pull fluid across.

CONVECTION – Solute transfer with ultrafiltration

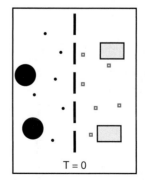
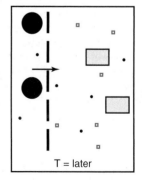

T = 0   T = later

Figure 13-4. Convection occurs when fluid movement drags solutes with it across the membrane, thereby changing the concentration on either side of the membrane.

physicians can tailor dialysis procedures to individual patients.

III. TYPES OF DIALYSIS

For dialysis to be successful, there must be access to blood with rapid blood flow, movement of the dialysate (preferably countercurrent to the blood), a gradient between the blood and the dialysate, and a semipermeable membrane separating the blood and the dialysate. Only with pure convective dialysis (e.g., CRRT) can solute clearance be achieved without diffusion. The different forms and methods of dialysis are based on variations of these four components. The two most frequently used dialysis modalities are hemodialysis and peritoneal dialysis.

A. Hemodialysis

Hemodialysis removes blood and passes it through an extracorporeal circuit and an artificial membrane, with dialysate running in countercurrent flow next to the blood in the membrane. After the blood is filtered through the membrane, it is returned to the body with a reduced quantity of metabolic waste products. Hemodialysis has the advantages of maintaining an efficient concentration gradient via rapid blood and dialysate flows as well as predictable transmembrane pressure between the blood and dialysate within the filter, thereby allowing for rapid solute and fluid removal (Fig. 13-5).

The *dialyzer* is a series of hollow fibers that are composed of special membranes that facilitate solute transfer (Fig. 13-6). The membranes are now made of various biocompatible materials (e.g., polysulfones). A large body of research has demonstrated that bioincompatible dialyzers (e.g., cellulosic dialyzers) activated leukocytes and contributed to complement generation during the dialysis procedure. Biocompatible membranes have significantly less complement

Dialyzers – Hollow Fiber

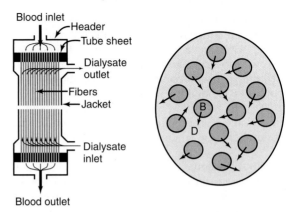

Figure 13-6. A cross-sectional view demonstrating how the hollow filters are placed within the dialyzer. Blood *(B)* moves through multiple small "straws" to increase surface area via diffusion into dialysate *(D)*.

generation. The tubes of the dialyzer membrane are surrounded by dialysate, with the countercurrent flow of dialysate and blood.

Dialysate is the fluid that is used in dialysis to adjust the extracellular fluid composition and to maintain body homeostasis. The dialysate is one of several variables that can be altered in a dialysis procedure to achieve certain patient care goals. For example, the dialysis prescription for a patient with a dangerously high level of potassium will be very different from that of a patient with edema and volume overload who has congestive heart failure but a normal serum potassium level. Dialysate includes bicarbonate and potassium. The potassium level in the dialysis is often lower than the desired final potassium level of the patient as a result of incomplete equilibration during the dialysis period. In an acute dialysis situation in which one particular electrolyte may be elevated, the dialysate concentration of that electrolyte can be lowered further or even removed completely to aid in the rapid removal of that electrolyte from the patient.

The standard buffer for dialysate includes bicarbonate, which has several important advantages. Bicarbonate induces far less hypotension than lactate, which is a buffer that had been used in the past. Moreover, there is evidence that buffering acid is beneficial for reducing bone loss.

Access for hemodialysis is established with either a dialysis catheter, which is most often used for temporary use and placed in a large vein (either the internal jugular or femoral vein); an arteriovenous shunt, such as an arteriovenous fistula; or an arteriovenous graft made of synthetic material such as polytetrafluoroethylene. Arteriovenous fistulas are preferred for long-term use in patients receiving hemodialysis (Fig. 13-7). These accesses can provide adequate blood flow with rates

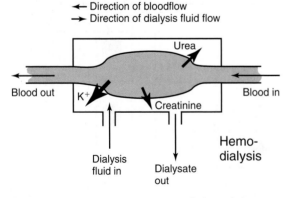

Figure 13-5. Schematic representation of a hemodialysis procedure. Blood runs through the dialysis membrane countercurrent to the dialysate, and various solutes are removed from the blood via diffusion down concentration gradients.

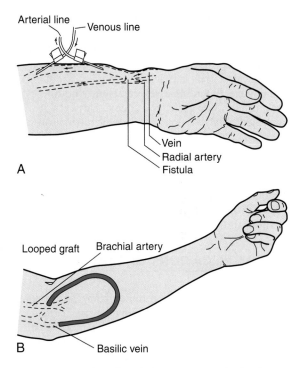

A

B

Figure 13-7. *A,* The radiocephalic arteriovenous fistula, showing blood flow and the usual position of access needles for dialysis. *B,* The common position of the loop arteriovenous graft placed between the brachial artery and the basilic vein. *(Modified from Daugirdas JT, Blake PG, Ing TS: The Handbook of Dialysis, 4th ed. Philadelphia, Lippincott Williams & Wilkins, 2007.)*

between 300 and 500 ml/min, and they also are less prone to complications such as infection and clotting.

The adequacy of hemodialysis for chronic dialysis patients is assessed on a monthly basis. Clinically, the patient is asked about signs and symptoms of uremia, including appetite, nausea, and neurologic symptoms such as restless legs. For solute clearance, the urea reduction ratio (URR) is one measure that can be used to estimate whether the dialysis treatments are effective. By assessing the difference between blood urea nitrogen levels before and after a dialysis session, the URR value can be calculated. An optimal URR is >70%. Adequacy can also be determined using the Kt/V formula, where K is clearance, t is the time on dialysis, and V is the volume of distribution of the patient's extracellular space. Recent studies have found that the value for Kt/V for a patient on hemodialysis should be >1.2, but there is little added benefit if this value exceeds 1.55 to 1.6.

Clinical assessment is most important for assessing volume status, although recent advances in technology have led to the inclusion of blood volume monitors as part of the dialysis machinery itself. High blood pressure or edema indicates hypervolemia. Low blood pressure may reflect hypovolemia, the

effect of medications (e.g., antihypertensive agents), infection, or even poor cardiovascular function. In each instance, it is important to assess the patient to make sure that the dialysis treatment achieves its goals.

B. Peritoneal Dialysis

Peritoneal dialysis uses the natural lining of the peritoneum as the semipermeable membrane for solute and fluid removal. The peritoneal membrane has a monolayer of mesothelial cells, and it separates the peritoneal cavity from the blood and the lymphatic vessels. The visceral layer of the peritoneum covers the abdominal organs, whereas the parietal layer lines the abdominal cavity. Access to blood is through the peritoneal blood vessels, and the dialysate solution is placed in the peritoneal cavity to provide a concentration gradient across this natural membrane.

A patient must undergo a surgical procedure to have an access catheter placed within his or her abdomen before undergoing peritoneal dialysis (Fig. 13-8).

The dialysate flows into the peritoneal space, where it then dwells for one to several hours as the

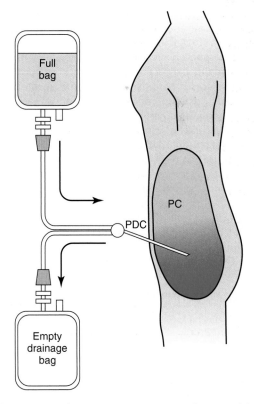

Figure 13-8. A diagrammatic representation of peritoneal dialysis via a continuous ambulatory peritoneal dialysis system. *PC,* Peritoneal cavity; *PDC,* peritoneal dialysis catheter. *(Modified from Greenberg A, Cheung AK, Falk RJ, et al [eds]: Primer on Kidney Diseases, 4th ed. Philadelphia, Saunders, 2005.)*

solute flows down the concentration gradients. When adequate time has elapsed, the solution is removed. Solute removal in peritoneal dialysis is by the process of diffusion. Solutes such as urea nitrogen and potassium move from the blood in the peritoneal capillaries across the peritoneal membrane to the dialysate in the peritoneal cavity. Solutes such as lactate can move from the peritoneal dialysis fluid in the opposite direction. Peritoneal dialysis is very effective for the removal of low-molecular-weight substances such as creatinine, urea, and potassium. Larger molecules such as phosphate move across the membrane more slowly. Albumin can be removed by peritoneal dialysis, perhaps through the lymphatics. During peritoneal dialysis, the dialysate is often hyperosmotic as a result of an increased glucose concentration. Glucose is the most commonly used osmotic agent in peritoneal dialysis. The hyperosmotic peritoneal dialysis fluid facilitates the movement of fluid from the blood into the dialysate (ultrafiltration; Fig. 13-9).

Increasing the glucose concentration creates an osmotic gradient that "pulls" salt and water out of the mesenteric circulation. The volume of ultrafiltration can thus be increased by increasing the osmotic gradient and using dialysis solutions containing higher concentrations of glucose. If the dialysis solution is left in the peritoneal cavity for a longer period of time (i.e., a longer dwell time) with increasing glucose absorption, there is diminished glucose concentration in the dialysis fluid and less fluid removal. Although glucose is effective as an osmotic agent, it can also cause peritoneal inflammation that can eventually lead to ultrafiltration failure. Newer substances (e.g., icodextrin) continue to be evaluated for their efficacy in peritoneal dialysis.

There are two types of peritoneal dialysis. *Continuous ambulatory peritoneal dialysis* involves manual fluid instillation and removal four to five times daily (i.e., four to five exchanges per day). In *continuous cycling peritoneal dialysis,* five to eight serial exchanges are provided by a machine during the night while the patient is sleeping.

Peritoneal dialysis is a continuous therapy. Although less efficient than hemodialysis, patients may do better in terms of solute clearance because it is ongoing 7 days per week. The adequacy of peritoneal dialysis is based on several different parameters, including assessments of symptoms, weight, blood pressure, and edema. However, as with hemodialysis, there is a specific calculation that can be used to assess adequacy. It is possible to measure the dialysate and urinary clearance of creatinine and urea (with a 24-hour collection of the dialysate as well as the urine if the patient has residual kidney function), which results in a weekly Kt/V value. The goal level for a patient receiving peritoneal dialysis is at least 2.0.

IV. COMPLICATIONS OF DIALYSIS

A. Hemodialysis
Hypotension is the most common complication that occurs while a patient is receiving dialysis, particularly when an effort is being made to remove large amounts of volume. With the use of polysulfone rather than cellulosic membranes, reactions to dialyzer membranes are now rare. Bacteremia is not uncommon because of infection from needle sites or dialysis catheters. Arrhythmias can occur because of the underlying cardiovascular disease in combination with rapid fluid volume and electrolyte shifts. Bleeding complications certainly do occur when patients require anticoagulation with heparin during the procedure, especially if the vascular access has a stenosis at the venous anastomosis.

B. Peritoneal Dialysis
Common complications of peritoneal dialysis include infection and the malfunctioning of the dialysis catheter. Infections can occur in the peritoneal fluid, the catheter tunnel, and at the site in the skin where the catheter exits. Patients are trained to look for signs of infection, such as abdominal pain, cloudy dialysate, or purulent discharge at the exit site. These infections are, in general, successfully treated at home with antibiotics. About 80% of these infectious complications are the result of gram-positive organisms such as *Staphylococcus* and *Streptococcus,* with the remaining 20% predominantly caused by gram-negative organisms and, rarely, by fungal infections. Because of the high protein losses that occur with peritoneal dialysis, patients often have trouble maintaining their nutritional status, which is indicated by low serum albumin levels. Finally, patients who undergo peritoneal dialysis will sometimes have gradual failure of this therapy as a result of changes in the peritoneal membrane. This can occur through scarring or repeated infection (peritonitis). Patients may develop volume overload, edema, and even congestive heart failure or uremic complications. When this

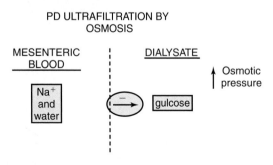

PD ULTRAFILTRATION BY OSMOSIS

Figure 13-9. The osmotic role of glucose in peritoneal dialysate helps to achieve fluid removal.

occurs, patients will need to be transitioned to hemodialysis or receive kidney transplants.

V. MORTALITY ON DIALYSIS

Patients on dialysis have an average mortality rate of 20% to 23% during the first year and of nearly 75% by 5 years. Many patients die from comorbid diseases (e.g., cardiovascular disease) or infection as a result of their immunocompromised status. Age and the cause of kidney failure are two important factors that seem to influence the risk of death.

VI. CONCLUSIONS

In summary, dialysis has been very successful for prolonging the survival of patients with kidney failure with a reasonable quality of life. Dialysis is based on the principles of diffusion and convection for solute clearance and ultrafiltration for fluid removal. Hemodialysis is primarily performed at a health care facility, although it can also be a daily home therapy in selected patients. Peritoneal dialysis is exclusively a home therapy; it allows the patient to manage his or her care at home, and it has the advantage of being administered 7 days a week.

Quality and quantity of life can be good on dialysis, but the mortality rate remains high, primarily as a result of comorbid conditions and infection.

Clinical Case

A 56-year-old man with stage 5 chronic kidney disease had a peritoneal catheter placed to initiate dialysis. After 6 weeks of peritoneal dialysis, his blood pressure is 170/100 mm Hg, and he has 2+ edema; however, his nausea has resolved, and his appetite is better. He currently does four exchanges of 2 L every 6 hours. He is using two peritoneal dialysis fluid bags of 1.5% glucose and two of 2.5% glucose daily. His serum albumin level is 3.4 g/dl.

What can you do to improve this patient's edema?

Increasing the concentration of glucose in the dialysate will remove more fluid as a result of the increased osmotic pressure provided by the increased glucose concentration. In addition, patients receiving peritoneal dialysis often have residual kidney function, and thus they may still be responsive to high doses of diuretics.

Why is his serum albumin level low?

The peritoneal dialysis fluid that is removed from the patient after dwelling in the peritoneal cavity can contain a significant amount of protein. This is an important cause of low serum albumin level in patients receiving peritoneal dialysis. Decreased appetite and poor intake of dietary protein may be another cause of low levels of serum albumin in some patients.

Are there other treatment options for the patient if he does not improve?

Patients who do not do well on peritoneal dialysis can transition to hemodialysis or possibly undergo kidney transplantation.

Suggested Readings

Daugirdas JT, Blake PG, Ing TS: *The Handbook of Dialysis*, 4th ed. Philadelphia, Lippincott Williams & Wilkins, 2007.
Gokal R: Peritoneal dialysis in the 21st century: An analysis of current problems and future developments. *J Am Soc Nephrol* 13(Suppl 1):S104–S116, 2002.

PRACTICE QUESTIONS

1. A 56-year-old man with known chronic kidney disease and a glomerular filtration rate of 20 ml/min noted 3 months earlier presents to the emergency department with sharp chest pain of 2 days' duration. He has had a poor appetite, and he has been vomiting for the last 2 weeks. On examination, his blood pressure is 160/95 mm Hg, and his pulse rate is 90 beats per minute. Auscultation of the chest reveals bilateral basal rales and a pericardial friction rub. Laboratory results are a blood urea nitrogen level of 90 mg/dl, a creatinine level of 6.5 mg/dl, a serum potassium level of 6.0 mmol/L, a serum calcium level of 8.4 mg/dl, and a phosphorus level of 7.2 mg/dl. He is hospitalized and, after the placement of a dialysis catheter in the femoral vein, he is started on hemodialysis. Hemodialysis is likely to effectively remove all of the following, except which one?

   A. Potassium
   B. Blood urea nitrogen
   C. Uremic toxins causing the pericarditis
   D. Phosphorous

2. A 75-year-old man on peritoneal dialysis for kidney failure as a result of longstanding hypertension presents to the emergency department with increasing shortness of breath of a few days' duration. He has been less than compliant with the dietary restrictions. He has increased jugular venous pressure and 2+ pedal edema. His weight has increased from its usual level by 6 lb, and on auscultation widespread rales are heard in his chest. Laboratory tests reveal the following electrolyte levels: sodium, 130; potassium, 5.9; chlorine, 100; bicarbonate, 15 mmol/L; and blood urea nitrogen, 75 mg/dl. This patient is likely to have which of the following?

   A. An increase in total body sodium
   B. A decrease in total body sodium
   C. A decrease total body potassium
   D. A decrease in total body water

Replacement Therapy for Kidney Failure: Transplantation

14

Milagros D. Samaniego
Yolanda T. Becker
Joshua David Lindsey

OUTLINE

I. Introduction
II. Pathophysiology of Kidney Transplantation
   A. Immediate Nonspecific Inflammation
   B. Surgical Complications and Their Contribution to Renal Transplant Pathophysiology
   C. Acute Antigen-Specific Responses
   D. Histocompatibility Antigens
III. Pathophysiology of Rejection
   A. Hyperacute Rejection
   B. Acute Rejection

C. Chronic Rejection
D. Tissue (Human Leukocyte Antigen) Typing and Cross Matching
E. The Basics of Immunosuppression
IV. Recurrence of Native Kidney Disease in the Allograft

Objectives

- Recognize that kidney transplantation is an important consideration for kidney replacement therapy and that it may be the therapy of choice for some patients.
- Describe the nonimmune and immune mechanisms of injury that contribute to the pathophysiology of kidney transplantation and that are important determinants of early and late kidney transplant function.
- Name the three phases of response elicited by kidney transplants if the transplant acts as a source of foreign proteins (i.e., donor proteins).
- Understand that immunosuppressants inhibit each of the three immune signals involved in transplant rejection.
- Know the primary kidney disease that may recur in the transplanted kidney.

Clinical Case

A 46-year-old woman with kidney failure as a result of type 2 diabetes mellitus receives a deceased donor kidney transplant. Surgery goes well, and she is discharged home 5 days after transplant with a serum creatinine level of 0.9 mg/dl. Two months after the transplant, she starts feeling ill over a period of 1 week. No precipitating factor was noted. However, she has noticed increased fatigue, nausea, vomiting, and poor appetite. She also mentions decreased urination. She may have had chills, but she denies having had fevers and diarrhea, and she says that she is not taking any other drugs. Her husband mentions that she has been taking her antirejection drugs appropriately. On physical examination, the patient's blood pressure is at 210/120 mm Hg without orthostatic changes. Her pulse is 98 beats per minute, and her respirations are 23 breaths per minute. The patient appears to be tired, but she is not in distress. The skin examination is normal, the heart sounds are regular, and the lungs are clear to auscultation. The allograft area in the right lower quadrant is nontender. There is 2+ pitting edema. The patient's blood laboratory values reveal a serum creatinine level of 3.9 mg/dl.

What are the possible causes of acute kidney transplant dysfunction in this patient?

I. INTRODUCTION

The year 2004 marked the 50th anniversary of the first successful kidney transplant, which was performed at Harvard University by Dr. Joseph Murray. It was an isograft from a healthy man to his genetically identical twin brother (Box 14-1). A genetically identical isograft from a living donor represents the ideal transplant, because it overcomes two of the main barriers for the survival of the transplant:

1. The immediate nonspecific inflammatory response elicited by the procurement, preservation,

- *Autologous graft:* The transplantation of one's own tissue to another or the same site (e.g., autologous skin graft, autologous bone marrow transplant).
- *Isograft or syngeneic graft:* A graft that is transplanted between two genetically identical individuals (i.e., between identical twins).
- *Allograft or allogeneic graft:* A graft that is transplanted between two genetically different individuals of the same species.
- *Xenograft or xenogeneic graft:* A graft that is transplanted between members of different species (e.g., baboon to human, pig to human).
- *Donor:* The person from whom the graft is obtained. There are deceased and living donors.
- *Recipient or host:* The patient who receives the transplant.

and storage of the organ (i.e., cold ischemia). (This phase is primarily ischemic in nature, and its pathophysiology is very similar to that of acute tubular necrosis.)
2. The acute immune response that is generated against antigens (i.e., human leukocyte antigens [HLAs]) that are recognized as foreign in allografts and that results in rejection

Kidney transplantation is the treatment modality of choice for patients with kidney failure. It increases a patient's lifespan by approximately 10 years (range, 3 to 17 years) as compared with dialysis, with diabetic patients between the ages of 20 to 59 years deriving the greatest benefit. The most frequent diagnoses of kidney failure in transplant patients are diabetes mellitus, hypertension, and chronic glomerular diseases, according to the United States Renal Data

System. As of May 2006, more than 68,000 patients were waiting for a kidney transplant. From January through December 2005, more than 17,000 kidney transplants were performed in the United States, according to the United Network for Organ Sharing. Most of these transplants were from deceased donors.

II. PATHOPHYSIOLOGY OF KIDNEY TRANSPLANTATION

Clinical transplants elicit three phases of response (Table 14-1):
1. An immediate non–antigen-specific inflammatory response that is mediated by elements of the innate immune system.
2. An acute antigen-specific immune response that is mediated by lymphocytes against the HLAs expressed on the transplant cells.
3. A chronic repair and remodeling response that involves antigen-specific and non–antigen-specific mechanisms.

A. Immediate Nonspecific Inflammation
The initial inflammatory response elicited by a kidney transplant is related to the surgical procedure of transplantation. It involves events that occur in the donor during organ procurement and organ preservation and in the recipient during the reimplantation and reperfusion of the organ.

All transplants are subjected to periods of warm ischemia (i.e., in the donor), cold ischemia (i.e., during preservation), and reperfusion injury (i.e., during the reimplantation of the transplant into the recipient). The impact of ischemic injury on the recovery of kidney function depends on the length of ischemia:
- Kidney damage is reversible only if warm ischemia lasts for less than 30 minutes.

Table 14-1. The Three Phases of Response to Transplants

	Innate inflammation	Antigen-specific immunity	Tissue remodeling
Cells	Polymorphonuclear leukocytes, macrophages	Lymphocytes	Macrophages, fibroblasts, smooth muscle cells
Mediators	Complement system, adhesion molecules, chemokines, cytokines	T lymphocytes, antibodies, cytokines	Chemokines, cytokines
Antigen dependence	Antigen independent	Antigen dependent	Both antigen independent and antigen dependent
Timing to treatment event	0–72 hours	0–10 days	Months to years
Clinical correlate	Delayed graft function	Acute rejection	Chronic allograft dysfunction and failure

- The recovery of kidney function is predictable in organs that are preserved for 3 days or fewer; it becomes less reliable after 5 days.

The effects of ischemia on kidney cellular metabolism are shown in Figure 14-1. The main targets of ischemic injury in the transplant are the tubular epithelial cells and the endothelium of the arteries and the veins.

In the tubule, ischemic injury results in the perturbation of the cytoskeleton, which is indistinguishable from ischemic injury of the native kidney. There is a loss of the brush border and a sloughing of viable and nonviable tubular cells into the tubular lumen, which results in tubular cast formation and obstruction. Clinically, the loss of brush border and polarity results in sodium wasting (i.e., increased fractional excretion of sodium). Tubular obstruction and cast formation reduce the glomerular filtration rate, which results in azotemia and delayed graft function.

In the endothelium, ischemia activates complement and upregulates receptors that attract inflammatory and noninflammatory cells (i.e., chemokines and cell adhesion molecules). This results in vasoconstriction, the trapping of platelets, red and white blood cells in the vessel lumen, and inflamed tissue causing hypoxia in the medulla.

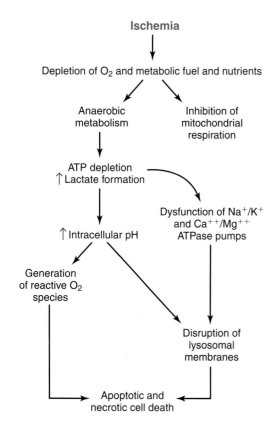

Figure 14-1. The effects of ischemia on kidney cell metabolism. *(Compliments of Agnes Fogo, MD.)*

The injured endothelial cells and infiltrating inflammatory cells (i.e., polymorphonuclear leukocytes and macrophages) produce acute-phase cytokines such as tumor necrosis factor-α and interferon-γ that facilitate immunologic responses against the transplant and initiate the events that are responsible for the second phase.

B. Surgical Complications and Their Contribution to Renal Transplant Pathophysiology

Surgical complications related to the transplant procedure may contribute to pathology in the allograft. The most common complications involve the urologic outflow of the kidney and include urinary leaks and obstructions. The pathophysiology and clinical presentation of these patients is identical to that of patients with postrenal acute kidney injury. Although easy to treat and recognize, chronic urinary leaks or obstruction can lead to chronic infection and interstitial fibrosis (scarring) of the transplant, thereby resulting in transplant failure.

Complications of the vasculature of the new transplant are less common and can result in the acute loss of the allograft if they are not attended to promptly. The most common complications include renal artery and/or vein thrombosis and renal artery stenosis. Patients with thrombosis of the renal artery or vein present with acute oliguria and have characteristics of both prerenal and intrarenal acute kidney dysfunction. Transplant renal artery stenosis is a subacute complication that is usually associated with severe hypertension. As in unilateral native renal artery stenosis, the arterial perfusion to the renal transplant is compromised, which results in the activation of the renin–angiotensin–aldosterone system. The activation of this system leads to increased sodium reabsorption, edema, and hypertension.

C. Acute Antigen-Specific Responses

The second response to clinical transplants develops within minutes to weeks after transplantation. The central event in this response is the reaction of the recipient's immune system to donor cells in the transplanted graft. This reaction involves the recognition of specific proteins on the surface of the parenchymal and endothelial cells of the transplant by T- and B-lymphocytes and antibodies of recipient origin and the generation of immune responses against the transplant (i.e., rejection). In many ways, the rejection of a transplant is very similar to the immune response elicited by viral infections. In a viral infection, the viral proteins are recognized by the immune system as foreign. In the transplant scenario, the histocompatibility antigens of the donor are recognized as foreign. To maintain the viability of the transplant, immunosuppressive drugs must be used to inhibit this response of the recipient's immune system.

D. Histocompatibility Antigens

Histocompatibility antigens are the target of the rejection response. They were initially discovered and named for their capacity to induce transplant rejection. However, their principal immunologic function is to present foreign proteins (i.e., viral, bacterial, parasitic, animal, and human proteins) to the immune system by forming complexes with the T-lymphocytes through specific receptors. In eukaryotic species, these proteins are produced by a set of genes that are clustered over a short stretch of a single chromosome (i.e., the short arm of chromosome 6 in humans); they are called the *major histocompatibility complex* (MHC). In humans, the MHC is called the HLA because these antigens are easily detectable on leukocytes.

HLAs are glycoproteins that can be divided into two classes:

1. Class I (in humans, HLA-A, HLA-B, and HLA-C):
   a. Expressed codominantly on all nucleated cells
   b. Interact with CD8, which is expressed by cytotoxic T-lymphocytes
2. Class II (in humans, HLA-DR, HLA-DQ, and HLA-DP):
   a. Expressed codominantly on dendritic cells, macrophages, B-lymphocytes, some vascular endothelial cells, and thymic epithelial cells
   b. Expression is induced by the cytokine-mediated activation of T-lymphocytes and tubular epithelial cells
   c. Interact with CD4, which is expressed by helper T-lymphocytes

MHC class I and II antigens are inherited in a codominant pattern from both the mother and the father (Fig. 14-2). Patients waiting for transplants are tissue-typed for their MHC antigens. Tissue typing will be discussed later in this chapter.

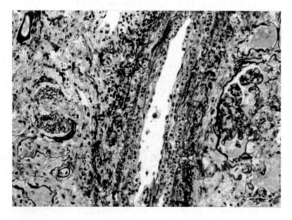

Figure 14-2. An example of vascular acute rejection. There is severe subendothelial and transmural lymphocytic infiltrate in this medium-sized artery. *(Copyright © 2000, National Kidney Foundation. Compliments of Agnes Fogo, MD.)*

III. PATHOPHYSIOLOGY OF REJECTION

Clinically, rejection is classified according to the rate at which it occurs. This in turn reflects to some degree the underlying immune response and histology (Table 14-2).

A. Hyperacute Rejection

Hyperacute rejection is characterized by the thrombotic occlusion of the transplant vessels that begins within minutes to hours after the vascular anastomosis is completed. Preexisting host antibodies against endothelial cell antigens (ABO or MHC antigens) mediate this type of rejection. The binding of antibodies to endothelium activates the classical pathway of complement, thereby leading to endothelial cell injury and the subsequent activation of platelets and the coagulation cascade. These processes contribute to thrombosis and vascular occlusion, and the transplanted organ suffers irreversible ischemic and inflammatory damage. A typical biopsy reveals neutrophil infiltration of the allograft with areas of hemorrhage and necrosis. The performance of pretransplant tissue and ABO blood typing has contributed to a reduction in the incidence of hyperacute rejection.

B. Acute Rejection

Acute rejection is a process of vascular and parenchymal injury that is mediated by T-cells and antibodies. It usually begins during the first week after transplantation. In acute rejection, the T-cells develop during a few days or weeks in response to the transplant itself. In antibody-mediated rejection, anti-HLA antibodies can be present at the time of transplant and result in hyperacute or accelerated acute rejection within minutes or days after transplantation. Acute rejection is diagnosed by correlating organ function with pathologic findings on biopsy usually manifested by a mononuclear cell infiltrate. The main targets of injury are endothelial and parenchymal cells that express HLA molecules. Anti-HLA T-cells cause direct lysis of transplant cells (e.g., CD8+ T-cells) or produce cytokines (e.g., CD4+ T-cells) that recruit and activate inflammatory cells that in turn injure the graft. In vascularized grafts such as kidney transplants, endothelial cells are the earliest targets of acute rejection (Fig. 14-2), followed by the tubular epithelial cells (Fig. 14-3). Clinically, the patient presents with acute kidney dysfunction, a high fractional excretion of sodium, mild proteinuria, and sterile pyuria. Antibodies can also mediate acute rejection if the recipient develops a humoral response to HLAs in which antibodies bind the vessel wall and activate complement (Fig. 14-4).

C. Chronic Rejection

Chronic rejection is characterized by fibrosis and vascular abnormalities with a loss of transplant function that occurs during a prolonged period. The pathogenesis

Table 14-2. Types of Allograft Rejection

	Hyperacute	Acute		Chronic
Duration	Minutes to hours	Days	Weeks	Months to years
Mediators	Preformed antibodies	Antibodies (memory)	Activated T-cells	Tissue response
Incidence	Rare	Less common	More common	Universal
Pathology	Graft thrombosis	Vasculitis	Parenchymal injury	Vascular remodeling
Prevention	Cross matching	Avoiding risk factors	Optimizing match (tissue typing)	Decreasing early injury (questionable)
Therapy	Avoid transplant	Plasmapheresis and intravenous immunoglobulin	Increase or change in immunosuppression	None

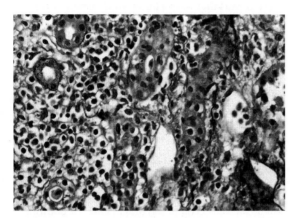

Figure 14-3. An example of tubulointerstitial acute rejection. There are numerous lymphocytes infiltrating the tubules and the interstitium. *(Copyright © 2000, National Kidney Foundation. Compliments of Agnes Fogo, MD.)*

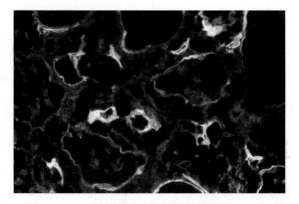

Figure 14-4. The presence of C4d (a breakdown product of complement) staining in the peritubular capillaries (bright fluorescence). This is a marker of antibody-mediated rejection. *(Copyright © 2000, National Kidney Foundation. Compliments of Agnes Fogo, MD.)*

of chronic rejection is less well understood than that of acute rejection. The fibrosis of chronic rejection may result from immune reactions and from the production of cytokines that stimulate fibroblasts (i.e., transforming growth factor-β), or it may represent wound healing after the parenchymal cellular necrosis of acute rejection. The hallmark of chronic rejection is accelerated graft arteriosclerosis in the transplant. This is an arterial occlusion that results from the proliferation of the smooth muscle cells of the vascular media layer. This proliferation of smooth muscle cells may represent a specialized form of immune reaction in which lymphocytes that are activated by HLAs in the transplant vessel wall induce macrophages to secrete smooth muscle cell growth factors (Fig. 14-5). Anti-HLA antibodies can also develop months and years after transplant and cause late transplant rejections.

The term *chronic rejection* implies an underlying chronic immune process. Chronic rejection is thus different from chronic fibrotic changes in allografts, which are characterized by tubular atrophy and interstitial fibrosis. This was previously called *chronic allograft nephropathy.* Nonimmune mechanisms of allograft injury (e.g., uncontrolled hypertension, diabetes, dyslipidemia, drug toxicity) all contribute to these chronic tubular and interstitial changes. Chronic tubular atrophy and interstitial fibrosis with a loss of function and patient death with a functioning graft are the two principal causes of late allograft loss.

D. Tissue (Human Leukocyte Antigen) Typing and Cross Matching

Patients waiting for transplants are tissue typed for their MHC antigens. Currently, HLA-A and B and HLA-DR are assessed. Kidney donors are HLA typed prospectively, and donor kidneys are HLA matched to recipients. For living related kidney transplants, the maternal and paternal sources of HLAs can be surmised, and the HLAs can be assigned to haplotypes.

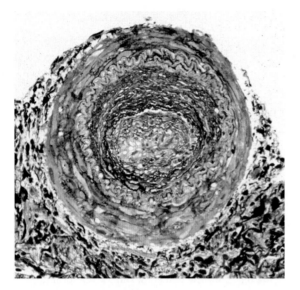

Figure 14-5. A classic image of accelerated graft arteriosclerosis with the occlusion of the vascular lumen from the proliferation of the smooth muscle cells of the vascular media. Kidney tissue distal to the site of occlusion suffers chronic ischemic damage. *(Copyright © 2000, National Kidney Foundation. Compliments of Agnes Fogo, MD.)*

Antigens coded on one chromosome constitute a haplotype (Fig. 14-6).

The microcytotoxicity test developed by Paul Terasaki has been used for more than 30 years for cross matching. The goal of this test is to prevent hyperacute rejection. Lymphocytes from the donor are used as donor tissue because they are easily obtained and express HLA. Donor lymphocytes are incubated with sera from potential recipients to test for antibodies against the potential donor. If an antibody directed against the donor HLA is present in the recipient's sera, then the lymphocytes are destroyed by the lysis that results from complement activation. This is interpreted as a positive cross match and is a contraindication for transplantation.

E. The Basics of Immunosuppression
The rejection response is a natural immune mechanism that must be inhibited to ensure the survival of the graft. Thus, because immunosuppression results in the inhibition and control of the rejection response, it also interferes with other natural immune mechanisms that have evolved to eliminate foreign antigens such as viral and bacterial proteins as well as tumor antigens. Thus, it is not surprising that immunosuppressed patients are at increased risk for developing various infectious complications and malignancies. Table 14-3 summarizes some of the most commonly used immunosuppressive agents, their cellular and humoral targets, and the infections and malignancies to which they have been linked.

IV. RECURRENCE OF NATIVE KIDNEY DISEASE IN THE ALLOGRAFT

The recurrence of primary kidney disease in the transplant is a well-recognized complication of transplantation, and it constitutes the third most common cause of kidney transplant failure.

Tissue Typing for MHC Antigens

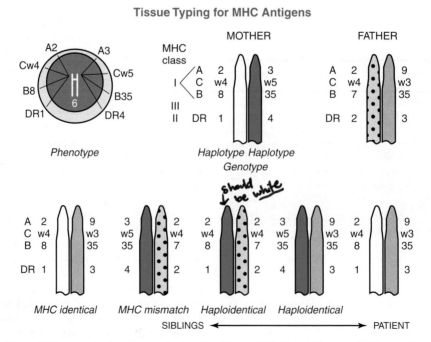

Figure 14-6. Tissue typing of human leukocyte antigens. *MHC,* Major histocompatibility complex.

Table 14-3. Immunosuppressant Targets and Associated Infections and Malignancies

Drugs	Examples	Targets	Infections and malignancies
Calcineurin inhibitors	• Cyclosporine • Tacrolimus	• T cells • T and B cells	• Cytomegalovirus, Epstein-Barr virus, polyoma virus • Bacterial infections • Skin cancers • Head and neck cancers • Posttransplant lymphoproliferative disorder • Colon cancer
Antiproliferative agents	• Azathioprine • Mycophenolate • Sirolimus	• T and B cells • T and B cells • T cells and fibroblasts	• Papilloma virus • Cytomegalovirus, Epstein-Barr virus, polyoma virus • Skin cancers, posttransplant lymphoproliferative disorder
Steroids	• Prednisone	• T cells, polymorpho-nuclear leukocytes • Fibroblasts	• Bacterial infections • Tuberculosis, fungal infections
Antilymphocyte antibodies	• OK-T3 • Thymoglobulin • Alemtuzumab	• T cells only • T and B cells • T and B cells	• Cytomegalovirus, Epstein-Barr virus, herpes simplex virus, posttransplant lymphoproliferative disorder • Cytomegalovirus, Epstein-Barr virus, herpes simplex virus, posttransplant lymphoproliferative disorder • Cytomegalovirus, herpes simplex virus • Other: fungal infections, listeria, nocardia

Not all primary diseases of the kidney recur after transplantation. For example, genetic diseases that result in defective renal morphogenesis (i.e., autosomal dominant polycystic kidney disease or Alport syndrome) do not recur in the transplant. However, diseases such as Goodpasture syndrome or antiglomerular-basement membrane (anti-GBM) mediated idiopathic crescentic glomerulonephritis can recur in the allograft if the patient has anti-GBM antibodies in his or her circulation at the time of transplantation. It is recommended that these patients wait to receive a kidney transplant until anti-GBM antibodies are no longer detectable in their circulation.

In patients with systemic metabolic diseases (e.g., diabetes mellitus) or immunologic diseases of the kidney (Goodpasture syndrome, ANCA vasculitis, membranous nephropathy, among others), glomerular disease recurs in the transplant at different frequencies. In these diseases, kidney disease is the result of systemic disease. Unless the systemic disease itself is cured, the initial mechanism of kidney injury would persist and eventually result in the damage of the transplanted kidney.

The recurrence of primary kidney disease in the transplant and the risk of kidney transplant loss as a consequence of recurrence are highly variable. This variability is intimately related to the pathophysiology of the kidney injury. In descending order of frequency, the diseases that most commonly recur in the kidney transplant are as follows:

- Hemolytic uremic syndrome
- Focal segmental glomerulosclerosis
- Immunoglobulin A nephropathy
- Membranoproliferative glomerulonephritis
- Antineutrophil cytoplasmic antibody vasculitis
- Diabetic nephropathy
- Membranous nephropathy

Diabetic nephropathy recurs in almost all diabetic kidney transplant recipients who do not also receive a pancreas transplant. Thickening of the glomerular basement membrane and mesangial expansion are seen by 2 years, and this is followed by the hyalinization of the afferent and efferent arterioles by 4 years after transplantation. The classic nodular glomerulosclerosis of native diabetic nephropathy rarely recurs in the transplant. The pathogenesis of recurrent or de novo diabetic nephropathy in the transplant is similar to that of the native disease; however, the rate of disease progression is somewhat slower. Good glycemic control and the prolonged maintenance of normoglycemia are important to prevent diabetic nephropathy of the transplant.

In some forms of primary or idiopathic focal segmental glomerulosclerosis, the injury of the podocyte results from a circulating factor. The full characterization of this factor has been difficult. Recurrence occurs in 30% to 40% of patients with primary focal segmental glomerulosclerosis.

In patients with the hemolytic uremic syndrome without the preceding symptom of diarrhea, recurrence has been noted in 80% to 100% of patients who are deficient in complement regulatory proteins such as Factor I, Factor H, or membrane cofactor protein-1. Combined liver and kidney transplantation reduces the risk of recurrence significantly.

The recurrence of glomerular disease in the allograft is puzzling, yet insights into why this occurs continue to develop. The treatment of the renal transplant recipient, even with newer and more potent immunosuppressive medications, has not influenced the recurrence of glomerular diseases in the allograft. One potential explanation for this paradox may reside in the nature of the immune response underlying glomerular diseases.

Clinical Case

A 46-year-old woman with kidney failure as a result of type 2 diabetes mellitus receives a deceased donor kidney transplant. Surgery goes well, and she is discharged home 5 days after transplant with a serum creatinine level of 0.9 mg/dl. Two months after the transplant, she starts feeling ill over a period of 1 week. No precipitating factor was noted. However, she has noticed increased fatigue, nausea, vomiting, and poor appetite. She also mentions decreased urination. She may have had chills, but she denies having had fevers and diarrhea, and she says that she is not taking any other drugs. Her husband mentions that she has been taking her antirejection drugs appropriately. On physical examination, the patient's blood pressure is at 210/120 mm Hg without orthostatic changes. Her pulse is 98 beats per minute, and her respirations are 23 breaths per minute. The patient appears to be tired, but she is not in distress. The skin examination is normal, the heart sounds are regular, and the lungs are clear to auscultation. The allograft area in the right lower quadrant is nontender. There is 2+ pitting edema. The patient's blood laboratory values reveal a serum creatinine level of 3.9 mg/dl.

What are the possible causes of acute kidney transplant dysfunction in this patient?

The major causes of acute kidney injury early (i.e., during the first 3 months) after the transplant are many and include decreased renal blood flow as a result of arterial vasoconstriction by calcineurin inhibitors and volume contraction of any cause, including emesis, diarrhea, bleeding, and so on. Surgical complications include urinary tract obstruction and hypoperfusion as a result of vascular anastomosis. Urinary tract infections are common because the patients are immunosuppressed. Acute rejection occurs mainly during the first year after the transplant. Approximately 15% to 25% of patients experience an episode of acute rejection, and these episodes may be nearly asymptomatic (like in this case). The diagnosis is made on the basis of the biopsy of the allograft after having ruled out all of the above possibilities.

Suggested Readings

Pascual M, Theruvath T, Kawai T, et al: Strategies to improve long-term outcomes after renal transplantation. *N Engl J Med* 346(8):580-590, 2002.

Patel R, Terasaki PI: Significance of the positive crossmatch test in kidney transplantation. *N Engl J Med* 280(14): 735-739, 1969.

Suthanthiran M, Strom TB: Renal transplantation. *N Engl J Med* 331(6):365-376, 1994.

United Network for Organ Sharing home page (website): www.unos.org. Accessed February 29, 2008.

PRACTICE QUESTIONS

1. If rejection is diagnosed in the patient who presented in the clinical case, which of the following statements is incorrect?

   A. Acute cellular rejection and antibody-mediated rejection are both possible.
   B. $CD8^+$ cells recognize donor HLA as foreign in the parenchymal and endothelial cells of the transplant and release enzymes that destroy the cells (cytotoxicity).
   C. An inflammatory infiltrate composed of mononuclear cells is observed invading the tubules and the interstitial space.
   D. The glomeruli are damaged by the rejection process.

2. Which of the following statements about the initial response to a kidney transplant is/are correct? (Choose all that apply.)

   A. It is closely related to ischemic injury and surgical events.
   B. Ischemic injury of the transplant is always reversible.

   C. It is nonspecific and independent of the HLA type of the recipient or the donor.
   D. The clinical presentation is that of acute renal failure with oliguria and a high fractional excretion of sodium.

3. Which of the following statements is true about a patient who receives a haploidentical kidney transplant from his brother? (Choose all that apply.)

   A. The chance of having a haploidentical sibling is 50%.
   B. Haploidentical siblings share both maternal and paternal haplotypes.
   C. Haploidentical siblings are HLA identical.
   D. Immunosuppression is necessary because the recipient can develop a rejection response to the nonshared HLA that is expressed in the transplant.

Essential Hypertension

15

Theodore L. Goodfriend
Kristin M. Lyerly

OUTLINE

I. Definitions and Epidemiology
  A. Essential Hypertension
  B. Subclassifications within Essential Hypertension
II. Epidemiology of Hypertension
III. Epidemiology of Hypertensive Sequelae
IV. Evolution of Hypertension in Individuals
  A. Early Stage (High Cardiac Output)
  B. Adult Stage (High Peripheral Resistance)
  C. Late Stage (Complications)
V. Cause of Essential Hypertension
  A. Facts Concerning the Cause of Essential Hypertension
  B. Hypotheses Concerning the Cause of Essential Hypertension
VI. Pathologic Consequences of Hypertension
  A. Effect of Hypertension on the Arteries
  B. The Heart in Hypertension

C. The Kidney in Hypertension
D. The Kidney in Malignant Hypertension
E. The Brain in Hypertension
F. The Retina in Hypertension
G. Causes of Death
VII. Management of the Patient with Essential Hypertension
  A. Lifestyle Changes
  B. Therapies That Influence Salt and Water Balance
  C. Drugs That Block the Renin–Angiotensin–Aldosterone System
  D. Drugs That Block the Autonomic Nervous System
  E. Drugs That Block Vascular Smooth Muscle Contraction
  F. Combinations of Antihypertensive Therapies

Objectives

- Know the definitions of labile hypertension, isolated systolic hypertension, and malignant hypertension, and the categories of hypertension as defined by the Seventh Report of the Joint National Committee on Prevention, Detection, Evaluation, and Treatment of High Blood Pressure.
- Learn the epidemiologic parameters that are associated with the increased prevalence of hypertension in certain populations.
- Appreciate the factors that multiply the cardiovascular risk associated with hypertension.
- Be able to describe how sodium handling by the kidney can affect blood pressure.
- Learn the common pathologic changes that hypertension induces or aggravates in its target organs.
- Learn the clinical findings that indicate the presence of the most common pathologic changes that are caused by hypertension in its target organs.
- Understand the lifestyle changes that are the most likely to lower the blood pressure of typical adult hypertensive patients.
- Know the classes of commonly used antihypertensive drugs, and understand how they work to lower the blood pressure.

Clinical Case

A 45-year-old African-American man presents to a neighborhood urgent care office complaining of a nasal discharge. Routine measurements by office staff reveal a blood pressure of 160/105 mm Hg, a heart rate of 82 beats per minute, a temperature of 98.6°F, a respiratory rate of 20 breaths per minute, a height of 69 inches, and a weight of 210 lbs (body mass index, 31). He reports no known previous elevations in his blood pressure, but he has rarely sought medical care as an adult. He has no symptoms that are indicative of renal or cardiac disease. His family history includes a father who died of "heart disease" at the age of 55 years and a mother who died of a stroke at the age of 60 years. He is recently divorced, eats most of his meals at restaurants, enjoys 2 to 4 drinks with dinner, and smokes one pack of cigarettes every 2 days.

The examining clinician records a blood pressure of 156/102 mm Hg. The patient's nasal turbinates are pale

179

and swollen with clear exudate. The ophthalmoscopic examination is unremarkable. No carotid bruits are heard, and the lungs are clear. No cardiac murmurs are heard, but there is a barely audible presystolic S_4 at the apex. The abdominal examination is unremarkable except for obesity. The extremities have barely palpable pulses below the femorals, a trace of pitting edema over the lower half of both tibias, and normal deep tendon reflexes.

A complete blood count is normal. Urinalysis shows trace proteinuria. Chest x-ray reveals a "boot-shaped" heart and no evidence of pulmonary disease.

A tentative diagnosis of seasonal allergic rhinitis is made, and a prescription is written for a nonsedating antihistamine. The patient is advised to find a primary care clinician for further evaluation of his blood pressure and other risk factors.

What is the likely underlying cause of the elevated blood pressure, if it can be established that the pressure is chronically elevated (i.e., "fixed")? What is the differential diagnosis? Which features of the patient's habits, history, heritage, and habitus might be contributing to his elevated pressure? Which are contributing to his risk of cardiovascular disease? What should this patient's primary caregiver recommend as nonpharmacologic approaches to use to improve his cardiovascular health? If drugs were necessary to lower this patient's blood pressure, which ones should be used?

I. DEFINITIONS AND EPIDEMIOLOGY

A. Essential Hypertension
Essential hypertension is also called *primary hypertension* to differentiate it from secondary hypertension, which is the elevated pressure that accompanies identifiable causes like renal artery stenosis. About 90% to 95% of all hypertension arises from an unknown cause, so the vast majority of hypertension is "essential" (Box 15-1).

The demarcation between normal and hypertensive blood pressure is defined by committees. Life expectancy is inversely proportional to arterial pressure, and there is no point at which the pressure has no effect. The cut point has been defined at lower and lower levels over the years as treatment to lower blood pressure has become more practical.

The current consensus is that, in adults 18 years old and older who have no other diseases that can be aggravated by hypertension (most notably diabetes and renal diseases), pressures of 140/90 mm Hg or higher are considered hypertensive (Box 15-2). Either a

---

Box 15-1. Essential Hypertension

About 90% to 95% of all hypertension arises from an unknown cause; this is essential hypertension.

Box 15-2. Definition of Hypertension

Hypertension is defined by pressures of 140/90 mm Hg and higher in adults without comorbidity.

---

systolic pressure of at least 140 mm Hg or a diastolic pressure of at least 90 mm Hg is considered abnormal. Using these levels, about 15% to 25% of American adults have hypertension. Normal pressures in preadolescent children are lower, and there are grids that define the distribution of pressures at different ages. After puberty, adult criteria apply.

The average pressure of populations in developed countries tends to rise with age, so the border between normal blood pressure and hypertension used to be defined at higher levels in older people than in younger people. It is now known that, in many primitive cultures, there is no increase with age; in all cultures, higher pressures shorten life expectancies, whatever the starting age. Thus, the cut points between normal and abnormal are no longer shifted upward with age. Although age is often associated with higher pressures, that is no longer considered normal or inevitable.

B. Subclassifications within Essential Hypertension
1. Labile Hypertension
Labile hypertension is the presence, in one patient, of normal and abnormal pressures at different examinations. Everyone's pressure varies from time to time, but not all variations extend into the abnormal range.

2. Borderline Hypertension
Borderline hypertension is often called *high normal pressure* or *prehypertension*. This term refers to pressures in the gray zone between clearly normal and clearly abnormal levels. The Seventh Report of the Joint National Committee on Prevention, Detection, Evaluation, and Treatment of High Blood Pressure defined prehypertension as pressures in the range from 120 to 139/80 to 89 mm Hg. Although that range includes the population average blood pressure of 120/80 mm Hg, the Committee wanted to raise public awareness of the need to prevent the common progression of normal pressures into the abnormal range during life and to encourage healthier lifestyles in an attempt to prevent this progression.

3. Sustained (Fixed or Established) Hypertension
Sustained hypertension is the garden variety of hypertension, which is usually defined as blood pressure readings that exceed the appropriate norm during three consecutive measurements on 3 different days. The severity of fixed hypertension is defined by two broad ranges: stage 1 and stage 2. (This replaces

previous divisions into the three categories of mild, moderate, and severe.) Stage 1 denotes a systolic pressure between 140 and 159 mm Hg or a diastolic pressure between 90 and 99 mm Hg; stage 2 denotes a systolic pressure of at least 160 mm Hg or a diastolic pressure of at least 100 mm Hg. If a patient has a systolic pressure in one category and a diastolic pressure in another, then the higher category is used to characterize the situation (Box 15-3).

4. Isolated Systolic Hypertension
Isolated systolic hypertension exists when the systolic pressure is above normal but the diastolic pressure is normal. Two groups of hypertensive patients tend to have this condition: people with hyperkinetic or hyperdynamic hearts (sometimes caused by hyperthyroidism) and those elderly patients with sclerotic, noncompliant arteries. Isolated systolic hypertension has become extremely common as the population has aged.

5. Malignant Hypertension
Malignant hypertension is a medical emergency. Also called *accelerated hypertension*, this condition is marked by the following:
- Rapidly rising blood pressure
- Very high pressure readings, usually over 120 mm Hg diastolic (although there is no definite pressure cutoff between malignant and nonmalignant hypertension)
- Hemorrhages and exudates in the retina
- Neurologic changes that can vary in location and severity over time
- Red cells and protein in the urine, frequently with a history of reduced urine output
- Edema of the optic disk (papilledema), which reflects edema of the brain

II. EPIDEMIOLOGY OF HYPERTENSION

Although the actual cause of hypertension is not known, much is known about the epidemiology of essential hypertension. The frequency (prevalence) of hypertension is related to the following (Box 15-4):
1. *Age.* The prevalence of hypertension rises with age. At ages over 60 years old, 30% of white Americans

> **Box 15-3.** The Seventh Report of the Joint National Committee on Prevention, Detection, Evaluation, and Treatment of High Blood Pressure Classification of Blood Pressure Readings
>
> | | |
> |---|---|
> | <120/80 mm Hg | Normal |
> | 120/80 to 139/89 mm Hg | Prehypertension |
> | 140/90 to 159/99 mm Hg | Stage 1 hypertension |
> | ≥160/100 mm Hg | Stage 2 hypertension |

> **Box 15-4.** Epidemiologic Risk Factors for Hypertension
> - Old age
> - Male gender
> - African-American ethnicity
> - Obesity
> - High sodium intake
> - Low potassium intake
> - Genetic (family) predisposition
> - Excess alcohol intake

and 50% of African Americans have pressures of more than 165/95 mm Hg. The rate of increase in pressure with age is proportional to the starting pressure; relatively high pressures in early life predict very high pressures later in life. The pathogenesis of the age-related increase in pressure is complex. The elevated systolic component is related in part to the rigidity and noncompliance of the large arteries. The large arteries (also called the *capacitance arteries*) absorb some of the force and volume of blood ejected from the heart during systole. When these vessels become noncompliant, their buffering of systole is diminished, and more of the force generated by the heart is delivered directly downstream. In addition, noncompliant arteries in the periphery reflect the pressure wave that is generated by the heart back from the periphery toward the heart; when the vessels are stiff, this reflected wave travels so rapidly that it combines with the outgoing wave, thus adding to peak systolic pressure. Finally, some of the increase with age may be related to the simultaneous development of obesity. As mentioned later in this list, increased body fat leads to high arterial pressure, both systolic and diastolic.
2. *Gender.* Until the age of 45 years, more men than women have hypertension. After menopause, the relative immunity for females disappears. The cause of the gender difference is unknown.
3. *Ethnicity.* At all ages and in both sexes, a higher percentage of African Americans have hypertension than white Americans. However, this racial difference is not true worldwide. For example, it is not as pronounced in the rural areas of the predominantly black nations of Africa as it is in Western countries or in the major cities of Africa. The cause of the racial difference is unknown. However, there is evidence that favors roles for genetics, diet, and stress.
4. *Weight.* Obese people are more likely to be hypertensive than nonobese people. When obese people begin to eat less than their usual intake, their pressure falls much faster than their weight. This has led to hypotheses built around the hormones that increase when people eat, such as

insulin. Insulin may contribute to hypertension by its salt-retaining effect on the kidney and/or its trophic effect on blood vessels. There is a constellation of findings that includes hypertension and obesity called *syndrome X, metabolic syndrome,* or *dyslipidemic hypertension.* Hallmarks of this condition include hypertension, abdominal (visceral or upper-body) obesity, insulin resistance, low high-density lipoprotein cholesterol, high triglycerides, and subclinical inflammation (Box 15-5). Associated laboratory abnormalities include high plasminogen activation inhibitor-1 and uric acid levels. Another common sequela of obesity, obstructive sleep apnea, is one cause of hypertension, and it may account for part of the association between weight and pressure.

5. *Salt intake.* The incidence of hypertension correlates directly with sodium chloride intake when different groups of humans are compared with one another. Within groups, not every individual suffers a rise in pressure with increased salt intake. In other words, "salt sensitivity" is not universal. About 25% of Americans are "salt-sensitive" individuals, which means that their blood pressure rises significantly when they eat a high-salt diet and that it drops significantly when they eat very little salt. Salt sensitivity is a product of genetics (although which genes are involved is not known) and hormones (e.g., the salt-retaining steroid aldosterone).

6. *Potassium.* Blood pressure varies inversely with potassium intake. A low intake of potassium favors high blood pressure. Most food processing both adds sodium chloride and removes potassium, so many of the correlations of pressure with dietary sodium may actually be correlations with the absence of potassium. How dietary potassium could decrease pressure is unclear, although it is known that oral potassium supplements cause mild diuresis in humans.

7. *Genetics.* Hypertension clearly runs in families. Its association with race also points to a genetic basis. Roughly speaking, 50% of the average hypertensive patient's elevation in pressure is determined genetically, and 50% is determined environmentally; this has been demonstrated by studies of identical twins who are raised in different homes.

Arterial pressure is almost certainly determined by many different genes, but the identity of the most common genes is unknown. There are a few families with hypertension that is caused by mutations of genes that have been identified; this is called *monogenic* hypertension. All of the identified culprits are genes that directly or indirectly increase sodium retention by the kidney; they are described in Chapter 16.

8. *Alcohol intake* (Box 15-6). Alcohol is listed here as a contributor to essential hypertension, although it could also be considered a known cause of one form of secondary hypertension. When all dietary ingredients are examined for their relationship to blood pressure in large population studies, alcohol shows the best correlation, even better than salt. The mechanism by which alcohol raises blood pressure is not known.

9. *Other factors.* There are some weak correlations between hypertension and psychologic stress, uterine fibroids, and gout. With respect to the first item, most situations that are recognized as stressful raise the blood pressure acutely but not chronically. When stress raises blood pressure chronically, it is usually from internalized stresses that are difficult for an outside observer to detect, like those that strain marriages or worry the parents of difficult children.

III. EPIDEMIOLOGY OF HYPERTENSIVE SEQUELAE

It is clear that death and disease from cardiovascular pathology occur more frequently in hypertensive than normotensive individuals, and the incidence of the sequelae is proportional to the height of the pressure. It is equally clear that the harmful effects of hypertension on the cardiovascular system, like the pressure, are influenced by genetic and environmental factors apart from those that affect the pressure. For example, at any given pressure, African Americans suffer the ill effects of hypertension more than Caucasians. As another example, hypertensive patients in Japan have relatively more strokes as compared with Americans, whereas hypertensive patients in the United States have relatively more coronary artery disease.

In addition to genetics, factors that influence the dire outcomes that are associated with hypertension include cigarette smoking, high low-density lipoprotein and low high-density lipoprotein cholesterol levels, diabetes, and abdominal obesity (Box 15-7).

Box 15-5. Metabolic Syndrome Hallmarks

- Hypertension
- Insulin resistance
- Low high-density lipoprotein cholesterol level
- High triglyceride level
- Abdominal obesity

Box 15-6. Alcohol Intake

Excessive alcohol intake is more closely associated with hypertension than excessive salt intake.

- Genetic predisposition and ethnicity
- Cigarette smoking
- High low-density lipoprotein cholesterol level
- Low high-density lipoprotein cholesterol level
- Diabetes
- Abdominal obesity

Each major risk factor, including blood pressure, multiplies the risk. Thus, people with moderate hypertension are twice as likely as those with normal blood pressure to die of cardiovascular problems. If they also smoke cigarettes, they are four times as likely.

IV. EVOLUTION OF HYPERTENSION IN INDIVIDUALS

A. Early Stage (High Cardiac Output)
In its early stages (e.g., in patients who are 15 to 30 years old), hypertension is characterized by high cardiac output and normal peripheral resistance. This is the hemodynamic picture one would see after a dose of epinephrine, and increased β-adrenergic activity can be documented among many young hypertensive patients. They are labeled *hyperkinetic* or *hyperdynamic*. Hyperdynamic hypertensive patients are unusually sensitive to catecholamines' effects on the heart. They are also readily treated with β-blockers.

B. Adult Stage (High Peripheral Resistance)
Hypertensive patients who are 40 years old and older are hemodynamically characterized by high total peripheral vascular resistance and normal or below-normal cardiac output. The excess arterial resistance is unevenly distributed among vascular beds. A large part of the elevated resistance is in the renal vessels. The arteries of adult hypertensive patients are hyperresponsive to pressor substances such as norepinephrine and angiotensin. It is unknown whether this hypersensitivity is the cause of the hypertension, the result of vascular hypertrophy that follows increased pressure, or both the cause and the result.

C. Late Stage (Complications)
During the late stage of hypertension, peripheral resistance is high, cardiac output may be below normal, and the left ventricle is hypertrophied. The walls of the peripheral arteries are hypertrophic, noncompliant, and atherosclerotic; the density of capillaries in various beds is attenuated; and renal function is measurably decreased.

V. CAUSE OF ESSENTIAL HYPERTENSION

There are many theories about the cause of essential hypertension, and there are a few well-established facts.

A. Facts Concerning the Cause of Essential Hypertension
The well-established facts include the following three:
1. Many factors influence blood pressure. Pressure is the product of cardiac output and total peripheral arterial resistance (Box 15-8). Cardiac output and peripheral resistance are affected by many factors, including blood volume, oxygen and nutrient supplies, the contractile apparatus within the vascular smooth muscle and the myocardium, the metabolism that supports contraction, and a host of hormones and mediators, including catecholamines, angiotensin, prostaglandins, and nitric oxide and the signal transduction mechanisms that mediate their action. It is not yet clear whether any one element of this complex array is solely responsible for the added increment of pressure that distinguishes essential hypertension, but it is almost certain that many factors contribute to the sum total (normal plus abnormal) of arterial pressure.
2. Everyone seems to have a setpoint. Most important for understanding hypertension would be knowledge of the integration of all of the influences that can bear upon cardiac output and peripheral resistance. Each individual seems to have a setpoint of arterial blood pressure. This suggests the existence of a "barostat," by analogy with a thermostat. There must be a sensor somewhere in the circulation that is sensitive to the mean arterial pressure. From this sensor, signals must emanate that affect the various regulatory mechanisms. The sensor (barostat) uses both cardiac output and peripheral resistance to maintain the characteristic pressure, whether normal, high, or low. Possible barostat mechanisms are discussed later in this chapter.
3. Hypertension is a chronic disease. Many of the best-known regulatory reflex arcs that affect blood pressure, like those involving the carotid baroreceptors and the autonomic efferent impulses they control, are not candidates for the barostat because their effects are transient and wane (accommodate) within hours or days, whereas blood pressure is held at a steady level for years.

Pressure = Cardiac output × Total peripheral arterial resistance

B. Hypotheses Concerning the Cause of Essential Hypertension

1. A Functional Flaw in the Kidney

This is essentially the hypothesis of the late Professor Arthur Guyton at the University of Mississippi. It is based on the concept that arterial pressure in the kidney determines the net excretion of salt and water by a process called *pressure natriuresis*. The barostat is therefore envisioned to be in the kidney. Exactly how the kidney senses pressure is unknown, but the way sodium excretion affects pressure can be described as follows: if the kidney requires high pressure to excrete a given load of salt, then, at lower pressures, sodium and water are retained, and the blood volume rises. An increased blood volume returns more blood to the heart, thereby increasing cardiac output. The increased output is sensed by the peripheral vessels, which do not like increased flow and constrict in response (i.e., autoregulation of flow), and autoregulation increases arterial resistance. The reverse occurs when pressure rises: more salt and water are excreted, and that lowers blood volume, which reduces cardiac output. Sensing lesser flow, arterioles autoregulate by dilating, which reduces peripheral resistance. These congruent changes in cardiac output and peripheral resistance together affect blood pressure. This theory has been difficult to prove, because it is hard to measure the relationship between arterial pressure and natriuresis in humans. In animals with spontaneous hypertension, in isolated perfused kidneys, and in a few experiments on humans, the Guyton formulation has been shown to be operative. Although the dominance of pressure natriuresis in essential hypertension is debated, its importance in patients with severe renal disease is indisputable.

2. Too Much Vasoconstrictor Activity

As endogenous pressors have been discovered, each has been postulated as the cause of essential hypertension. The list includes norepinephrine, angiotensin, aldosterone, thromboxane, and endothelin (Box 15-9). It is clear that no one of these can be blamed for more than a small proportion of hypertension, but it is equally clear that they all contribute in some circumstances to pressure regulation.

Ironically, one fourth to one third of all patients with essential hypertension have low plasma-renin activity that responds sluggishly to standard stimuli such as upright posture. Despite the low plasma-renin activity in low-renin essential hypertension, plasma aldosterone is normal. It looks like there is another adrenal stimulus at work, but it is not currently known what it is. Theories involving pressors beg the question of the location of the barostat (i.e., the site that regulates the release of the pressors as a function of pressure).

3. Too Little Vasodilator Activity

As each new endogenous vasodilator has been discovered, it too has been considered as a player whose deficiency may lead to essential hypertension. This list includes dopamine, bradykinin, prostacyclin, atrial natriuretic peptide, and nitric oxide (Box 15-10). In some animal models, blockade of these vasodilators causes increased arterial pressure, but that does not prove their critical role in essential hypertension in humans. Again, where is the barostat that regulates release?

4. Hypersensitive Arterioles

One hallmark of hypertension is vascular smooth muscle hypertrophy and hyperresponsiveness. This suggests that the primary problem in essential hypertension is vascular supersensitivity. Exaggerated responsiveness may involve any element of the contractile mechanism or signal transduction, including receptors, intracellular calcium release, phospholipases and their products (e.g., inositol phosphates), and protein kinases. Trophic (growth) factors may participate by growing vascular smooth muscle. Although there is no doubt that peripheral blood vessels help to regulate blood pressure, there is no good evidence that they are the site of the barostat.

5. Faulty Ion Pumps and Channels

Because of their central role in the kidney and because every cell has a membrane loaded with them, ion pumps and channels get a lot of play in the hypertension literature. The existence of Liddle syndrome, in which hypertension is caused by excessively active sodium-reabsorbing channels in the kidney, encourages the view that flawed pumps can cause more common types of hypertension. In addition to their obvious role in sodium reabsorption,

Box 15-9. Endogenous Pressors
• Norepinephrine
• Angiotensin
• Aldosterone
• Thromboxane
• Endothelin

Box 15-10. Endogenous Vasodilators
• Dopamine
• Bradykinin
• Prostacyclin
• Atrial natriuretic peptide
• Nitric oxide

ion pumps affect transmembrane potential and intracellular ion concentrations, all of which play important roles in cell responsiveness and signal transduction. Therefore, they could be the basis of hyperresponsive vascular smooth muscles and defective pressure regulators.

6. A Defective Central Barostat

One durable theory of the cause of essential hypertension is probably the most difficult to test: the fault lies not in the kidneys or the vessels but in the brain. Specifically, there may be a cerebral setpoint that is too high. This raises two more questions: where in the brain is the barostat, and what set it so high? The best evidence for this hypothesis is the dramatic efficacy, in some patients, of antihypertensive drugs that only act on the brain and the hypotensive response of most patients to sleep, hypnosis, and operant conditioning.

VI. PATHOLOGIC CONSEQUENCES OF HYPERTENSION

Pathologic aspects of hypertension include those conditions that cause hypertension and the pathologic effects of hypertension. This section focuses on the effects.

The pathologic effects of prolonged hypertension are not equally distributed. Those organs that suffer the most are called *target organs*, and the damage that results is called *target organ damage*. The target organs that are most commonly damaged by hypertension are the peripheral arteries (including the aorta), the heart, the kidneys, the brain, and the retina (Box 15-11). These targets are damaged by a combination of the pressure itself, the decreased blood flow that results from vascular disease, and the direct cellular effects of mediators of growth and inflammation. Some of the mediators of growth and inflammation are the same as those that increase blood pressure (e.g., angiotensin, aldosterone). In hypertension, the vessels and heart synthesize more of themselves, which leads to hyperplasia and hypertrophy. These responses may be adaptive in some ways, accommodating to the high hydrostatic pressure, but they eventually become maladaptive and contribute to morbidity and mortality.

> **Box 15-11.** Target Organs that are Damaged by Hypertension
>
> - Peripheral arteries
> - Heart
> - Kidneys
> - Brain
> - Retinas

A. Effect of Hypertension on the Arteries
1. General
Hypertension induces changes in the arteries that are marked by the thickening of various layers. It almost looks like the vessels are arming themselves to withstand the stress of increased pressure. Note how the normal components of the vessel wall increase in hypertension: collagen, elastin, smooth muscle, and the cells of the intima. When the hypertension becomes malignant, elements of inflammation and necrosis are added to those of hypertrophy.

2. Large Arteries
Atherosclerosis is accelerated by hypertension, particularly in the aorta and its major branches and most importantly in the coronary, cerebral, and renal vessels. This is marked by the accretion of intimal cells infiltrated with smooth muscle and amorphous deposits of cholesterol. In the larger arteries and the branches of the aorta, elastic hyperplasia occurs, with reduplication of the internal elastic laminae. This reduplication causes decreased compliance (i.e., "stiff pipes"). The change is detected on physical examination by the palpable rigidity of the arteries. In the case of the brachial and radial arteries, they may become so stiff that they are still palpable when a blood pressure cuff placed proximal to them is inflated above arterial pressure (Osler's sign). As the arteries become stiffer, the pulse pressure widens, because the capacitance vessels cannot buffer the left ventricular impulse, which raises systolic pressure. In addition, they cannot propel much blood downstream during diastole, which lowers diastolic pressure.

3. Small Arteries and Arterioles
Hyperplastic arteriolosclerosis is the most common lesion in hypertension. It begins with the hypertrophy of the smooth muscle in the media, and it is accompanied by the reduplication of elastic laminae, the growth of new cells in the intima, and the deposition of collagen (Fig. 15-1A). These layers give rise to a microscopic appearance called *onion skin* (Fig. 15-1B). Hyperplastic arteriolosclerosis may severely limit flow and eventually result in the obliteration of the lumen. This would be detected on physical examination by the weakness or absence of the peripheral pulses. Hyaline sclerosis is another change in the vessels of hypertensive patients: the vessel wall becomes thickened with collagen.

4. Aneurysms
Hypertension predisposes patients to aneurysms and accelerates the growth of aneurysms. Abdominal aortic aneurysms are very dangerous. They may be palpated through the abdominal wall. When detected early, abdominal aortic aneurysms can be replaced by surgical grafts or reinforced with stents. The detection of aortic aneurysms begins with palpation and is

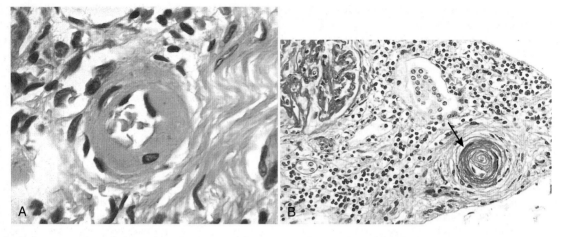

Figure 15-1. Vascular pathology in hypertension. *A,* Hyaline arteriolosclerosis. The arteriolar wall is hyalinized, and the lumen is markedly narrowed. *B,* Hyperplastic arteriolosclerosis (onion skinning) causing luminal obliteration *(arrow),* with secondary ischemic changes that are manifested by the wrinkling of the glomerular capillary vessels at the upper left (periodic acid–Schiff stain). *(From Kumar V, Abbas A, Fausto N:* Robbins & Cotran Pathologic Basis of Disease, *7th ed. Philadelphia, Saunders, 2005.)*

confirmed by imaging techniques like ultrasound. Wall stress is proportional to the radius of a hollow vessel (the law of LaPlace). Thus, the larger that aneurysms become, the more stress is placed on their walls and the more likely they are to rupture. In other words, bad things tend to progress more rapidly as the aneurysm grows larger (Fig. 15-2).

Hypertension aggravates the aortic lesion of cystic medionecrosis, which is the precursor of dissecting aortic aneurysm. After dissection has begun, it is accelerated by hypertension; this is a medical emergency. The new channel within the wall of the aorta distorts the openings to branches like the carotid, renal, and celiac arteries, often occluding them, with dire consequences. Unlike most other vascular changes, dissecting aortic aneurysms are almost always excruciatingly painful.

Hypertension predisposes individuals to the rupture of saccular cerebral aneurysms (often called *berry aneurysms*) in the circle of Willis and its branches at the base of the brain. Hypertension may or may not cause these little balloons, but it definitely promotes their rupture. These aneurysms are the leading cause of spontaneous subarachnoid hemorrhage. They may be detected before they rupture if they are large enough to cause neurologic changes from the pressure that they exert on a cranial nerve or the brain. Hypertension causes microaneurysms in small cerebral arteries; these are known as *Charcot–Bouchard aneurysms,* and they are discussed in further detail later in this chapter.

B. The Heart in Hypertension

Concentric left ventricular hypertrophy is the classic change in the hypertensive heart; this involves a thickening of the myocardium without any enlargement of the ventricular chamber (Fig. 15-3). The normal upper limit of heart weight for women is 350 to 375 g, and for men it is 375 to 400 g. The heart weight of patients with hypertensive heart disease is

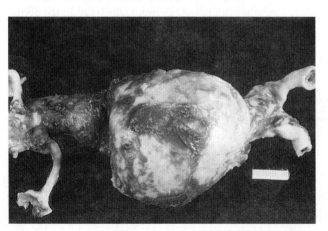

Figure 15-2. A large aortic aneurysm, often found in patients with longstanding hypertension, complicated by atherosclerosis. The leakage or rupture of these aneurysms is often fatal, but they can be treated if they are discovered early. *(From Silver MD, Gotlieb AI, Schoen FJ:* Cardiovascular Pathology. *Philadelphia, Churchill Livingstone, 2001.)*

blood supply predisposes these patients to ar-rhythmias.

4. Increased arterial pressure leads to the more rapid atherosclerosis of the coronary arteries and an increased incidence of myocardial infarction. Hypertension is an important risk factor for myocardial infarction at all ages and in both sexes.

5. Hypertensive heart disease may be the underlying condition in some cases of unexplained cardiomyopathy. When a previously hypertensive patient is seen for the first time with a dilated heart, heart failure may have reduced the blood pressure, so the patient has some hallmarks of left ventricular hypertrophy but normal pressure. When a diagnosis of idiopathic dilated cardiomyopathy is made, the cause may be previous longstanding hypertension.

6. Hypertension aggravates the poor function of a heart that is affected by any pathology. By demanding more work, high arterial pressure drives the heart to consume more oxygen and nutrients, and it may induce heart failure if the coronary circulation is compromised or the myocardium is diseased. Pressure work is more demanding of the heart than output work, consuming more oxygen as a result of the increased wall tension. High arterial pressure is a severe stress for a diseased heart, whatever the nature of the cardiac disease.

C. The Kidney in Hypertension

Hypertension causes the same vascular lesions in the kidneys that it causes in all peripheral vessels, but, in the kidney, this is called *nephrosclerosis*. The specific arteriolar lesions include those mentioned previously: hyperplastic arteriolosclerosis and hyaline sclerosis (see Fig. 15-1). When severe or longstanding, these changes occlude vessels and cause small infarcts of renal parenchyma. Grossly, kidneys with long-standing nephrosclerosis have a cobblestone appearance: a granular surface pitted by multiple areas of fibrotic scars between areas of healthy tissue.

D. The Kidney in Malignant Hypertension

Malignant hypertension is defined as a rapidly increasing pressure (also called *accelerated hypertension*) with severe, sudden damage to the brain, the eyes, and the kidneys. Several histologic manifestations of inflammation and necrosis characterize malignant hypertension and differentiate it from nonmalignant hypertension:

1. Fibrinoid necrosis of the arterioles occurs. *Fibrinoid* is a term that is given to an eosin-staining substance, fibrin, that is extruded into the blood vessel wall under the extreme pressures of malignant hypertension (Fig. 15-4).

2. In malignant hypertension, the glomeruli may show areas of thrombosis and areas of necrosis. The hemorrhages into the kidney parenchyma cause the spotty, red, "flea-bitten" appearance of the surface.

3. The arteriolar and arterial lesions result in the considerable narrowing of all vascular lumina, with ischemia and infarctions distal to the abnormal vessels.

The question of cause and effect enters into all discussions of renal pathology in hypertension, whether benign or malignant. Diseases of the renal arteries can cause hypertension either by impairing sodium excretion, by stimulating renin release, or both. In turn, the hypertension itself damages renal vessels, so there is a vicious cycle. In malignant hypertension, the vascular damage is acute, and renin release is a very important part of the pressure increase. In benign, essential hypertension, vascular damage is chronic, and its most important pressure-raising influence is sodium retention.

E. The Brain in Hypertension
1. Stroke

Hypertension predisposes individuals to strokes (cerebrovascular accidents) in several ways:

1. Hypertension accelerates atherosclerosis, damages the endothelium, and activates platelets. As a result, the diseased vessels may occlude,

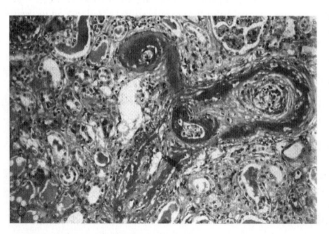

Figure 15-4. Fibrinoid necrosis of vessels in a kidney from a patient with malignant hypertension. The amorphous material is protein that has been extruded from vessels under high pressure. *(From Silver MD, Gotlieb AI, Schoen FJ:* Cardiovascular Pathology. *Philadelphia, Churchill Livingstone, 2001.)*

thereby causing infarction of the brain. These are called *thrombotic* or *ischemic strokes* as distinct from hemorrhagic strokes. The cerebrovascular consequences of hypertension account for 80% of all strokes.

2. Elevated pressure clearly increases the risk of the rupture of berry aneurysms of the circle of Willis.

3. Hypertension predisposes individuals to the rupture of tiny microaneurysms in small cerebral arteries, called *Charcot–Bouchard aneurysms.* These tiny aneurysms occur principally in small perforating arteries that are less than 1 mm in diameter, especially in the basal ganglia and cortical regions (lenticulostriate vessels). The aneurysms result from the loss of the media layer of the artery. Although the vessels are small, the rupture of these aneurysms can cause intracerebral hemorrhages larger than one might predict from the size of the aneurysm because the brain is so soft.

4. Hypertension may cause a series of changes in the brain that make it look like Swiss cheese at autopsy, with multiple fluid-filled cysts or lacunae. This is the end result of small infarctions caused by the occlusion of small vessels. The lacunae are commonly found in the region of the basal ganglia, and the fully developed condition is sometimes described as *multiple lacunar infarcts.*

Clinically, strokes are marked by one or more neurologic deficits, including a loss of motor and/or sensory function, and cognitive changes, which may be obvious or subtle.

2. Transient Ischemic Attack

Transient ischemic attacks (TIAs) are brief episodes of focal cerebral ischemia that cause the transient loss of some cerebral functions. Manifestations may include a brief loss of consciousness, slurred speech, visual changes, confusion, dizziness, weakness, numbness, or paresthesias. TIAs are probably caused by microemboli from arteriosclerotic plaques or platelet pileups in narrowed vessels. If a firm clot does not form, then the platelet aggregates can break up, and blood flow resumes. Hypertension aggravates TIAs, probably because the pressure damages the vascular endothelium and provides a site for platelet adhesion, or because the process that raises the pressure also causes arterial spasms so that platelet aggregates can plug the circulation.

F. The Retina in Hypertension

Arteries of the retina in hypertension show several changes, most of which are actually atherosclerotic in nature rather than pathognomonic for hypertension. These include the following:

1. The arterial wall thickens. During life, the hypertensive retina displays apparent narrowing of arterioles as viewed through the ophthalmoscope. This apparent narrowing of the vessel is illusory, because the red streak that is seen is actually the column of blood in the vessel rather than the vessel wall. In fact, the walls of the arterioles are thicker rather than thinner in hypertension. The thicker walls sometimes become more prominent and resemble silver or copper wire.

2. Thick-walled arteries carrying high pressure press on the softer veins where the two vessels cross each other. This causes arteriovenous nicking or crossing defects, which are seen on ophthalmoscope examination.

3. Hemorrhages into the retina result from ruptured arterioles.

4. Exudates, which are composed of partially reabsorbed hemorrhages, can be seen in the retina of some hypertensive patients. They can appear as cottony or waxy smudges on the retina.

5. The retinal sign that is the most characteristic of hypertension is arteriolar spasm (segmental narrowing). It gives the arteries the appearance of a string of sausages. Unlike the other changes, arteriolar spasm is not seen with atherosclerosis alone.

6. In malignant hypertension, there is edema of the retina and of the optic nerve that leads to papilledema.

G. Causes of Death

The most common causes of death related to hypertension are as follows:

1. Congestive heart failure: 45%
2. Coronary insufficiency or infarction: 35%
3. Cerebral vascular accident: 15%
4. Chronic kidney disease: 5%

VII. MANAGEMENT OF THE PATIENT WITH ESSENTIAL HYPERTENSION

The cause of essential hypertension is unknown, so therapy cannot be as specific as the selection of an antibiotic on the basis of a blood culture. However, the damage from hypertension comes from the pressure itself (aided and abetted by other risk factors, of course). Therefore, the goal of therapy for most hypertensive patients is simply to lower the arterial pressure to a level that is less damaging to the target organs. Not knowing the specific cause of the patient's blood pressure, one aims to lower the overall pressure by undermining one or more normal mechanisms of arterial pressure maintenance (Box 15-13). Some of those mechanisms may be hyperactive in some patients, but that is not the presumption on which therapy is based.

A. Lifestyle Changes

Epidemiologic data show that changes in lifestyle can lower blood pressure if they modify those habits and characteristics, such as a large body habitus, that are associated with elevated blood pressure. Lifestyle

changes are commonly called *nonpharmacologic therapies.* These helpful changes include reduced alcohol, calorie, and salt intake as well as aerobic exercise. Reducing alcohol intake to two drinks per day or fewer lowers the blood pressure of most people who consume more than two drinks per day. Reducing calorie intake to reduce body fat, especially visceral fat, lowers the blood pressure of most obese patients. Aerobic exercise can lower the pressure of sedentary hypertensive patients, partly by reducing body fat but also by other mechanisms that affect autonomic nervous traffic. These approaches are difficult for most patients to follow, and they are difficult to maintain. Adherence to therapy, whether nonpharmacologic or pharmacologic, is the key to the successful treatment of hypertension, and the required duration of therapy is lifelong.

B. Therapies That Influence Salt and Water Balance

A principal prop that supports arterial blood pressure is intravascular volume, because it directly affects cardiac output. Intravascular fluid is essentially saltwater. When salt is excreted in amounts that are larger than intake or when intake is very low, intravascular volume is reduced, cardiac output decreases, and blood pressure drops. The two therapeutic modalities that directly affect salt and water balance are dietary salt restriction and diuretics (Box 15-14). Reductions in salt intake have more or less efficacy based on the salt sensitivity of the patient. Depending on how much salt it takes to raise the blood pressure and how much of an elevation is considered significant, about 25% to 50% of humans are considered to be salt sensitive. Almost every hypertensive person can

enjoy some drop in pressure if he or she restricts his or her salt intake sufficiently, but it may require Spartan restraint.

Diuretics attack sodium-reabsorbing mechanisms in the renal tubules. Thiazide diuretics are the most commonly used, and they inhibit reabsorption by the distal tubule. Loop diuretics do the analogous thing in the ascending limb of the loop of Henle. Potassium-sparing diuretics inhibit the aldosterone-sensitive sites in the distal tubule. Each of these classes inhibits a different sodium pump. All of these are effective hypotensive agents, and diuretics are the cornerstone of therapy for most hypertensive patients.

One characteristic of therapy with dietary salt restriction and diuretic drugs is the compensatory mechanisms that they induce, because the body has many ways to maintain circulation when intravascular volume shrinks. The renin–angiotensin–aldosterone system (RAAS) is stimulated, and if intravascular volume is shrunken sufficiently, then the sympathetic nervous system may be activated. These counterregulatory mechanisms limit the efficacy of volume-directed therapy. They also suggest two good ways to amplify the response to diuretics: adding drugs that block the RAAS or adding those that block the sympathetic nervous system.

The most worrisome side effect of diuretics is the disturbance of blood electrolyte concentrations, especially potassium, which is lowered by thiazides and loop diuretics and elevated by potassium-sparing drugs. The combination of a thiazide and a potassium-sparing diuretic offers added diuretic efficacy while avoiding potassium depletion or accumulation.

C. Drugs That Block the Renin–Angiotensin–Aldosterone System

There is always some renin in the circulation, some angiotensin being formed, and some aldosterone being secreted. This tonic activity of the RAAS participates in the support of arterial blood pressure to a greater or lesser degree in virtually all humans. It is least important in low-renin essential hypertension and in subjects who eat large amounts of salt, and it is most important in those who eat little salt or who are being treated with diuretics. Drugs that block this system are effective for lowering arterial blood pressure in most humans to a degree that is proportional to the activity of the RAAS (Box 15-15).

One class of RAAS blockers inhibits the angiotensin-converting enzyme (ACE); these drugs have names that end in -pril. Another class blocks the type 1 receptor for angiotensin II; these drug names end in -sartan. As suggested in the preceding section, these agents are extremely effective when added to diuretics.

As a result of angiotensin's ability to protect glomerular filtration by stimulating efferent glomerular arterial constriction, a reduction in angiotensin production or the blockade of its receptor can aggravate renal functional impairment, thereby further reducing glomerular filtration in patients in whom it is already compromised by dehydration or glomerular disease. Therefore, the most worrisome side effect of these drugs is renal impairment. This reduction in glomerular filtration, by decreasing injury to the glomerular capillaries, serves to preserve renal function over the long term in patients with several glomerular diseases, including diabetic nephropathy. The glomerular filtration drops initially, but it deteriorates more slowly, so the kidneys of treated patients outlast those of untreated patients.

Because angiotensin is a principal stimulus of aldosterone release, ACE inhibitors and angiotensin receptor blockers (ARBs) lower aldosterone levels. Reduced aldosterone and reduced glomerular filtration can both predispose patients to potassium accumulation, and that is another feared side effect of these blockers. Aldosterone antagonists are inhibitors of the second effector hormone of the RAAS, but they are usually considered as members of the class of potassium-sparing diuretics. They, too, can cause dangerous increases in plasma potassium.

The newest inhibitor of the RAAS is a direct inhibitor of the enzyme renin that is marketed under the name Aliskerin (Novartis, Cambridge, MA). Clinical experience with this drug is limited at the present time.

D. Drugs That Block the Autonomic Nervous System

Activation of the sympathetic nervous system increases cardiac output (β_1 adrenergic effect) and total peripheral arterial resistance (α_1 adrenergic effect), thus clearly supporting blood pressure in both normal and hypertensive patients. Drugs that block this system at the level of the brain, the nerve terminals, or the receptors undermine a key support and lower arterial pressure (Box 15-16).

The easiest antiadrenergic agents to understand are the α_1-blockers, which have names that end

in -azosin. They block the vasoconstrictive effects of norepinephrine. The principal side effect of α-blockers is postural hypotension; patients may feel faint when they stand up.

β-Blockers, with names that end in -olol, reduce cardiac output and renin release. β-Blockers exert subtle effects on the central nervous system, and those central effects contribute to the drugs' hypotensive efficacy. However, effects on the brain also account for an annoying side effect, which is the flattening of emotional experience. By blocking β_2 receptors, nonspecific β-blockers impair bronchodilation and predispose patients to worsening asthma and other bronchospastic conditions. Some β-blockers are relatively specific for β_1 receptors and cause fewer pulmonary side effects.

The most difficult autonomic blockers to understand are the α_2-agonists. These drugs, which were originally designed to constrict nasal mucosal arterioles, act in the central nervous system to reduce sympathetic output from the brain, thereby lowering both cardiac output and peripheral arterial resistance. They also inhibit norepinephrine synthesis by sympathetic nerves. The most commonly used agent of this class is clonidine. (α-Methyldopa, rarely used these days, also belongs to this class.) These drugs are most predictably effective when hypertension clearly comes from the brain (e.g., in alcohol withdrawal); they are also effective in many other situations.

Among the oldest antihypertensive drugs is reserpine. It interferes with sympathetic nervous function by depleting nerve terminals of their catecholamine transmitters. This action in the basal ganglia results in parkinsonism, which is a side effect of high doses of reserpine. High doses can also cause emotional changes, including depression.

E. Drugs That Block Vascular Smooth Muscle Contraction

One common pathway of pressure regulation in adult hypertensive patients is peripheral arterial resistance; the effector organ is vascular smooth muscle surrounding resistance arterioles. Relaxation of vascular smooth muscle is the mechanism of many antihypertensive drugs. Some vasodilators were described previously; they work by blocking vasoconstrictors like norepinephrine and angiotensin. The following paragraphs describe vasodilators that act directly on vascular smooth muscle (Box 15-17).

Box 15-16. Drugs That Block the Autonomic Nervous System

Drugs that block the autonomic nervous system include α_1-blockers, β-blockers, and α_2-agonists.

Box 15-17. Drugs That Dilate Resistance Vessels

Drugs that dilate resistance vessels include calcium-channel blockers, nitrovasodilators, hydralazine, and potassium-channel agonists

Calcium-channel blockers, especially those of the dihydropyridine class (with names that end in -ipine, such as amlodipine and nifedipine), block the entry of calcium into vascular smooth muscle cells. They work primarily on arteries rather than veins, and they work better when the smooth muscle is contracting than when it is idle, so they lower hypertensive pressure better than they lower normal pressure.

Calcium-channel blockers of the nondihydropyridine class (i.e., diltiazem and verapamil) combine moderate vasodilation with direct cardiac effects that lower cardiac output, thereby reducing both factors that determine arterial pressure.

Another class of vasodilators is called *nitrovasodilators*, because they are transformed into nitric oxide, which is a potent but short-lived vasodilator. Nitric oxide stimulates the formation of cyclic guanosine monophosphate, the universal intracellular relaxant. The most powerful vasodilator is sodium nitroprusside, which decays in plasma into nitric oxide and cyanide. It is available only for intravenous use, and its use is limited by the effects of cyanide, so it is administered primarily in hypertensive crises. The oldest nitrovasodilator drugs are the nitrates, like nitroglycerine. They work better on veins than on arteries, so their role in the treatment of hypertension is less prominent than their role in unloading the heart in patients with angina pectoris.

Hydralazine is a potent arterial vasodilator with an unknown cellular mechanism of action. It has the salubrious quality of selectively dilating renal arteries so that renal perfusion pressure is less affected by the drop in systemic pressure than it is when other antihypertensive drugs are administered. Hydralazine is frequently used when hypertensive patients with impaired renal function experience a fall in glomerular filtration every time their pressures are lowered. It is also a drug of choice for pregnancy-associated hypertension.

Vascular smooth muscles contract when their membranes are depolarized. Anything that increases membrane potential makes it harder to depolarize, harder to activate the cell, and harder for vascular smooth muscle to contract. Drugs that increase potassium permeability through potassium channels hyperpolarize the membrane potential; in arterioles, they act as vasodilators. The best-known potassium-channel agonist/vasodilator is minoxidil. Its value as an antihypertensive is limited by its propensity to increase the growth of hair. Because of that side effect, it is seldom prescribed for women, but, in its topical formulation, (e.g., Rogaine [Minoxidil; McNEIL-PPC, Inc., Fort Washington, PA]), it can ameliorate baldness.

Vasodilators as a class have side effects that are attributable to their actions on arterial smooth muscle. By lowering pressure suddenly, vasodilators activate compensatory physiologic mechanisms that try to restore pressure to pretreatment levels. One response is the activation of the RAAS with consequent salt and water retention. Another compensatory reflex arc triggers sympathetic nervous system activity, thereby causing increased heart rate and palpitations. Excessive vasodilation can cause an excessive fall in pressure, especially when patients rise from a lying to a standing posture (i.e., postural or orthostatic hypotension). There may also be facial flushing and headache.

F. Combinations of Antihypertensive Therapies

As mentioned at the beginning of this therapy section, the treatment of hypertension is directed at lowering arterial pressure by eroding the known supports of pressure, whether they are the etiologic culprits in individual patients or not. When any one pressure support is attacked, the others tend to compensate and to attenuate the pressure drop. For that reason, combinations of drugs are often used (Box 15-18).

The most consistent compensatory mechanism involves increased sodium and water retention by the kidney when arterial pressure is lowered. Diuretics block this compensatory effect, and they are often combined with drugs from all other classes. Vasodilators trigger increased activity of the sympathetic nervous system and the RAAS and also increased sodium retention by the kidney, so they are often combined with β-blockers, ACE inhibitors, and/or diuretics. ACE inhibitors or ARBs lower pressure by mechanisms that are distinct from those affected by calcium-channel blockers, so RAAS blockers and calcium-channel blockers are often used together. Many of these combinations are conveniently formulated in single tablets that contain two drugs. The efficacy of these combination tablets can be assumed, because pharmaceutical companies only invest in the tortuous process of US Food and Drug Administration approval when they are sure that the combination works.

The selection of therapy for individual patients is somewhat of an art. One of the best guides is the existence of comorbidities. For example, the presence of prostatism in a hypertensive man would encourage the use of an α-adrenergic blocker to address both conditions. The existence of diabetes would encourage the use of ACE inhibitors or ARBs, and so on. To obtain the optimum correction of hypertension, trial

---

Box 15-18. Common Drug Combinations

- A thiazide + a potassium-sparing diuretic
- A thiazide + an angiotensin-converting enzyme inhibitor or an angiotensin receptor blocker
- A calcium-channel blocker + an angiotensin-converting enzyme inhibitor or an angiotensin receptor blocker
- A vasodilator + a β-blocker

and error is usually needed. Conventional wisdom calls for the use of multiple drugs, each in modest doses, to avoid troublesome side effects.

Clinical Case

A 45-year-old African-American man presents to a neighborhood urgent care office complaining of a nasal discharge. Routine measurements by office staff reveal a blood pressure of 160/105 mm Hg, a heart rate of 82 beats per minute, a temperature of 98.6°F, a respiratory rate of 20 breaths per minute, a height of 69 inches, and a weight of 210 lbs (body mass index, 31). He reports no known previous elevations in his blood pressure, but he has rarely sought medical care as an adult. He has no symptoms that are indicative of renal or cardiac disease. His family history includes a father who died of "heart disease" at the age of 55 years and a mother who died of a stroke at the age of 60 years. He is recently divorced, eats most of his meals at restaurants, enjoys 2 to 4 drinks with dinner, and smokes one pack of cigarettes every 2 days.

The examining clinician records a blood pressure of 156/102 mm Hg. The patient's nasal turbinates are pale and swollen with clear exudate. The ophthalmoscopic examination is unremarkable. No carotid bruits are heard, and the lungs are clear. No cardiac murmurs are heard, but there is a barely audible presystolic S_4 at the apex. The abdominal examination is unremarkable except for obesity. The extremities have barely palpable pulses below the femorals, a trace of pitting edema over the lower half of both tibias, and normal deep tendon reflexes.

A complete blood count is normal. Urinalysis shows trace proteinuria. Chest x-ray reveals a "boot-shaped" heart and no evidence of pulmonary disease.

A tentative diagnosis of seasonal allergic rhinitis is made, and a prescription is written for a nonsedating antihistamine. The patient is advised to find a primary care clinician for further evaluation of his blood pressure and other risk factors.

What is the likely underlying cause of the elevated blood pressure, if it can be established that the pressure if chronically elevated (i.e., "fixed")? What is the differential diagnosis?

Odds favor a diagnosis of essential hypertension. This diagnosis is based on probability and on the absence of any obvious cause of secondary hypertension. The differential diagnosis would need to include diseases of the kidneys, such as renal artery stenosis. Other diseases that cause hypertension include primary hyperaldosteronism, obesity, alcoholism, and obstructive sleep apnea.

Which features of the patient's habits, history, heritage, and habitus might be contributing to his elevated pressure? Which are contributing to his risk of cardiovascular disease?

Alcohol intake of three drinks per day or more and obesity can both contribute to elevated pressure. Genetics most probably predisposes this man to hypertension; his ethnicity carries increased risk, and his family history is strongly suspicious of hypertension. It is likely that his diet is rich in salt. Contributing to his risk of cardiovascular disease are his smoking habit, his sedentary lifestyle, and the probable high salt and saturated fat content of restaurant meals.

What should this patient's primary caregiver recommend as nonpharmacologic approaches to use to improve his cardiovascular health?

Fewer cigarettes, fewer calories, fewer alcoholic beverages, more aerobic exercise would all improve the patient's life expectancy.

If drugs were necessary to lower this patient's blood pressure, which ones should be used?

A conservative approach to drug therapy would begin with a thiazide diuretic; an ACE inhibitor could then be added, if needed. For a third drug, a calcium-channel blocker would be logical. Side effects would need to be addressed as they arose, but they would likely include hypokalemia from the diuretic and cough from the ACE inhibitor. Hypokalemia can be ameliorated by adding potassium supplements or a potassium-sparing diuretic, and cough can be circumvented by switching from an ACE inhibitor to an ARB.

Suggested Readings

Messerli FH, Williams B, Ritz E: Essential hypertension. *Lancet* 18:370:591-603, 2007.

Flack JM, Peters R, Shafi T, et al: Prevention of hypertension and its complications: Theoretical basis and guidelines for treatment. *J Am Soc Nephrol* 14(7 Suppl 2):S92-S98, 2003.

Israili ZH, Hernández-Hernández R, Valasco M: The future of antihypertensive treatment. *Am J Ther* 14:121-134, 2007.

The Joint National Committee: The Seventh Report of the Joint National Committee on Prevention, Detection, Evaluation, and Treatment of High Blood Pressure (JNC 7) (website): www.nhlbi.nih.gov/guidelines/hypertension/. Accessed March 3, 2007.

PRACTICE QUESTIONS

1. Which one of the following demographic and historic characteristics of a hypertensive patient helps the physician to decide whether to search further for a curable cause of hypertension?

   A. Gender
   B. Race
   C. Age at onset
   D. Occupation

2. Which of the following statements about the heart in chronic hypertension is correct?

   A. There is concentric hypertrophy of the left ventricle that may be difficult to detect by x-ray.
   B. There is concentric hypertrophy of the left ventricle that appears on x-ray as a widened cardiac silhouette.

   C. There is both left and right ventricular hypertrophy that is difficult to see on x-ray.
   D. The early changes of hypertension in the heart are marked by increased numbers of cells.

3. Which of the following drugs lowers the circulating level of angiotensin II and aldosterone?

   A. Dihydropyridine calcium channel blockers (e.g., nifedipine)
   B. Thiazide diuretics (e.g., hydrochlorothiazide)
   C. Angiotensin-converting enzyme inhibitors (e.g., lisinopril)
   D. Direct vasodilators (e.g., hydralazine)

Secondary Hypertension

16

Kristin M. Lyerly
Theodore L. Goodfriend

OUTLINE
  I. Introduction
 II. Conditions That Cause Hypertension
    A. Renal (Kidney) Diseases
    B. Estrogens and Eclampsia/Preeclampsia
    C. Coarctation of the Aorta
    D. Aldosteronism
    E. Pheochromocytoma
    F. Sleep Apnea
    G. Alcohol
    H. Brain Lesions
    I. Cushing Syndrome
    J. Drugs
    K. Endocrine Disorders
III. Conclusions

Objectives

- Understand the distinction between secondary hypertension and essential hypertension.
- Be familiar with the following causes of secondary hypertension and when to suspect them:
  - Renal artery stenosis
  - Estrogens and eclampsia/preeclampsia
  - Coarctation of the aorta
  - Aldosteronism
  - Pheochromocytoma
  - Sleep apnea
  - Alcoholism
  - Brain lesions
  - Cushing syndrome
  - Drugs
  - Endocrine diseases

Clinical Case

A 42-year-old married woman presents to the emergency department with a headache. The headache began abruptly while she was watching television. She reports that she was watching a television program that was marked by violence, and she noted that her heart was pounding, which she attributed to the drama. Her history is unremarkable, although she has been bothered by a cold for the past week. Her recent physical examinations have been reported to her as completely normal. She has never been pregnant, but she has missed one period this month, which she thinks could be the result of menopause. She works as a secretary, uses alcohol occasionally, and has smoked one pack of cigarettes per day for 20 years. On physical examination, the patient's blood pressure is found to be 165/110 mm Hg.

Her heart rate is 80 beats per minute. She is 5 feet and 2 inches tall, and she weighs 140 lbs. She is noted to be sweating profusely. Examinations of the head and eyes and a quick neurologic examination are negative except for swollen nasal turbinates. Examination of the heart reveals a grade 3/6 systolic murmur. The remainder of the physical examination is normal. Laboratory tests show a normal blood count, but the urinalysis shows 1+ protein. Blood chemistry shows normal serum electrolytes, creatinine, and blood urea nitrogen levels. A pregnancy test is positive.

What aspects of the history suggest the presence of secondary hypertension as opposed to essential hypertension? Which aspects of the patient's clinical picture favor a renal cause of hypertension? Which aspects of the patient's picture favor or argue against preeclampsia? Could the patient have a coarctation of the aorta? Is pheochromocytoma a plausible explanation for the patient's hypertension? What other forms of secondary hypertension should be considered for this patient?

I. INTRODUCTION

Although most human hypertension arises from unknown causes and is called *essential hypertension* or *primary hypertension*, about 5% to 10% of cases arise from a known cause. These are, as a group, called *secondary hypertension* (Box 16-1). These cases can be managed more intelligently and sometimes cured if they are identified.

It may be helpful to use a mnemonic aid to remember the classical causes of secondary hypertension, such as *RECAPS ABCDE* (Box 16-2). In this

chapter, each type of secondary hypertension will be considered in the sequence dictated by that mnemonic.

II. CONDITIONS THAT CAUSE HYPERTENSION

A. Renal (Kidney) Diseases

The kidneys are powerful regulators of blood pressure over the short and long term, and diseases of the kidneys are often accompanied by hypertension. There are at least two ways in which the kidneys can raise blood pressure:

1. *Via the retention of excess sodium and water, which increases blood volume.* This may be considered *volume-dependent hypertension.*
2. *Via the secretion of greater than normal amounts of renin.* This is the principal way in which renal artery stenosis raises pressure.

Volume-dependent hypertension arises when the kidney fails to excrete all of the sodium that has been ingested. The retained sodium and water raise blood pressure by increasing extracellular (including intravascular) volume. Increased blood volume raises cardiac output by increasing the volume of blood that is returned to the heart. Increased cardiac output sends more blood through the arteries. Some arteries constrict to maintain a constant blood flow (autoregulation of flow), and that constriction raises peripheral resistance. Thus, increased blood volume raises both determinants of blood pressure: cardiac output and peripheral resistance.

First, there is a discussion of the second broad category of kidney diseases that cause hypertension: arterial

diseases that reduce blood flow to the juxtaglomerular apparatus and stimulate renin release. These arterial diseases are all subsumed under the term *renal vascular disease,* of which the most easily recognized is *renal artery stenosis.*

1. Renal Artery Stenosis

A. Pathophysiology

Renal artery stenosis is the cause of hypertension in 1% to 3% of all patients with elevated blood pressure. To cause hypertension (i.e., to be physiologically or hemodynamically significant), the lesion must have just the right effect on blood flow. Renin is released from the kidneys only when renal blood flow is reduced significantly. Slight stenosis fails to release renin because it does not diminish renal blood flow. Blood flow is dependent on the total resistance offered by all of the vessels in the kidney, and most of the total resistance is contributed by the small arterioles within the kidneys. As stenosis of the main renal artery gets progressively tighter, the downstream renal arterioles autoregulate (dilate) in a compensatory effort to maintain constant flow. As a result, total vascular resistance in the kidney remains constant, flow is maintained at a constant level, and there is no stimulus for renin release. Only when autoregulatory capacity is exceeded will further stenosis of the renal artery cause renin release.

There is a limit to the degree of stenosis that causes renin release, because excessive stenosis kills the kidney, and dead kidneys produce no renin. There must be precisely the right amount of stenosis to cause renin release and hypertension. Thus, there are more patients with some degree of narrowing of their renal arteries than there are patients who have hypertension as a result (Box 16-3).

There are many possible pathologic causes of stenosis:

- Atherosclerosis is the most common pathologic process that narrows the renal arteries. Atherosclerosis usually affects more than one site in the renal circulation (Fig. 16-1). Sometimes, the plaque is in the aorta itself, and it impinges on the origin of the renal artery for a so-called "ostial" stenosis.
- Especially common in young to middle-aged females is fibromuscular dysplasia. Spotty overgrowth of connective tissue in the arterial media causes a series of alternating constrictions and dilations that look like a string of beads in an arteriogram.

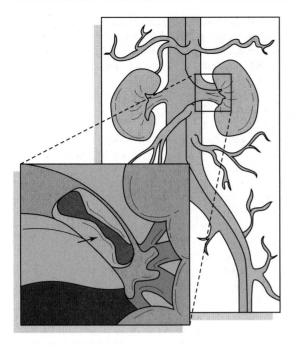

Figure 16-1. A visual representation of renal artery stenosis from atherosclerosis. *(Modified from Pacific Vascular:* About vascular diseases *(website): http://www.pacificvascular.com/ vasculardisease.htm. Accessed March 3, 2008.)*

- In children, one cause of renal artery stenosis is neurofibromatosis.
- Renal circulation can also be impaired by emboli, inflammatory lesions, extrinsic pressure from tumors or cysts, kinking after transplantation, or trauma.

The ischemic kidney produces an excessive amount of renin, an enzyme that releases angiotensin I from its precursor, angiotensinogen. Angiotensin I is converted into angiotensin II by the action of the converting enzyme. Angiotensin II is a potent vasoconstrictor and raises blood pressure. It also stimulates the adrenal release of aldosterone with the resultant retention of sodium. This further increases extracellular fluid volume and increases the blood pressure.

B. Diagnosis

Clues from the clinical history that point toward renal artery stenosis include the following:

- Onset of hypertension before the age of 25 years or after the age of 50 years, especially when there is no family history of hypertension
- A rapid worsening of preexisting hypertension, especially when there is vascular disease elsewhere
- Very severe hypertension requiring multiple drugs (among severely hypertensive patients, the proportion that have renal artery stenosis is as high as 30%)

- Coexistence of severe hypertension and impaired renal function, especially if there is a rapid worsening of function when arterial pressure is reduced by a drug
- Recurrent pulmonary edema without obvious cardiac cause (i.e., "flash pulmonary edema")

On physical examination, abdominal bruits are valuable clues to renal artery stenosis. Renal artery bruits are best heard in the midline, just below the xiphoid process. The classic bruits of renal artery stenosis are audible in both systole and diastole. (Irregularities of the abdominal aorta usually cause bruits in systole only.) However, only about 40% of patients with renal artery stenosis have a characteristic bruit.

Several screening and diagnostic tests are available to assist with the diagnosis of renal artery stenosis and to identify the relatively rare patient with renal hypertension among the large number of patients with essential hypertension.

Arteriography (injecting contrast into the aorta or renal arteries) is the diagnostic gold standard for anatomic renal artery stenosis (Fig. 16-2). On the downside, it is invasive, it requires the injection of contrast media that can damage the kidneys, and it does not perfectly differentiate between simple anatomic stenosis and hypertension-inducing ("functionally significant") stenosis. For example, among normotensive people who were more than 50 years old who were studied for other reasons, 30% had anatomic stenosis of their renal arteries. Obviously, most anatomic stenotic lesions do not cause hypertension. There are additional clues on the arteriogram that suggest that the stenosis is significant:

- A reduction of diameter by 75% or more
- A decrease in the overall length of the affected kidney that is caused by reduced blood flow, making it at least 1.5 cm shorter than the normal side
- The presence of collateral vessels supplying the parenchyma of the kidney on the stenotic side
- Poststenotic dilatation, which is a widening of the vessel distal to the stenosis, as if the narrow vessel were trying to expand itself

Magnetic resonance angiography is probably the most widely used screening test for renal artery stenosis. Although its powers of resolution are less than those of an arteriogram, magnetic resonance angiography can visualize most of the vessels that would be accessible to repair. The contrast medium, gadolinium, presents less danger to renal function than the iodine-rich contrast media that are usually used in classic arteriograms. Magnetic resonance angiographs also reveal information about the renal parenchyma.

Computed tomography (CT) angiography uses the same contrast as arteriography, but the injection is through a peripheral vein. This is a test of growing prominence because of its convenience, but the contrast medium could be toxic to the kidney, so this test

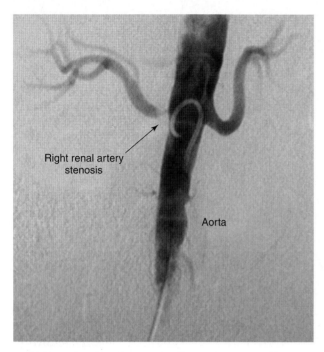

Figure 16-2. Arteriogram showing stenosis of the right renal artery with some poststenotic dilatation. The catheter delivering the contrast medium is curled in the aorta. *(From Surowiec SM, Davies MG: Endoluminal therapy for renal artery ostial stenosis, VascularWeb (online resource provided by the Society for Vascular Surgery): www .vascularweb.org/professionals/Clinical_Information/ Images_Cases/Renal_stenosis_Davies.html. Accessed March 3, 2008.)*

Right renal artery stenosis

Aorta

is only done in patients with reasonable overall kidney function.

Ultrasonography, which is also called *duplex sonography* or *duplex ultrasonography*, is noninvasive and devoid of radiation exposure. It uses two physical modalities: sound waves for echolocation of the artery and Doppler techniques to measure flow. It is especially useful for patients with impaired kidney function because it requires no contrast medium. By measuring the increase in the velocity of blood as it passes through a stenosis, the Doppler transducer indicates the degree of narrowing, which is a clue to the functional significance of the stenosis. The success of sonography depends on the size of the vessel and the ability of the technician to visualize it through intestinal gas, feces, and fat. Obese subjects are very difficult to examine by this technique.

Renograms (also called *kidney scans* or *scintirenography*) are nuclear medicine procedures in which injected, radiolabeled compounds are taken up from the blood by the kidney and excreted into the urine. While in the kidney parenchyma, these compounds emit radioactivity that is detected by an assembly of Geiger counters that together construct a picture. Because renogram dyes can be very radioactive and can be composed of atoms like technetium rather than iodine, very little potentially nephrotoxic substance is injected. This makes the procedure safer for patients who are sensitive to iodine or who have impaired renal function. In renograms, one looks for the delayed appearance, as well as the delayed washout, of the dye from the kidney with the stenosed artery. The images one retrieves from nuclear medicine

scans have less resolution than other kinds of images, so renograms are poor for localizing stenoses of small arteries.

Because the renin–angiotensin system may compensate for a stenosed renal artery, the administration of angiotensin-converting enzyme (ACE) inhibitors can reveal physiologically significant stenoses. Physiologically significant stenoses are indicated by the worsening of the renogram image of the kidney with the stenosed artery after ACE inhibitor administration (Fig. 16-3).

Renal vein renin measurement is useful to assess the significance of renal artery stenosis. If the stenosis is contributing to elevated blood pressure, it is probably stimulating the release of renin, certainly more than the normal kidney. To perform this test, a radiologist threads a catheter from the femoral vein up the inferior vena cava to the level of the renal veins. The catheter tip is inserted sequentially into each of the renal veins, and some venous blood is collected for the measurement of renin activity. If there is a suspicious stenosis and the venous renin from that side is high, there is a high likelihood that the stenosis is physiologically significant. In addition, plasma samples are taken from the vena cava below and above the renal veins. This allows for an estimate of the overall contribution of the stenosis to the systemic renin levels. There may well be a shrunken kidney with very little blood flow, but each drop of blood could be rich in renin. That kidney would be sick, but it would not necessarily be affecting systemic renin levels or blood pressure.

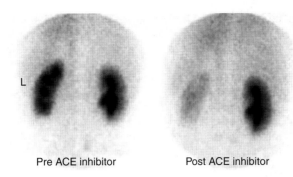

L

Pre ACE inhibitor   Post ACE inhibitor

✱ See errata

Figure 16-3. Renograms before and after the use of an angiotensin-converting enzyme (ACE) inhibitor. These images were created by injecting a radioactive compound filtered at the glomerulus and recording radioactivity by an array of detectors over the abdomen. The first image was made before giving the patient any medication; the image on the right was from a study on the same patient after the administration of an ACE inhibitor. ✱ The first study appears normal, but the second shows ~~less~~ *more* radioactivity over the ~~left~~ R kidney. This indicates that the left kidney depends on the local release of renin and the formation of angiotensin to sustain glomerular filtration. After ACE inhibitor administration, this function of locally released angiotensin is lost, so less radioactive dye is filtered into the renal tubules. *(Data from Wenting GJ, Tan-Tjiong HL, Derkx MHM, et al: Split renal function after captopril in unilateral renal artery stenosis.* Br Med J (Clin Res Ed) *288:886–890, 1984.)*

C. Treatment

The most widely used treatment of renal artery stenosis is balloon dilatation, which is also called *percutaneous transluminal renal angioplasty.* A double-lumen catheter with a balloon near the tip is inserted into a femoral artery and threaded up to the renal artery. If the lumen is sufficiently large to permit catheter passage, it is placed in the stenotic area, and the balloon is inflated to squash the occluding plaque. After ballooning the plaque, the interventional radiologist inserts a stent, which is a hollow sleeve that holds the vessel open.

Surgery is often preferred when the stenosis is at the aortic root of the renal arteries (ostial), when the artery is so stenotic that a balloon cannot be passed through the lesion, or when the stenosis is beyond the reach of balloon catheters. The vascular surgeon can remove the stenosis and reconstruct the artery, insert a graft, or connect the kidney to a healthy vessel like the splenic artery.

Medical therapy for the high blood pressure of renal artery stenosis is possible as a result of powerful antihypertensive drugs, but there are caveats. It is worth recognizing the survival value of systemic hypertension in renal artery stenosis: it ensures renal perfusion beyond the stenosis. Any intervention that lowers blood pressure without relieving the stenosis will threaten the function of the downstream kidney. Therefore, the first rule of drug management is to monitor renal function. ACE inhibitors and angiotensin receptor blockers work extremely well to lower blood pressure in unilateral renal artery stenosis. In one study, 80% of patients with unilateral renal artery stenosis were successfully treated with ACE inhibitors. However, ACE inhibitors and angiotensin receptor blockers are contraindicated in bilateral stenosis because they block the angiotensin-mediated efferent glomerular arteriolar vasoconstriction that maintains glomerular filtration (Box 16-4). If both kidneys are using the renin–angiotensin–aldosterone system to compensate for their stenoses, total renal function will be compromised by drugs that block it (Box 16-5).

Box 16-4. Renal Artery Stenosis Therapy

Angiotensin-converting enzyme inhibitors and angiotensin receptor blockers work well for the treatment of unilateral renal artery stenosis, but they are contraindicated for bilateral renal artery stenosis.

Box 16-5. Renal Artery Stenosis Summary

- Renal artery stenosis causes 1% to 3% of hypertension cases.
- Physiologically significant blockage is suggested by a 75% to 90% decrease in renal artery diameter.
- Atherosclerosis is the most common cause of renal artery stenosis in adults.
- Noninvasive screening tests for renal artery stenosis include magnetic resonance angiography, computed tomography angiography, captopril renogram, and duplex ultrasonography. The gold standard imaging technique is contrast arteriography.
- The presence of a stenosis does not prove that it causes hypertension.
- Treatment can be with drugs, intra-arterial balloon, or vascular surgery.

2. Other Kidney Diseases that Cause Hypertension

Acute kidney diseases (e.g., glomerulonephritis) are often accompanied by damage to the juxtaglomerular cells. Such damage causes the juxtaglomerular cells to release renin into the circulation at levels that are either frankly elevated or inappropriately high for the patient's blood volume. Hypertension usually subsides as the acute disease clears.

Chronic kidney disease that results from conditions such as glomerulonephritis, nephrosclerosis (diffuse atherosclerosis of the very small renal arteries), and diabetic nephropathy commonly causes a higher incidence of hypertension than is seen in a normal population of the same age. The pathogenesis of hypertension with these diseases is not always clear. A defect in sodium excretion may be too subtle to be detected by current methods, and the release of renin may only be high relative to the level of volume expansion. Complicating the picture is the fact that hypertension from any cause results in disease of the renal arterioles, which is called *nephrosclerosis*. This creates a vicious cycle of worsening hypertension and worsening kidney function. Therefore, it is almost impossible to tell how much kidney disease is the cause of, and how much is the effect of, hypertension.

When chronic kidney disease causes hypertension, it is usually because the kidneys fail to excrete normal amounts of sodium. Arterial pressure in this condition is dramatically modified by sodium intake (i.e., volume-dependent hypertension). These patients have pressure elevations that respond dramatically to changes in blood volume effected by hemodialysis using an artificial kidney or diuresis induced by drugs.

Whatever initiates hypertension, when it is severe enough (e.g., in malignant hypertension), it can acutely damage the kidney parenchymal cells, including the arterioles and the juxtaglomerular apparatus. This can start another vicious cycle of events that includes sodium retention, worsening hypertension, and excessive release of renin.

Renin-secreting tumors, specifically hemangiopericytomas or Wilms' tumors, may cause hypertension by releasing huge quantities of renin into the blood. These tumors are usually seen in children. Liddle syndrome is a genetically determined abnormality of the epithelial sodium channels in the cortical collecting duct of the nephron that are held in the "open" position by an amino acid replacement. This results in excessive sodium reabsorption, volume expansion, and hypertension. The clinical picture resembles that of hyperaldosteronism, but aldosterone levels are very low.

B. Estrogens and Eclampsia/Preeclampsia

1. Estrogens

Exogenous estrogen in high doses may cause hypertension. The magnitude of the rise in arterial pressure depends on the dose of estrogen and on individual susceptibility to its effects. About 5% of all women taking large doses of estrogen become clinically hypertensive during the first year. Older age, obesity, and a family history of hypertension raise the odds of becoming hypertensive with estrogens. At most estrogen doses in use today, blood pressure is not elevated by the hormone in the vast majority of women. Contraceptive pills containing progestational steroids alone are not as likely to induce hypertension as those that contain estrogens. Progesterone is a diuretic; it interferes with aldosterone action (Box 16-6).

The mechanism of estrogen-induced hypertension is complex. Some known factors include the following:

- Estrogens have sodium-retaining effects on the kidney.
- Estrogens stimulate the hepatic synthesis of renin substrate, thereby raising its concentration in the plasma, with a consequent increase in plasma renin activity and angiotensin production.
- Estrogens potentiate the actions of catecholamines, in part by inducing an increased number of catecholamine receptors.

2. Eclampsia/Preeclampsia

A. Pregnancy and Blood Pressure

The average woman who becomes pregnant experiences a fall in arterial blood pressure (5 to 15 mm Hg) by the second trimester. This drop is caused in part by a reduction in total peripheral vascular resistance and in part by the aldosterone-antagonizing property of progesterone. The blood pressure usually returns to baseline before delivery.

Hypertensive disorders during pregnancy are divided into two large classes: chronic (preexisting) hypertension in a pregnant woman, and hypertension that occurs as a result of pregnancy. In this chapter, the focus will be on the latter, a syndrome called *preeclampsia/eclampsia*.

B. Preeclampsia

Preeclampsia is characterized in its classic form by the following triad:

1. *Hypertension.* A diastolic pressure of more than 90 mm Hg is significant at any time, especially

---

Box 16-6. Estrogen Summary

- Exogenous estrogen in high doses raises blood pressure in a minority of people. At the doses seen in today's oral contraceptives or postmenopausal hormone replacement therapy, estrogen rarely causes hypertension.
- Additional risk factors for estrogen-induced hypertension include advanced age, obesity, and a family history of hypertension.

before the 38th week. Another criterion is a pressure during pregnancy that is 30/15 mm Hg higher than prepregnant pressures.

2. *Proteinuria.* Significant proteinuria is defined as excretion of more than 300 mg per 24 hours. Another criterion is a urine protein concentration of 100 mg/dl in two specimens. Using a dipstick, 1+ is suspicious and 2+ is very suspicious of significant proteinuria.

3. *Edema.* Edema of the lower extremities occurs in 80% of all pregnancies, and it is not by itself a predictor of dire outcome; it is usually caused by the pressure of the uterus on the veins that drain the legs. A better indicator of preeclampsia is edema of the hands or face (i.e., generalized edema), which almost never occurs without underlying pathology.

Essential hypertension usually shows itself early during gestation, whereas preeclampsia usually arises after the 20th week of pregnancy. Differentiating essential hypertension from preeclampsia can be aided by looking for signs of longstanding hypertension, such as left ventricular hypertrophy. Proteinuria can occur in essential hypertension or in renal diseases that cause hypertension, and trace proteinuria is not uncommon during pregnancy, so its presence is not pathognomonic of preeclampsia. By contrast, generalized edema is rare in essential hypertension, so its presence strongly suggests preeclampsia (Box 16-7).

C. Eclampsia

Eclampsia is the most severe hypertensive complication of pregnancy. It is a combination of preeclampsia (hypertension, proteinuria, edema) and convulsions, coma, or death. It is usually superimposed on preeclampsia during or just after labor; in only 25% of cases do convulsions begin before labor.

The only thing that is known for sure about the cause of preeclampsia/eclampsia is that it arises in the uteroplacental unit. Delivery is followed by a reversal of the disease, although hypertension and the risk of convulsions persist for a few hours after delivery. Postulated causes include the underperfusion of the uteroplacental unit with the release of factors that constrict vessels and/or increase sensitivity to pressors. There may be reduced production of vasodilators like nitric oxide and dilating eicosanoids. The search for the humoral mechanisms of eclampsia is one of the ongoing treasure hunts of modern medical science.

The fetal complications of eclampsia/preeclampsia include prematurity, low birth weight, deformity, and death. It is the leading cause of prematurity; one in three premature deliveries is marked by preeclampsia. All of these consequences are probably caused by the underperfusion of the fetoplacental unit.

Box 16-7. Preeclampsia Summary

- Hypertension during pregnancy may be either preexisting and possibly aggravated by the pregnancy or new and caused by the pregnancy.
- Preeclampsia is characterized by hypertension, proteinuria, and edema, and it is usually noted after the 20th week of pregnancy.

C. Coarctation of the Aorta

Coarctations (also called *coarcts*) are fibrous narrowings of the aorta. They represent the failure of a segment of the aorta to grow along with the rest, so they become more and more noticeable as childhood progresses (Fig. 16-4). The constriction can occur anywhere along the aorta. The closer a constriction is to the heart, the more dangerous it is. Coarctation is often accompanied by other congenital defects.

1. Pathogenesis of Hypertension in Coarctation

Pressure is elevated in arteries that are proximal to the constriction. Although this may seem easy to explain by the constriction alone, there are actually two contributors to the hypertension of coarctation: one is the resistance imposed by the narrowing itself, and the other is humoral. In an animal model of coarctation, systemic arterial pressure was normalized by transplanting the kidneys to a region that is proximal to the constriction. This and other evidence strongly suggest that one contributor to hypertension in coarctation is the activation of the renin–angiotensin–aldosterone system. In other words, coarctation proximal to the renal arteries is a form of bilateral renal artery stenosis.

2. Clinical Findings and Diagnostic Tests

It is incumbent on clinicians to look for coarcts in all young patients with hypertension and in anyone with elevated blood pressure and paradoxically low blood

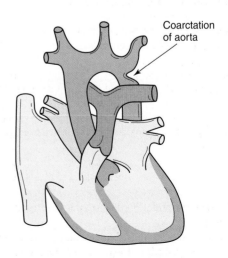

Coarctation of aorta

Figure 16-4. Diagram of a coarctation of the aorta.

pressure in the legs. The cardinal finding in coarctation is a lower measured blood pressure in the legs as compared with the arms (Box 16-8). Normally, blood pressure in the thighs is slightly higher than the pressure in the arms because the vessels are larger and offer less resistance and also because there is a reflected pressure wave from the periphery that meets the forward pressure wave in the femoral arteries. Neither reason applies when there is a major obstruction to flow in the proximal aorta, so thigh pressure is lower than arm pressure. Some patients may give a history of pain or weakness in the legs during exercise that reflects the impaired blood flow to the lower extremities. The pulse felt in the ankle may be delayed as compared with the wrist. A systolic murmur caused by the coarctation itself can be heard over the chest (both front and back), and it is usually loudest between the scapulae. As described in the following, there are usually large intercostal arteries, and these can cause bruits in the chest wall.

The chest x-ray often shows two diagnostic features: a dent along the left side of the aortic shadow, between a bulge above the constriction and poststenotic dilatation below, and notching of the undersides of the ribs, caused by enlarged intercostal vessels that act as collaterals carrying blood around the coarct. CT scanning and magnetic resonance imaging (MRI) yield unmistakable images of coarcts. Doppler sonograms not only confirm the diagnosis of coarctation, they can also define the degree of narrowing (Box 16-9).

D. Aldosteronism

Increased plasma levels of the salt-retaining steroid aldosterone can raise blood pressure. Aldosterone is the principal mineralocorticoid that is secreted by the adrenal cortex. Increased aldosterone is responsible for somewhere between 1% and 15% of all hypertension. Secondary hyperaldosteronism is a condition in which renin and angiotensin are increased by kidney disease or by contracted plasma volume. The increased renin, angiotensin, and aldosterone may be appropriate, and they may serve to compensate for

stresses like dehydration or hemorrhage. In those situations, the blood pressure may not be elevated. In primary hyperaldosteronism, the increased secretion of aldosterone is inappropriate, pathogenic, and not accompanied by elevated renin; in fact, renin levels are very low, and blood pressure is usually high (Box 16-10).

1. Pathogenesis of Primary Hyperaldosteronism

Aldosterone stimulates sodium reabsorption by the distal tubule of the nephron. At the same time, aldosterone stimulates the excretion of potassium ions and protons. One can think of this as a "trade" of sodium for potassium and hydrogen. The reabsorbed ("retained") sodium brings water with it into the extracellular space and thereby increases the blood volume, the cardiac output, and, ultimately, the peripheral resistance.

Although primary aldosteronism starts as a volume-expanded state, sodium retention and volume expansion reach a limit despite increased levels of aldosterone. This is called *mineralocorticoid escape* (Box 16-11). Escape is the result of the high arterial pressure that increases pressure natriuresis and the release of atrial natriuretic peptide from the heart in response to intravascular volume expansion. Pressure natriuresis and atrial natriuretic peptide flush more sodium down the tubule than the distal site can completely reabsorb, no matter how much aldosterone is present. At that point, sodium intake and output are equal, no net retention occurs, and the extracellular volume reaches equilibrium at its expanded level.

Even after "escape," potassium loss continues in cases of hyperaldosteronism. As the increased flux of sodium flows down the tubule under the impulse of high arterial pressure and natriuretic peptide, the distal site, which is driven by aldosterone, heroically excretes potassium while trying to catch every last sodium ion. The tubular flow of sodium is too great to allow net sodium retention, but potassium loss continues. Therefore, one laboratory finding in hyperaldosteronism is a low serum potassium level. If the patient is not ingesting much sodium, there is less

---

Box 16-8. Coarctation of the Aorta: Clinical Finding

In coarctation of the aorta, the blood pressure in the legs is lower than the blood pressure in the arms.

Box 16-9. Coarctation of the Aorta: Summary

- Coarctation of the aorta is a congenital narrowing of the aorta.
- CT and MRI techniques detect coarctations.

Box 16-10. Primary Hyperaldosteronism

In primary hyperaldosteronism, renin secretion is suppressed by salt retention, fluid retention, and the expansion of the blood volume.

Box 16-11. Mineralocorticoid Escape

Elevated aldosterone → increased extracellular volume → new equilibrium established (No further sodium retention occurs.)

"trade" for potassium, and the serum potassium level will be normal.

The two most common causes of primary hyperaldosteronism are adrenal adenomas and adrenal hyperplasia. Adrenal adenomas arising in cells of the glomerulosa zone (i.e., Conn syndrome) are benign tumors that usually occur in one gland only. Adrenal hyperplasia (idiopathic hyperaldosteronism) involves the glomerulosa zones of both glands.

2. Clinical Findings in Primary Hyperaldosteronism

Clinical features of primary hyperaldosteronism include hypertension that may be quite severe, with levels as high as 280/140 mm Hg and weakness and muscle cramps that can be attributed to a loss of potassium. Perhaps surprisingly, there is no edema in primary hyperaldosteronism, probably as a result of the mineralocorticoid escape explained previously (Box 16-12).

Characteristic laboratory findings in primary hyperaldosteronism include high blood and urine aldosterone, low plasma renin activity (despite upright posture, salt restriction, and diuretics, all of which should raise renin), high urine potassium excretion, low serum potassium, and metabolic alkalosis (Box 16-13). The alkalosis can be explained by the excretion of both potassium and protons into the urine under the influence of high aldosterone. The most sensitive laboratory test is the ratio of plasma aldosterone to plasma renin activity, which is called the *aldosterone/renin ratio*. This ratio is not very specific for primary aldosteronism, but when it is normal (below 20), the diagnosis is unlikely. Because primary aldosteronism is defined as the excessive secretion of aldosterone despite low renin activity, another important test is the persistence of high plasma aldosterone levels and high urinary aldosterone excretion despite high salt intake. The high salt intake will suppress renin (and angiotensin) levels even further, so persistent high residual aldosterone secretion will strongly suggest primary aldosteronism.

Other tests to use in suspicious cases with abnormal laboratory findings include MRI and CT scanning of the abdomen, which can localize adenomas as small as 0.7 cm, and ^{131}iodocholesterol scans. The scan uses a radioactive derivative of cholesterol that localizes in the adrenal gland. It is taken up as if it were cholesterol, ready to be transformed into steroids, but it cannot be metabolized, so it stays in the gland, emitting detectable radioactivity. Because iodocholesterol is a false precursor of all steroids, it could localize in all zones of the adrenal cortex. To focus on aldosterone-producing tissue, it is necessary to suppress the activity of the fasciculata and reticularis zones with an adrenocorticotropic-hormone (ACTH)–suppressing dose of exogenous glucocorticoid (e.g., dexamethasone). Aldosteronomas continue to take up steroid precursors whether they are stimulated or not. Continuous uptake by *both* adrenal glands, despite the presence of dexamethasone, suggests hyperplasia rather than tumor (Boxes 16-14 and 16-15).

Other less common adrenal causes of hypertension include congenital adrenal hyperplasias that are caused by defects in the enzymes that catalyze cortisol synthesis. Defective cortisol synthesis results in a lack of suppression of ACTH. Increased ACTH in the presence of defective steroid synthesis causes the increased production of cortisol precursors, some of which are salt retaining and lead to high blood pressure. This condition responds to treatment with a synthetic steroid that turns off pituitary ACTH production, thereby decreasing production of the abnormal steroids.

Box 16-12. Clinical Features of Hyperaldosteronism

- Hypertension
- Weakness
- Muscle cramps
- No edema

Box 16-13. Laboratory Findings in Hyperaldosteronism

- High blood and urine aldosterone levels
- Low plasma renin levels
- High urine potassium excretion
- Low serum potassium levels
- Alkalosis

Box 16-14. Summary of the Diagnostic Scheme for Checking for Primary Hyperaldosteronism

- Is the serum potassium low? This could be the result of excessive excretion or inadequate intake. Check the urine potassium.
- Is the urine potassium high? If so, draw plasma to measure the aldosterone and renin levels to assess for hyperaldosteronism. If not, consider low potassium intake.
- Is the plasma aldosterone level high and the renin activity low? If so, primary hyperaldosteronism is a possibility. Repeat measurements after an infusion of saline or after the ingestion of large amounts of salt. Normal adrenal glands suppress secretion with salt; adenomas and hyperplastic adrenal glands do not. If these results are consistent with adenoma, look for it with imaging techniques.
- Perform imaging with the use of magnetic resonance imaging, computed tomography scanning, or ^{131}iodocholesterol scanning.

E. Pheochromocytoma

Pheochromocytomas are tumors that secrete pressor catecholamines. Pheochromocytomas are the cause in less than 1 in 1000 cases of elevated blood pressure, but they are a well-studied example of curable hypertension.

1. Pathogenesis of Pheochromocytoma

Pheochromocytomas are derived from the chromaffin cells of the sympathetic nervous system and other cells of neural crest origin. Most pheochromocytomas arise in the adrenal medulla (70% to 90%), some arise in the abdominal sympathetic chains, and rare ones occur in the bladder, neck, chest, ear, eye, and other places. In the rare instance of a malignant pheochromocytoma, bone is a common site of metastasis. The elevated blood pressure in pheochromocytoma results from the ability of catecholamines to increase the two classic components of pressure: cardiac output and peripheral resistance. However, the level of the pressure does not correlate precisely with the measured levels of catecholamines in the blood or urine.

2. Clinical Findings in Pheochromocytoma

Because catecholamines are secreted from pheochromocytomas in bursts, the syndrome is characterized by paroxysms of one or more of the following: hypertension, headache, sweating, alpitations, pallor, nervousness, tremor, nausea, and vomiting. The triad of headache, sweating, and palpitations in a hypertensive patient strongly suggests pheochromocytoma (Box 16-16). Paroxysms usually last 15 minutes or less and rarely longer than an hour, but the hypertension is more persistent and may be constant.

The best laboratory tests for pheochromocytoma measure catecholamines or their metabolites in 24-hour urine samples (Box 16-17). The greatest sensitivity and specificity is obtained from a measurement of total metanephrines in a 24-hour collection. Another good test is the measurement of plasma catecholamines. Something as trivial as a needlestick will cause a burst of catecholamine release from normal adrenals, so blood should be drawn through an indwelling needle or catheter that has been inserted 30 minutes or more before the sample is taken. Measurement of urinary vanillylmandelic acid, which is the end product of catecholamine metabolism, is a screening test that can be falsely elevated by foods that contain vanilla, for example. It is the least specific test for pheochromocytoma.

Pheochromocytomas in the abdomen are most easily visualized by CT scanning or MRI. Of the two, MRI is probably preferable, because it requires no contrast medium and no radioactivity, and it can be used in pregnant women. Finally, the nature of the chromaffin tumor cells is such that its MRI image contrasts with surrounding tissue, which is helpful for making a diagnosis. Scintigraphy (nuclear scanning) is a very useful technique for picking up pheochromocytomas in odd places. An analogue of a catecholamine precursor (radioiodinated metaiodobenzylguanidine) is injected. It localizes primarily in chromaffin cell tumors, and it can be used to scan the whole body. It is also useful for finding recurrences or metastases (Box 16-18).

F. Sleep Apnea

Sleep apnea is a subset of a larger class of disorders called *sleep-disordered breathing*, which includes snoring at one end of the spectrum and repeated episodes

of totally obstructed breathing at the other. There is a remarkable epidemiologic coincidence between sleep apnea and hypertension. In some surveys as many as 50% of people with sleep apnea also had hypertension. Along with hypertension, people with sleep apnea have an unusually high incidence of many cardiovascular diseases.

The best guess about the pathogenesis of hypertension in patients with sleep apnea involves the periodic stimulation of the sympathetic nervous system by the recurrent episodes of hypoxia. Whatever the mechanism, it is short lived, because one can observe a rapid decline of blood pressure when the airway obstruction is treated by the application of a positive-pressure mask. The usual device applies positive pressure to the nose (nasal continuous positive airway pressure). When it works, this treatment can cure hypertension in a day. This is probably the most readily cured cause of hypertension. The key to diagnosis is a high index of suspicion: does your obese hypertensive patient make so much noise at night that it wakes up his or her spouse? Is he or she excessively sleepy during the day? If so, a sleep study should be performed. Obstructive sleep apnea is becoming more prevalent as our population becomes more obese (Box 16-19).

G. Alcohol

In worldwide epidemiologic surveys, there is a stronger correlation of blood pressure with alcohol than with salt intake. The effect is dose related; the dose of alcohol that is the most widely quoted as the threshold is three standard drinks per day. The mechanism of alcohol's hypertensive effect is unknown. Abstention from alcohol is an excellent treatment for hypertension among those who abuse the beverage, but it is not easy to achieve or sustain. Alternatively, reducing alcohol intake to two drinks per day may be effective, and it is easier to sustain (Box 16-20).

> **Box 16-19.** Sleep Apnea Summary
>
> - Up to 50% of people with sleep apnea have concomitant hypertension.
> - Sleep apnea is readily treated, and treatment often reverses hypertension.

> **Box 16-20.** Alcohol Summary
>
> - Drinking more than three alcoholic beverages per day has been shown to have a bigger impact on hypertension than salt intake.
> - Patients who are experiencing alcohol withdrawal may have an alarming burst of elevated blood pressure that resembles a pheochromocytoma attack.

H. Brain Lesions

Brain injury or brain tumors that result in increased intracranial pressure may elevate the blood pressure. The increased intracranial pressure deprives the cerebral pressor centers of blood, which triggers powerful discharges of sympathetic nerves. The hallmarks are a slow pulse, a high systolic pressure, and a wide pulse pressure.

I. Cushing Syndrome

Cushing syndrome is caused by excessive amounts of glucocorticoids (Box 16-21). The natural endogenous glucocorticoid is the adrenal hormone hydrocortisone (cortisol). Cushing syndrome may originate in adrenal tumors that make cortisol or in pituitary tumors that make ACTH, but it is actually more commonly caused by exogenous glucocorticoid medications like prednisone or dexamethasone, which are used for their antiinflammatory or immune-suppressing activities. The syndrome includes a long list of signs and symptoms, such as moon face, acne, purple striae on the abdomen, diabetes mellitus, and high blood pressure. The hypertension is probably a result of the intrinsic mineralocorticoid activity of the steroids, which is only manifested when large amounts of the glucocorticoids are present.

J. Drugs

Sympathomimetic drugs mimic or stimulate the adrenergic nervous system, and they can raise blood pressure to alarming heights, particularly in hypertensive patients. Many hypertensive patients are sensitive to all pressors, probably because they have hypertrophied vascular smooth muscles. Sympathomimetics include common nasal decongestants, appetite suppressants with amphetamine-like actions, stimulants prescribed for attention-deficit/hyperactivity disorder, and bronchodilators (Box 16-22).

Cocaine can elevate blood pressure by a direct vasoconstrictive effect. In combination with its ability to constrict coronary vessels and to contribute to arrhythmia, the pressor effects of cocaine have undoubtedly contributed to some well-publicized deaths among famous abusers of this drug.

Ergotamine is a vasoconstrictor that is used for the treatment of migraine. In susceptible patients, it can also elevate blood pressure.

Cyclosporine is an immunosuppressant drug that has revolutionized transplantation medicine. Unfortunately, it is a potentially hypertensive agent, and it

---

> **Box 16-21.** Cushing Syndrome
>
> Cushing syndrome is the result of excessive glucocorticoids.

Box 16-22. Drugs That Can Cause Hypertension

- Sympathomimetics (including nasal decongestants, appetite suppressants with amphetamine-like actions, and bronchodilators)
- Cocaine
- Ergot alkaloids
- Cyclosporine
- Monoamine oxidase inhibitors in the presence of foods that are high in tyramine
- Erythropoietin
- Glucocorticoids

Box 16-23. Endocrine Disorders

Hyperthyroidism: Systolic pressure is increased, whereas diastolic pressure is decreased.
Hypothyroidism: Diastolic pressure is increased.

can damage the kidneys. These untoward effects are dose-related. Hypertension is a common dose-related side effect that is caused by sympathetic activation, reduced production of vasodilators, and increased production of endothelin (a vasoconstrictor). Cyclosporine has renal toxicity; at high doses, the drug causes tubular damage and interstitial fibrosis, and it can lead to chronic kidney disease.

One of the best-recognized drug interactions in all clinical pharmacology is the potentially dangerous interaction between antidepressant monoamine oxidase inhibitors and either sympathomimetic agents or foods containing catecholamine precursors like tyramine (which is found in cheese and other foods). The monoamine oxidase inhibitors block the normal degradation pathway for the sympathomimetics, and the combination can result in dramatic bursts of hypertension. This interaction prompted the common warning to patients taking drugs like pargyline to avoid red wines and ripe cheeses.

Recombinant human erythropoietin is an extremely valuable component of the management of anemia among patients with chronic kidney disease. Some patients with chronic kidney disease who receive erythropoietin eventually develop hypertension. The pathogenesis of hypertension with erythropoietin is not clear, but it may in part be caused by an increase in hemoglobin and red blood cell volume.

K. Endocrine Disorders
In addition to hyperaldosteronism and Cushing syndrome, there are other endocrine disorders that can cause hypertension.

Hyperthyroidism can cause a classic example of "high-output hypertension." Cardiac output and pulse rate are increased. Peripheral resistance is decreased in most cases of hyperthyroidism; the skin feels warm because thermoregulators vasodilate the skin vessels to maximize heat loss. Systolic pressure is increased, whereas the diastolic pressure is decreased. Thyroxine affects the adrenergic receptors and potentiates circulating catecholamines. Most of the visible signs of hyperthyroidism, including hypertension, are the result

of this adrenergic action, which can be blocked by β-adrenergic blockers such as propranolol.

About 20% of patients with hypothyroidism have diastolic hypertension. Unlike patients with hyperthyroidism, those with hypothyroidism have increased peripheral resistance. They look like patients trying to retain their body heat and fluids. During treatment with a thyroid hormone, their vessels and kidneys open up (Box 16-23).

III. CONCLUSIONS

This chapter has described diseases and conditions that are often accompanied by hypertension. Because the hypertension is only one result of the disease, these elevations in blood pressure are called *secondary*. Hypertension is often the first manifestation of these diseases that comes to a clinician's attention. Because the treatment of the underlying disease can reduce blood pressure and because the disease merits attention for its own sake, every person who presents with hypertension should be examined with an eye toward finding or ruling out these conditions. The mnemonic *RECAPS ABCDE* is just one tool to use as part of this process.

Clinical Case
A 42-year-old married woman presents to the emergency department with a headache. The headache began abruptly while she was watching television. She reports that she was watching a television program that was marked by violence, and she noted that her heart was pounding, which she attributed to the drama. Her history is unremarkable, although she has been bothered by a cold for the past week. Her recent physical examinations have been reported to her as completely normal. She has never been pregnant, but she has missed one period this month, which she thinks could be the result of menopause. She works as a secretary, uses alcohol occasionally, and has smoked one pack of cigarettes per day for 20 years. On physical examination, the patient's blood pressure is found to be 165/110 mm Hg. Her heart rate is 80 beats per minute. She is 5 feet and 2 inches tall, and she weighs 140 lbs. She is noted to be sweating profusely. Examinations of the head and eyes and a quick neurologic examination are negative except for swollen nasal turbinates. Examination of the heart reveals a grade 3/6 systolic murmur. The remainder of the physical examination is normal. Laboratory tests show a normal blood count, but the

urinalysis shows 1+ protein. Blood chemistry shows normal serum electrolytes, creatinine, and blood urea nitrogen levels. A pregnancy test is positive.

What aspects of the history suggest the presence of secondary hypertension as opposed to essential hypertension?

The abrupt onset of hypertension, the level of the pressure, and the absence of a family history of hypertension all suggest that this is not the usual essential hypertension.

Which aspects of the patient's clinical picture favor a renal cause of hypertension?

The presence of proteinuria is suggestive, but anyone with a pressure as high as this patient's can have proteinuria as a consequence of hypertension. The absence of casts and cells in the urine sediment argues against an acute kidney disease. Renal artery stenosis is possible, especially the type caused by fibromuscular dysplasia, which is a relatively common cause in women. Normal serum creatinine and blood urea nitrogen levels do not rule out renal artery stenosis because the action of angiotensin and the function of the unaffected kidney would compensate for the stenosis of one renal artery or branch.

Which aspects of the patient's picture favor or argue against preeclampsia?

The patient reports missing only one menstrual period, so she is still in the early stages of her pregnancy; preeclampsia usually raises the blood pressure after 20 weeks of pregnancy. The presence of proteinuria favors preeclampsia, but the absence of edema argues against it. This pregnancy is considered high risk as a result of the blood pressure level, regardless of its cause.

Could the patient have a coarctation of the aorta?

Probably not, because she has lived 42 years without displaying a noticeable increase in pressure. The systolic murmur must have another explanation.

Is pheochromocytoma a plausible explanation for the patient's hypertension?

Pheochromocytoma is certainly possible, because the patient displays all three characteristic symptoms: headache, palpitations, and perspiration. All three are common in patients without a pheochromocytoma, and the measurement of urinary metanephrines is warranted.

What other forms of secondary hypertension should be considered for this patient?

All of them should be considered. Hyperaldosteronism is relatively common, and it is not always accompanied by hypokalemia. Sleep apnea is usually missed for the simple reason that clinicians forget to think about it. Alcohol abuse is unlikely in this patient, but even upstanding citizens have been known to underreport their intake. The patient's severe headache would encourage the consideration of a space-occupying brain lesion, but the rapid pulse argues against it. Endocrine disorders, including Cushing syndrome, are always possible. Hyperthyroidism is particularly common, and this patient has an elevated pulse rate, but her diastolic pressure is uncharacteristically high. Drug toxicity is a reasonable possibility, and the patient may have taken a nasal decongestant and forgotten to mention it, because it is not usually considered a drug by many laypeople. In brief, this patient could be affected by many diagnostic possibilities that only further tests can rule out. Playing the odds, one would guess that the patient has sinusitis, labile blood pressure, and an early pregnancy that needs careful observation.

Suggested Readings

Chiong JR, Aronow WS, Khan IA, et al: Secondary hypertension: Current diagnosis and treatment. *Int J Cardiol* 124:6–21, 2008.

Rossi GP, Seccia TM, Pessina AC: Clinical use of laboratory tests for the identification of secondary forms of arterial hypertension. *Crit Rev Clin Lab Sci* 44(1):1–85, 2007.

Krane NK, Hamrahian M: Pregnancy: Kidney diseases and hypertension. *Am J Kidney Dis* 49(2):336–345, 2007.

PRACTICE QUESTIONS

1. In a patient with bilateral renal artery stenosis, drugs that inhibit ACE inhibitors or that block angiotensin receptors can have a negative impact on renal function. Which renal function can be made worse?

   A. The ability to secrete renin
   B. The ability to concentrate urine
   C. Glucose-reabsorbing ability
   D. Glomerular filtration

2. Which of the following clinical signs or symptoms is not seen in patients with primary hyperaldosteronism?

   A. Edema of the ankles
   B. Weakness of the muscles
   C. Systolic blood pressure of more than
      180 mm Hg
   D. Muscle cramps

3. The initial physical examination of a hypertensive patient includes maneuvers that are designed to evaluate target-organ damage resulting from elevated pressure and to search for possible causes of primary hypertension. Which of the following is most likely to detect abnormalities that suggest a remediable cause of hypertension?

   A. Auscultation of the carotid and femoral arteries
   B. Auscultation of the heart and lungs
   C. Auscultation of the abdomen
   D. Palpation of the abdominal aorta

4. A physician is practicing in a third world region with no radiology or nuclear medicine support and a laboratory that can only measure blood counts, electrolytes, and simple blood chemistries. A young patient with hypertension who has no family history of hypertension presents to the clinic. Which of the following tests would the physician request to investigate the possibility that the patient has primary aldosteronism?

   A. Serum sodium concentration
   B. Serum and 24-hour urine potassium
   C. 24-hour urine sodium and creatinine
   D. Urine sodium concentration and pH

Chapter 1

1-1. Answer: C. This patient's estimated creatinine clearance, with the use of the Cockcroft–Gault equation, is as follows:

$$\frac{(140-age)(weight)}{72\,(serum\,creatine)} \rightarrow \frac{(140-50)(80)}{72(0.9)} = 111\,ml/min$$

1-2. Answer: D. Erythropoietin is a hormone produced by the kidney that stimulates the production of erythrocytes in the bone marrow. 1,25-Dihydroxyvitamin D_3 is a hormone that is activated by the kidney and that contributes to the body's calcium balance by increasing calcium uptake in the gastrointestinal tract. Renin is a hormone produced by the kidney in response to volume depletion, which then catalyzes the conversion of angiotensinogen produced by the liver to angiotensin I. Angiotensin I is then converted to angiotensin II by angiotensin-converting enzymes. Angiotensin II is a vasoconstrictor that increases sodium absorption by the kidney.

1-3. Answer: A. The blood flow through the glomerulus is kept constant by autoregulation and tubuloglomerular feedback. This is the result of a myogenic mechanism that varies the afferent arteriolar tone and the tubuloglomerular feedback. Tubuloglomerular feedback is the process by which the juxtaglomerular apparatus senses the concentration of sodium chloride in the tubular fluid and then regulates the renal blood flow (i.e., by decreasing pressure in the glomerulus if the sodium chloride concentration is high and by increasing it if the concentration is low).

Chapter 2

2-1. Answer, Part A: C. This patient has continued to lose water through the urine and the skin. The amount of water in his feeding has been inadequate to maintain the losses. Because of his stroke, he has been unable to increase his water intake in response to thirst. He needs an increase in the amount of water in the nasogastric feedings or an intravenous infusion of 5% dextrose in water.

Answer, Part B: A. This patient has lost blood from the vascular space. An isotonic fluid such as 0.9% (normal) saline is needed to maintain the extracellular volume while the patient waits for his blood transfusion.

Answer, Part C: ✗ This patient has lost hypotonic sweat (mostly water, but some sodium chloride). ~~Thus, he needs to receive a hypotonic fluid such as 0.45% (half-normal) saline.~~ Because his blood pressure is low, normal saline can be infused at first until his blood pressure normalizes, and then the water that has been lost through sweating can be replaced by 5% dextrose in water.

2-2. Answer, Part A: Increased. Given that osmolality equilibrates among the different body fluid compartments by the free movement of water across the cell membrane, a low serum sodium suggests a low osmolality in the intracellular fluid volume as well as an increase in the intracellular fluid volume.

Answer, Part B: Increased. Edema and an increase in the central venous pressure imply an increased extracellular fluid volume.

Answer, Part C: Increased. Edema is evidence of increased interstitial fluid volume.

Answer, Part D: Increased. This patient has expanded extracellular fluid volume in which resides all of the sodium in the body.

Chapter 3

3-1. Answer: C. Water losses exceed sodium losses. Therefore, hypernatremia is likely to develop.

3-2. Answer: D. The athlete has lost hypotonic sweat and thus his or her plasma osmolality is increased. Osmoreceptors detect this increase in plasma osmolality and stimulate antidiuretic hormone release from the posterior pituitary.

3-3. Answer: D. Assuming that the athlete has normal pituitary and kidney function, as the antidiuretic hormone secretion is increased, the urine osmolality will be higher than that of the plasma. This is the result of the antidiuretic-hormone–mediated retention of water by the kidneys, which in turn leads to increased solute concentrations in the urine.

3-4. Answer: D. Edema in both legs and ascites suggest extracellular fluid volume excess in this patient with cirrhosis of the liver. However, the

effective extracellular fluid volume is decreased in the patient with cirrhosis as a result of vaso-dilatation. This stimulates the baroreceptor-mediated antidiuretic hormone release, water retention with hyponatremia, and decreased water excretion.

3-5.   Answer: D. Although the low serum osmolal-ity leads to the inhibition of antidiuretic hormone release, the decreased effective extracellular fluid volume will overcome this inhibition and stimulate the antidiuretic hor-mone release through the baroreceptor. This patient's serum antidiuretic hormone level is most likely high.

3-6.   Answer: B. Decreased perfusion to the kidneys has led to the retention of sodium and the development of edema as well as to an increase in the level of serum creatinine.

Chapter 4
4-1.   Answer: B. Edema is a sign of excess salt (volume) accumulation. Because the cell wall membrane is freely permeable to water but not to salt, the excess salt builds up extracel-lularly. Within the extracellular space, volume distributes between the intravascular (where in excess it can result in elevated blood pres-sure) and interstitial (where it can manifest as edema) spaces.

4-2.   Answer: C. Loop diuretics, which act on the $Na^+/K^+/2Cl^-$ transporter in the ascending limb of the loop of Henle, are among the most powerful diuretics, and they are gener-ally used as the first-line agent for the treat-ment of edema. Of course, in reality the phy-sician is not limited to just a single agent when treating a patient such as the one de-scribed, and a combination of diuretics may be chosen for treatment (e.g., a thiazide di-uretic to block more distal reabsorption in addition to the loop diuretic).

Chapter 5
5-1.   Answer: B. Extremely low urine chloride (<10 mmol/L) with a relatively high urine potassium concentration (44 mmol/L) strongly suggests vomiting as the cause of potassium depletion. The mechanism of hypokalemia from vomiting is not so much from the loss of potassium in the gastric juice but rather from the kidney loss of potassium as a result of the development of metabolic alkalosis (serum bicarbonate

38 mmol/L), which increases kidney tubular potassium secretion directly and also indi-rectly from the distal delivery of poorly reabsorbable anion bicarbonate and the stimulation of aldosterone by extracellular fluid volume contraction.

5-2.   Answer: D. This patient has type 1 diabetes mellitus with evidence of diabetic ketoacido-sis. Increased kidney loss of potassium is in-dicated by a high urine potassium level at 53 mmol/L. This is caused by glycosuria (osmotic diuresis), ketonuria (poorly reab-sorbable anions), and volume contraction as a result of high urine sodium loss (stimula-tion of aldosterone). Poor intake of potas-sium from nausea and vomiting also adds to the potassium depletion. However, intracellu-lar fluid potassium depletion is masked by the outward shift of potassium from the cells to raise the extracellular fluid potassium level as a result of severe hyperglycemia (hyperos-molality) and metabolic acidosis. Hemocon-centration by dehydration usually causes only a minimal increase in serum potassium.

5-3.   Answer: C. Hyperkalemia in this case is caused by acute kidney injury (the reduced tubular secretion of potassium as a result of kidney failure and low urine output), meta-bolic acidosis (a shift of potassium out of the cells), and the potassium-retaining effect of an angiotensin-converting enzyme inhibitor (the inhibition of aldosterone-mediated kidney tubular potassium secretion). Increased aldo-sterone will promote the kidney loss of potas-sium; it does not contribute to hyperkalemia.

Chapter 6
6-1.   Answer: D. Although the kidneys work in par-allel with the lungs to regulate the acid–base balance, the mechanisms of acid–base han-dling by the kidneys do not depend on how well the lungs function.

6-2.   Answer: D. If acidemia is present, the kidneys must get rid of the extra acid on board. They do this by increasing ammoniagenesis and titratable acid formation.

6-3.   Answer: D. Please refer to Box 6-2.

Chapter 7
7-1.   Answer: A. The patient likely developed nor-mal anion gap metabolic acidosis as a result of lithium therapy.

7-2. **Answer: A.** Lithium therapy can induce a type I distal hypokalemic renal tubular acidosis.

7-3. **Answer: A.** In distal hypokalemic renal tubular acidosis, the urine pH is always more than 5.6 and typically more than 6.0.

Chapter 8

8-1. **Answer: B.** This history and presentation are consistent with thin basement membrane nephropathy. This condition often has a very benign course, presenting primarily with hematuria. However, it is closely related to Alport syndrome; they both arise from the same genetic abnormality, which is a mutation in the α_5 type IV collagen gene. This condition has a more severe course that features cochlear nerve deafness and lens dislocations and cataracts. Crescentic proliferation in the glomeruli can occur particularly in antiglomerular basement membrane disease, which is characterized by hematuria that rapidly progresses to renal failure and that is associated with antibodies against the α_3 type IV collagen. Evidence of schistocytes in the peripheral blood smears is found in patients with the hemolytic–uremic syndrome, which frequently has thrombocytopenia associated with it. Effacement of the podocytes from the glomerular basement membrane is found primarily in minimal change disease, and, although it also has a benign clinical course, it is associated with a nephrotic picture.

8-2. **Answer: D.** Diffuse effacement of the foot processes of glomerular podocytes is seen in patients with minimal change nephrotic syndrome. The other answer options are all characteristic findings of poststreptococcal glomerulonephritis.

8-3. **Answer: A.** The histologic findings are consistent with diabetic nephropathy, which fits the scenario of the man with uncontrolled diabetes who leaks small amounts of albumin into his urine. The scenario presented in option B is more consistent with Wegener's granulomatosis (a subset of antineutrophil-cytoplasmic-antibody–positive systemic vasculitis); the patient described in option C reflects a case of thrombotic thrombocytopenic purpura; and the patient in option D has symptoms that are consistent with minimal change nephrotic syndrome.

Chapter 9

9-1. **Answer: C.** These children could be given this information when they reach the age of 30 years.

9-2. **Answer: C.** Alport syndrome famously involves the triad of renal failure, hearing loss, and vision problems, all of which are caused by a defect in type IV collagen. Thin basement membrane nephropathy (option A) also presents with hematuria, but this is typically the sole symptom. Autosomal dominant polycystic kidney disease (option D) often has hematuria as a feature, but it typically presents with other renal and extrarenal symptoms as well as hypertension, urinary tract infection, and massively enlarged kidneys; hearing loss is not a feature of this condition. von Hippel–Lindau syndrome (option B) is also associated with a famous triad: hemangioblastomas, pheochromocytomas, and visceral cysts. However, hearing loss and hematuria are not features of this syndrome.

Chapter 10

10-1. **Answer: D.** A dipstick test showing 4+ proteinuria suggests a nephrotic range of proteinuria with more than 3.5 g of protein per 1 g of creatinine on quantitative testing. This patient is likely to have a disorder of the glomerulus rather than of the renal tubule.

10-2. **Answer: B.** In an older patient with anemia, back pain, elevated serum creatinine, and fracture, the physician must suspect multiple myeloma, a malignancy of the plasma cells with the production of light chains. Urine light chains do not test positive on a dipstick as this is specific for albumin. Other methods of urine testing for the presence of light chains as implied by options A, C, and D must be used to diagnose multiple myeloma and the urinary excretion of light chains. Urine testing for microalbuminuria is diagnostic of kidney disease in a patient with diabetic nephropathy.

10-3. **Answer: B.** Red blood cell casts in the urine sediment suggest glomerular disease as a cause of this patient's hematuria. White blood cells in the urine sediment indicate urinary infection; eosinophils are seen in the urine sediment in patients with acute interstitial nephritis; and uric acid crystals are noted in a patient with gout or uric acid calculi with high urinary uric acid concentration.

Chapter 11

11-1. Answer: A. This patient's recent increase in creatinine indicates that this is an acute process. Clues that point to interstitial nephritis include the fact that the patient is taking antibiotics. He has a diffuse skin rash and the urinalysis shows 1+ protein, white blood cells, and white blood cell casts, which are diagnostic of acute interstitial nephritis. Special stains of the urine sediment to demonstrate eosinophils will be helpful, and a urine culture to exclude urinary infection is essential. A urinalysis in a patient with acute tubular necrosis would likely show proteinuria with renal tubular cells and casts and/or muddy brown casts.

11-2. Answer: D. This patient has not been able to urinate for a day. This acute urinary retention is likely caused by the diphenhydramine, with the contributing factor of the patient's benign prostatic hyperplasia. The insertion of a Foley catheter returns a significant amount of urine, which would point to a postrenal cause of the acute kidney injury (the normal postvoid residual is <100 ml). Postrenal kidney injury may be the result of bilateral ureteral obstruction (e.g., cervical carcinoma compressing the ureters, stones or a clot blocking the ureters), bladder obstruction (e.g., structural diseases such as carcinoma of the bladder, functional disorders after the use of anticholinergic medications), or urethral obstruction (e.g., benign prostatic hypertrophy, prostate cancer).

Chapter 12

12-1. Answer: B. The patient has nephrotic syndrome, likely as a result of diabetic nephropathy. She has a long history of diabetes and hypertension, and she has diabetic retinopathy. Her estimated glomerular filtration rate is 112 ml/min, which places her in stage 1 chronic kidney disease.

12-2. Answer: A. Elevated blood pressure of more than 125/75 mm Hg, poor diabetes control with a glycosylated hemoglobin value of more than 7.0%, and significant proteinuria are all likely to increase the progression of chronic kidney disease in this patient. Male and female patients with chronic kidney disease and these other findings have no differences in outcome.

12-3. Answer: C. The progression of chronic kidney disease is increased by all of the listed factors except for decreased glomerular hydrostatic pressure. Actually, it is the increased glomerular hydrostatic pressure (called *glomerular hypertension*) in the remaining nephrons in the patient with chronic kidney disease that leads to worsening kidney function.

Chapter 13

13-1. Answer: D. Hemodialysis is effective for the removal of small-sized solutes such as urea and potassium. The exact nature of the uremic toxins is unknown. However, pericarditis that is noted in patients with kidney failure resolves with the initiation of dialysis and the amelioration of uremia. Phosphorous removal by dialysis is very limited, and patients on dialysis continue to require oral phosphate binders with food to limit the gastrointestinal absorption of phosphorous.

13-2. Answer: A. This patient has expanded extracellular fluid volume with increasing dyspnea. This is also confirmed by the increase in weight, the jugular venous pressure, the edema, and the rales in the chest. He is also likely to have increased total body water as shown by hyponatremia, although the acidosis (i.e., low serum bicarbonate) has caused a shift of potassium from the cells to the extracellular fluid, and this may have increased the serum potassium level. However, because this patient has minimal kidney function as well as a need for dialysis, his total body potassium is likely to be increased.

Chapter 14

14-1. Answer: D. Acute rejection could be caused by cellular rejection, in which the primary target of injury is the tubulointerstitial compartment of the kidney. In some cases, when rejection is severe, the vessels are also affected. In antibody-mediated rejection, the main target of injury is the vascular endothelium. In this process, the classic finding is the presence of C4d in the peritubular capillaries, which indicates the activation of the complement system by antihuman leukocyte antigens antibodies. An inflammatory infiltrate composed of mononuclear cells is often observed invading the tubules and the interstitial space. Glomerular damage is not a feature of acute rejection.

14-2. Answer: A and D. As stated in the chapter, the immediate nonspecific inflammatory response is elicited by the procurement, preservation, and storage of the organ (i.e., cold

ischemia). This phase is primarily ischemic in nature, and its pathophysiology is very similar to that of acute tubular necrosis. The initial response is closely related to the surgical procedure and to changes with reperfusion. Option D is also correct. The initial presentation is similar to that of acute tubular necrosis. The patient may present with oliguria, and the fractional excretion of sodium will be high. Option B is incorrect because warm ischemic injury becomes irreversible after 30 minutes. Option C is also incorrect. Although the initial response is closely related to the surgical procedure, the acute immunologic response is generated against the human leukocyte antigens that are expressed on the donor organ.

14-3. Answer: A and D. A haploidentical sibling may occur in 50% of cohorts. D is correct. Immunosuppression is required for haploidentical transplantation; the only patients who do not require immunosuppression are identical twins. B is incorrect. Haploidentical siblings share either maternal or paternal haplotypes, not both; major histocompatibility complex identical siblings share both haplotypes. C is incorrect; see the previous explanation.

Chapter 15

15-1. Answer: C. This question should really be a cause for reflection. Although there is a gender difference with regard to hypertension, it is not uncommon for either sex to develop hypertension. In addition, after menopause, the playing field is leveled, and hypertension is equally prevalent in men and women. African Americans tend to have more hypertension than other races, but hypertension is not uncommon in any race. Occupation has been weakly correlated with hypertension, but the connection is not strong enough to arouse clinical suspicion. The age at onset is critical for determining whether to search for a curable cause. People who present with hypertension when they are less than 25 years old or more than 50 years old warrant a closer look.

15-2. Answer: A. In chronic hypertension, the left ventricle is forced to pump blood into a high-pressure system, thereby causing the myocardium to thicken without enlargement of the ventricular chamber. Concentric left ventricular hypertrophy is the classic change in the hypertensive heart. Chest x-ray is often normal; therefore, echocardiography is often used to make the diagnosis. Microscopically, capillary density increases with the demand for oxygen as hypertrophy worsens. The number of cells does not change; rather, the cells themselves thicken and change.

15-3. Answer: C. Angiotensin-converting enzyme inhibitors reduce the production of angiotensin II. By lowering levels of angiotensin II, which is a stimulus to aldosterone release, they lower aldosterone as well. All of the other drugs listed stimulate the release of renin and the production of angiotensin II and aldosterone, largely as compensatory responses of the body to a perceived drop in the pressure of the intravascular volume. Pressure may fall with all of the other manipulations, but that pressure drop is blunted by the release of angiotensin II and aldosterone.

Chapter 16

16-1. Answer: D. Angiotensin-converting enzyme inhibitors and angiotensin receptor blockers are contraindicated in bilateral stenosis, because they block the angiotensin-mediated efferent glomerular arteriolar vasoconstriction that maintains glomerular filtration. If both kidneys are using the renin–angiotensin–aldosterone system to compensate for their stenoses, then the total renal function will be compromised by drugs that block it.

16-2. Answer: A. Clinical features of primary hyperaldosteronism include potentially severe hypertension as well as weakness and muscle cramps (both as a result of the loss of potassium). Surprisingly, there is no edema in primary hyperaldosteronism. Despite the presence of net fluid retention, there is no leakage of fluid into the tissue spaces. Do not confuse this with diseases such as cirrhosis of the liver and congestive heart failure in which the primary disease causes both edema and reduced effective perfusion of the kidneys, accompanied by renin release.

16-3. Answer: C. In 40% of patients with renal artery stenosis, auscultation of the abdominal midline just inferior to the xiphisternum will reveal bruits of the renal arteries that are audible during both systole and diastole.

16-4. **Answer: B.** A high aldosterone state would force the kidney to excrete potassium in the urine in exchange for sodium, thereby resulting in a high urine potassium level and causing a low serum potassium level. This scenario is also frequently seen with thiazide and loop diuretic use in which potassium is "wasted" in the urine. Some patients with low serum potassium are eating very little potassium, but they would excrete very little potassium in their urine.

Some Common Laboratory Tests and Their Normal Values as Reported by the Clinical Laboratory at the University of Wisconsin Hospital and Clinics

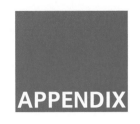

APPENDIX

BLOOD TESTS

Test	Normal values
Blood urea nitrogen	7–20 mg/dl
Serum creatinine	0.6–1.3 mg/dl
Serum calcium	8.5–10.2 mg/dl
Serum inorganic phosphate	2.5–4.5 mg/dl
Serum magnesium	1.7–2.3 mg/dl
Blood glucose	70–99 mg/dl
HbA1c	4.3–6.0%
Complete blood count	
Hemoglobin	Men: 13.6–17.2 g/dl Women: 11.6–15.6 g/dl
Hematocrit	Men: 40%–52% Women: 34%–46%
White blood cell count	3.8–10.5 K/µl
Platelet count	160–370 K/µl
Serum electrolytes	
Sodium	135–140 mmol/L
Potassium	3.8–4.8 mmol/L
Chloride	97–106 mmol/L
Carbon dioxide	22–32 mmol/L

Test	Normal values
Blood gases (arterial)	
pH	7.36–7.44
Partial pressure of oxygen	80–90 mm Hg
Partial pressure of carbon dioxide	34–46 mm Hg
Base excess	−2.5–+ 2.4 mmol/L
Actual bicarbonate	22–26 mmol/L
Serum lipids (after an overnight fast)	
Serum total cholesterol	Desired: <200 mg/dl
Serum triglycerides	Desired: <150 mg/dl
Serum high-density cholesterol	Low: <40 mg/dl High: >60 mg/dl
Serum low-density cholesterol	Optimal: 100–129 mg/dl
Miscellaneous blood tests	
Serum iron	50–160 µg/dl
Serum total iron binding capacity	250–450 µg/dl
Serum iron saturation	16–50%
Serum ferritin	20–300 ng/ml
Serum intact parathyroid hormone	15–65 pg/ml
Serum 25-hydroxyvitamin D_3	30–80 mg/ml

Serum albumin 3.4 - 5.4 g/dL

URINE TESTS

Test	Normal values
Urinalysis	
Specific gravity	1.005–1.030
pH	5.0–7.5
Protein	Negative to trace
Glucose	Negative
Ketones	Negative
Hemastix	Negative
Bilirubin	Negative
Leukocyte esterase	Negative
Nitrite	Negative
Urobilinogen	0.1–1.0 mg/dl
Urine microscopy	
White blood cells	0–5/hpf
Red blood cells	0–2/hpf
Epithelial cells	0–2 squamous cells/hpf
Crystals	Few calcium oxalate crystals
Casts	0–4 hyaline casts/hpf

hpf, *high power field.*

Index

A

AA amyloidosis, 97
Accelerated hypertension, 181, 188
ACE inhibitors, 12
Acid-base disorders, 83–85
  approach to, 83–85
  arterial blood gases, 83
  history and physical examination of, 83
  plasma electrolytes, 84
  stepwise approach to, 84–85
Acid-base homeostasis, 63–69
  acids/bases, 64, 64t
  bicarbonate reabsorption, 65–66
  Henderson-Hasselbalch equation, 64–65
  renal hydrogen excretion, 67–69
    aldosterone and, 68
    effective circulating volume, 67–68
    plasma pH, 67
    plasma potassium concentration, 68–69
  role of kidney, 65–66
  titratable acid formation, 66
  urinary ammonium formation, 66
Acidemia, 64f
Acute interstitial nephritis, 137–138
Acute kidney injury (AKI), 131–143
  acute interstitial nephritis, 137–138
  categories of, 132–133
  clinical history, 138
  definitions, 132
  diagnosis of, 138–139
  glomerulonephritis, 138
  incidence, 132
  intrinsic kidney disease, 132–133
  ischemic ATN, 133–136
  laboratory and radiologic testing, 139
  mortality/recovery, 140
  physical examination, 138–139
  postrenal disease, 132
  prerenal disease, 132
  toxic ATN, 136–137
  treatment, 140
Acute tubular necrosis (ATN), 123, 133–137
Addison's disease, 58
Adenoma sebaceum, 116
ADH. See Antidiuretic hormone
ADPKD. See Autosomal dominant polycystic kidney disease
Adynamic bone disease, 151
Afferent arteriole, 3
AGMA. See Anion gap metabolic acidosis
AKI. See Acute kidney injury
AL amyloidosis, 97
Alcohol, 207

Aldosterone, 45, 51, 68
  sodium dependent factors and, 68
  sodium independent factors and, 68
Aldosterone escape, 45
Aldosteronism, 204–205
Alkalemia, 64f
Allogeneic graft, 170b
Allograft, 170b
  rejection of, 173t
α-Actinin, 4
Alport syndrome, 4b, 100
Amiloride, 44
Amyloidosis, 97
Anatomy, 1–6
  glomerulus, 2–5
  kidney tubule, 2, 5–6
  nephron, 2
  vascular system, 2
ANCA. See Antineutrophil cytoplasmic antibody
Angiomyolipomas, 116
Angiotensin II, 11–12, 45, 73
Anion gap, 79–80
Anion gap metabolic acidosis (AGMA), 80–82
  AKI or CKD, 81–82
  ketoacidosis, 81
  high acid output, 80
  low acid output, 80
  lactic acidosis, 81
ANP. See Atrial natriuretic peptide
Antidiuretic hormone (ADH), 10–12, 30–32, 35b, 37–38
Anti-GBM disease. See Antiglomerular basement membrane disease
Antiglomerular basement membrane disease (Anti-GBM disease), 99
Antineutrophil cytoplasmic antibody (ANCA), 103–104
Anuria, 30b, 132
Arginine vasopressin (AVP), 45
ARPKD. See Autosomal recessive polycystic kidney disease
Arterial blood gas values, 84f
Arteriography, 199
Ascending loop of Henle, 8–9, 11b
Asymptomatic glomerulonephritis, 90–91
ATN. See Acute tubular necrosis
Atrial natriuretic peptide (ANP), 11, 45
Autologous graft, 170b
Autoregulation, 6, 6b, 44
Autosomal dominant polycystic kidney disease (ADPKD), 110–114
Autosomal recessive polycystic kidney disease (ARPKD), 114–115
AVP. See Arginine vasopressin
Azotemia, 132

B

Barostat, 183–185
Bartter syndrome, 53, 71
Benign familial hematuria, 100.
  See also Thin basement membrane nephropathy
Berger disease, 98. See also Immuno-globulin A nephropathy
Berry aneurysms, 186
Body fluid compartments, 17–25
  additions to compartments, 22–23
  body fluid regulation, 18–20
  losing fluid from body compartments, 21
  monitoring body fluid status, 20–21
  shifts from one compartment to another, 24
  Starling relationship, 19–20
Body fluid regulation, 18–20
Bone disease, 150–151
Borderline hypertension, 180
Bowman's capsule, 2–3, 3b
Bowman's space, 3–6, 3b
Bright's disease, 147b

C

C-ANCA. See Cytoplasmic antineutrophil cytoplasmic antibody
Calcitriol, 12
Capacitance arteries, 181
Carbonic anhydrase inhibitors, 43f, 44
Cardiac output, 32
Casts, 123, 124f, 124t
Cell lysis, 22
Central diabetes insipidus, 33, 37–38
Central venous pressure, 21
Charcot-Bouchard aneurysm, 189
Chronic allograft nephropathy, 174
Chronic kidney disease (CKD), 145–157
  altered excretory function, 149–150
  bone disease, 150–151
  cardiovascular consequences, 152–153
  defined, 145
  GFR, 146–147
  glomerular hypertension, 147–148
  hematologic consequences, 151–152
  history of, 147b
  incidence, 145–146
  neurologic consequences, 153
  other organ systems affected, 153–154
  pathophysiology of progression, 147–148
  signs/symptoms, 148–154
  slowing the progression of, 148
  stages of, 14b
  treatment, 154, 154b

Churg-Strauss syndrome, 103
CKD. *See* Chronic kidney disease (CKD)
Coarctation of the aorta, 203–204
Cocaine, 207
Cockcroft-Gault equation, 13, 13b, 146
Collapsing glomerulopathy, 96
Collecting duct, 9–11, 11b, 43
    cortical, 11b
    medullary, 11b
Concentration gradient, 161
Congenital nephrotic syndrome of the
    Finnish type, 4b
Continuous ambulatory peritoneal
    dialysis, 164
Continuous cycling peritoneal
    dialysis, 164
Continuous renal replacement therapy
    (CRRT), 161
Contraction alkalosis, 73
Convection, 161–162
Cor bovinum, 187
Cortical collecting duct, 11b
Creatinine clearance, 13
Crescents, 187
Crescentic GN, 138
CRRT. *See* Continuous renal replacement
    therapy
Cushing syndrome, 207
Cyclosporine, 207–208
Cystatin C, 14
Cystic diseases, 109–119
    ADPKD, 110–114
    ARPKD, 114–115
    hereditary polycystic kidney disease,
        110–115
    MCKD, 116
    miscellaneous hereditary, 116
    MSK, 116
    NPH, 115
    NPH-MCKD of the renal medulla,
        115–116
    TS, 116–117
    VHL, 117
Cytoplasmic antineutrophil cytoplasmic
    antibody (C-ANCA), 104

D
Dense deposit disease, 101
Descending loop of Henle, 8, 11b
Diabetes insipidus, 38
Diabetic glomerulosclerosis, 97
Diabetic nephropathy, 97. *See also*
    Diabetic glomerulosclerosis
Dialysate, 161–162
Dialysis, 159–167
    complications, 164
    convection, 161
    diffusion, 160–161
    hemodialysis, 162–163, 164
    historical overview, 159, 160b
    mortality, 165
    peritoneal dialysis, 163–164
        continuous ambulatory, 164
        continuous cycling, 164
    principles of, 160–161
    types of, 162–164
    ultrafiltration, 161
Dialyzer, 162
Diffusion, 160–161
Diluting segment of the nephron, 8

Dipstick urine testing, 121–122
Disorders of sodium metabolism,
    41–47
    diuretics, 44–45
    extracellular fluid compartment,
        45–46
    hypervolemia, 42
    hypovolemia, 42
    salt, 41
    sodium transport, 42–44
Disorders of water metabolism, 29–38
    assessment of patient, 32–33
    hypernatremia, 36–38
    hyponatremia, 33–36
    polyuria, 38
    water balance, 29–31
Distal convoluted tubule, 9–11, 11b, 43
Distal hyperkalemic RTA, 82, 83t
Distal hypokalemic RTA, 82, 83t
Distal sodium delivery, 53
Distal tubule diuretics, 43f, 44
Diuretics, 44–45
    carbonic anhydrase inhibitors,
        43f, 44
    loop, 43f, 44
    thiazide, 43f, 44
    potassium-sparing, 43f, 44
    osmotic, 43f, 44
Donor, 170b
Duplex sonography, 200
Duplex ultrasonography, 200
Dyslipidemic hypertension, 182
Dysmorphic erythrocytes, 123
Dyspnea, 42

E
ECF. *See* Extracellular fluid
Eclampsia, 203
Edema, 21, 42
    dependent, 42
    pulmonary, 42
Efferent arteriole, 3
Endocrine disorders, 208
Endocrine functions, 11–12
Ergotamine, 207
Erythropoietin, 12, 208
Essential hypertension, 179–195
    adult stage, 183
    arteries, effects on, 185–186
    brain, effects on, 188–189
    causes, 183–185
    combinations of antihypertensive
        therapies, 192–193
    common drug combinations, 192b
    death, 189
    definitions, 180
    drugs that block ANS, 191
    drugs that block RAAS, 190–191
    drugs that block vascular smooth
        muscle contraction, 191–192
    early stage, 183
    epidemiology, 181–182
    epidemiology of hypertensive
        sequelae, 182–183
    heart, effects on, 186–188
    hypotheses of causes, 184–185
    kidney, effects on, 188
    late stage, 183
    lifestyle changes, 189–190
    management of, 189–193

Essential hypertension (*Continued*)
    pathological consequences of,
        185–189
    retina, 189
    salt and water balance, 190
    stroke, 188–189
    subclassifications, 180–181
    TIAs, 189
Established hypertension, 180–181
Estrogen, 202
Extracellular fluid (ECF), 17–25, 30, 32
Extracellular fluid compartment, 45–46

F
Fanconi syndrome, 8, 82
Fibrinoid necrosis, 188
Fibrocystin, 114. *See also* Polyductin
Filtration barrier, 4
Fixed hypertension, 180–181
Fluid homeostasis, 17
Focal sclerosing glomerulopathy, 96
Focal segmental glomerulosclerosis, 96.
    See also Focal sclerosing glomeru-
    lopathy
Foot processes, 90

G
GBM. *See* Glomerular basement
    membrane
GFR. *See* Glomerular filtration rate
Gitelman syndrome, 53, 71
Glomerular basement membrane
    (GBM), 3–5
Glomerular capillary pressure, 147–148
Glomerular diseases, 89–107
    Alport syndrome, 100
    anti-GBM disease, 91b, 99
    antigens/antibodies, 93t
    asymptomatic glomerulonephritis,
        90–91
    chronic kidney disease, 91–92
    clinical findings, 90–93
    diabetic nephropathy, 97
    focal segmental glomerulosclerosis, 96
    glomerular physiology, 90
    immunoglobulin A nephropathy, 98
    laboratory studies, 92
    lupus nephritis, 100
    mechanisms of glomerular injury,
        93–94
    mechanisms of vascular injury, 102
    membranoproliferative glomerulone-
        phritis, 101
    membranous nephropathy, 95
    microscopic evaluation, 93
    minimal change nephrotic
        syndrome, 94
    mixed nephrotic/nephritic
        syndrome, 91
    nephritic syndrome, 91, 92b
    nephrotic syndrome, 91, 92b
    pathology, 94–102
        primary nephritic syndrome,
            98–100
        primary nephrotic syndrome,
            94–96
        secondary nephritic syndrome,
            100–102
        secondary nephrotic
            syndrome, 97

Glomerular diseases *(Continued)*
  physiology, 90
  poststreptococcal glomerulonephritis, 101–102
  renal amyloidosis, 97
  renal biopsy, 93
  systemic vasculitis, 102–104
  terminology, 90
  thin basement membrane nephropathy, 99–100
  TMAs, 104
  urinalysis, 92
Glomerular endothelium, 3
Glomerular epithelial cell, 3
Glomerular filtration, 6
Glomerular filtration barrier, 4, 6, 90, 90b
Glomerular filtration rate (GFR), 6, 12–14, 111, 146–147
Glomerular hypertension, 147–148
Glomerulonephritis, 132, 138
Glomerulus, 2–5, 3b
Glycosuria, 8, 122
Goodpasture antigen, 99
Goodpasture syndrome, 99, 126, 138
Guyton, Arthur, 184

H
Hematuria, 121–122, 126–127
Hemodialysis, 162–163, 164
  complications of, 164
Hemolytic uremic syndrome (HUS), 104, 126
Henderson-Hasselbalch equation, 64–65
Hereditary polycystic kidney disease, 110–115
High normal pressure, 180
Histocompatibility antigens, 172
Host, 170b
HLA. *See* Human leukocyte antigens
Human leukocyte antigens (HLA), 170, 172
HUS. *See* Hemolytic uremic syndrome
Hyperaldosteronism, 53
Hyaline casts, 123
Hypercalcemia, 71
Hyperchloremic metabolic acidosis, 57, 82
Hyperdynamic hypertension, 183
Hyperglycemia, 33
Hyperkalemia, 44, 56–58
Hyperkinetic hypertension, 183
Hyperosmotic, 17
Hypernatremia, 36–38
Hypertension. *See* Essential hypertension; Secondary hypertension
Hyperthyroidism, 208
Hypertriglyceridemia, 33
Hypervolemia, 42
Hypoalbuminemia, 91
Hypoaldosteronism, 56–57
Hypokalemia, 52–56, 73–74
  causes of, 53b
  consequences of, 54–55, 54b
  gastrointestinal loss of potassium and, 53
  kidney loss of potassium and, 53–54
  treatment of, 55–56, 55b
Hypoosmotic, 17
Hypotension, 42

Hyponatremia, 33–36
Hypothyroidism, 208
Hypovolemia, 36, 42

I
ICF. *See* Intercellular fluid
IgA nephropathy, 98
Immunoglobulin A nephropathy, 98
Insensible losses, 30
Intercellular fluid (ICF), 17–25
Interstitial fluid, 18
Interstitium, 133
Intravascular fluid, 18
Intravascular volume, 32
Intrinsic kidney disease, 132–133
Ischemic ATN, 133–136
Ischemic stroke, 189
Isograft, 170b
Isolated systolic hypertension, 181
Isomorphic RBCs, 122

K
Ketoacidosis, 81
Kidney ammonium excretion, 69f
Kidney bicarbonate reabsorption, 67f
Kidney failure, 56
Kidney scans, 200
Kidney titratable acidity function, 68f
Kidney transplant. *See* Transplantation
Kidney tubule, 2, 5–6
Kolff, Dr. Willem, 159

L
Labile hypertension, 180
Lactic acidosis, 81
Lisinopril, 12
Loop diuretics, 43f, 44
Loop of Henle, 5, 7–9, 43
  ascending, 8–9, 11b
  descending, 8, 11b
Looser zones, 151
Lupus nephritis, 100

M
Macula densa, 5
Major histocompatibility complex (MHC), 172
Malignant hypertension, 181
  kidney and, 188
Mannitol, 33, 38, 44
MCKD. *See* Medullary cystic kidney disease
MDRD formula. *See* Modification of diet in renal disease formula
Medullary collecting duct, 11b
Medullary cystic kidney disease (MCKD), 116
Medullary sponge kidney (MSK), 116
Membranoproliferative glomerulonephritis, 101
Membranous nephropathy, 95
Metabolic acidosis, 54, 79–83
  acute kidney injury, 81–82
  AGMA, 80–82
  anion gap, 79–80
  chronic kidney injury, 81–82
  diagnostic approach, 81f, 83
  differential diagnosis, 79–83
  ketoacidosis, 81
  lactic acidosis, 81

Metabolic acidosis *(Continued)*
  NAGMA, 82, 83t
  pathogenesis, 79
  treatment, 83
Metabolic alkalosis, 70–75
  alkali administration, 72–73
  chloride depletion, 73
  contraction alkalosis, 73
  diagnostic approach, 74
  diuretics, 71, 71f
  effective circulating volume depletion, 73
  gastrointestinal hydrogen loss, 71–72
  generation, 70–73
  hydrogen loss, 70–71
  hypokalemia, 73–74
  intracellular shift of hydrogen, 72
  maintenance, 73
  pathogenesis of, 70–74
  treatment approach, 74–75
Metabolic syndrome, 182
Metastatic calcification, 150
MHC. *See* Major histocompatibility complex
Microalbuminuria, 124–126
Microcytotoxicity, 174
Microscopic polyangiitis, 103
Milk-alkali syndrome, 71
Mineralocorticoid escape, 204
Minimal change nephrotic syndrome, 94
Mixed nephrotic/nephritic syndrome, 91
Modification of diet in renal disease (MDRD) formula, 13, 13b, 147
Monogenic hypertension, 182
Monomorphic RBCs, 122
MSK. *See* Medullary sponge kidney
Multiple lacunar infarcts, 189

N
NAE. *See* Net acid excretion
NAGMA. *See* Normal anion gap metabolic acidosis
Nephrin, 4
Nephritic syndrome, 91, 126–127
Nephrocystin-1, 115
Nephrogenic diabetes insipidus, 33, 37–38
Nephrogenic systemic fibrosis, 153
Nephron, 2
Nephronophthisis (NPH), 115
Nephrosclerosis, 188
Nephrotic syndrome, 91, 126
Net acid excretion (NAE), 65, 66
Normal anion gap metabolic acidosis (NAGMA), 82, 83t
  gastrointestinal causes of, 82, 83t
  kidney causes of, 82, 83t
Nonpharmacologic therapies, 189–190
NPH. *See* Nephronophthisis

O
Oliguria, 30b, 132
Oncotic pressure, 19–20
1,25-Dihydroxyvitamin D_3, 13
Onion skin, 185
Orthostasis, 42
Osler's sign, 185
Osmotic diuretics, 44
Osmotic pressure, 18
Osteitis fibrosa cystica, 150

P

P-ANCA, 104
Paraproteinemia, 33
Parietal epithelium, 3
Pauci-immune crescentic glomerulone-
     phritis, 103
Percutaneous transluminal renal
     angioplasty, 201
Peritoneal dialysis, 163–164
     complications of, 164
     continuous ambulatory, 164
     continuous cycling, 164
Pheochromocytoma, 206
PKD1, 110–111
PKD2, 111
PKHD1. *See* Polycystic kidney and
     hepatic disease 1
Plasma osmolality, 19, 32
Plasma solute concentration, 21
Podocin, 4
Podocyte, 3–4, 3b
Polycystic kidney and hepatic disease 1
     (PKHD1), 114
Polycystin-1, 111
Polycystin-2, 111
Polyductin, 114
Polyuria, 30b, 38
Posthypercapnic alkalosis, 71
Postrenal disease, 132
Poststreptococcal glomerulonephritis,
     101–102
Potassium
     balance of, 52
     body handling of, 51b
     gastrointestinal loss of, 53
     intake of, 50
     kidney handling of, 51–52, 51b
     kidney loss of, 53–54
     metabolism of, 49–52
Potassium balance, 52
Potassium metabolism, 49–61
     cellular uptake of potassium, 50
     excitability of neuromuscular tissues,
          50–51
     general measures, 58
     hyperkalemia, 56–58
     hypokalemia, 52–56
     kidney handling of potassium,
          51–52
     physiology, 49–52
     potassium balance, 52
     potassium intake, 50
     tubular secretion of potassium and,
          51b, 52
Potassium-sparing diuretics,
     43f, 44
Preeclampsia, 202–203
Prehypertension, 180
Prerenal disease, 132
Pressure gradient, 161
Pressure natriuresis, 184
Primary hyperaldosteronism, 204
Primary hypertension, 180. *See also*
     Essential hypertension
Protein AA, 97
Proteinuria, 122, 126
Proximal RTA, 82, 83t
Proximal tubule, 7–8, 11b, 43
Pseudohyponatremia, 34
Psychogenic polydipsia, 38

R

Rapidly progressive glomerulonephritis,
     99, 126, 138
RECAPS ABCDE, 198b
Recipient, 170b
Renal amyloidosis, 97
Renal artery stenosis, 198–201
Renin, 11
Renin-angiotensin-aldosterone system,
     11–12, 45
Renograms, 200
Resting membrane potential, 50

S

Salt, 41. *See also* Disorders of sodium
     metabolism
Scintirenography, 200
Secondary hyperaldosteronism, 73
Secondary hyperparathyroidism, 150
Secondary hypertension, 197–211
     alcohol, 207
     aldosteronism, 204–205
     brain injury, 207
     causes of, 198
     coarctation of the aorta, 203–204
     Cushing syndrome, 207
     drugs, 207–208
     eclampsia, 203
     endocrine disorders, 208
     estrogen, 202
     kidney disease, 198–202
     pheochromocytoma, 206
     preeclampsia, 202–203
     RECAPS ABCDE, 198b
     renal artery stenosis, 198–201
     sleep apnea, 206–207
Second hit, 111
Semipermeable membrane, 160–161
Serum osmolality, 22b
SLE. *See* Systemic lupus erythematosus
Sleep apnea, 206–207
Slit diaphragm, 3
Sodium escape, 45–46
Sodium metabolism. *See* Disorders of
     sodium metabolism
Sodium/potassium (Na^+/K^+)-ATPase,
     44–45
Sodium/potassium/2 chloride $(Na^+/$
     $K^+/2\ Cl^-)$ cotransporter, 44
Solutes, 18–19, 160
Specific gravity, 33
Spironolactone, 44
Starling forces, 6, 21, 24
Starling-Landis equation, 20, 20f
Starling relationship, 19–20
Steady-state condition, 18–19
Stroke, 188–189
Sustained hypertension, 180–181
Syndrome of inappropriate ADH, 38
Syndrome X, 182
Syngeneic graft, 170b
Systemic lupus erythematosus (SLE), 100
Systemic vasculitis, 102–104

T

TBW. *See* Total body water
Thiazide diuretics, 44
Thin basement membrane nephropathy,
     99–100
Threshold potential, 50

Thrombotic microangiopathies (TMAs),
     104, 126
Thrombotic stroke, 189
Thrombotic thrombocytopenic purpura
     (TTP), 104, 127
TIA. *See* Transient ischemic attack
Titratable acidity, 7
TMA. *See* Thrombotic microangiopathies
Total body water (TBW), 17–18
Toxic ATN, 136–137
Transient ischemic attack (TIA), 189
Transplantation, of kidney, 169–177
     acute antigen-specific responses, 171
     acute rejection, 172, 173t
     chronic rejection, 172–174
     cross-matching, 174
     histocompatibility antigens, 172
     hyperacute rejection, 172, 173t
     immediate nonspecific inflammation,
          169–171
     immunosuppression, 174, 175t
     ischemia and, 170–171
     pathophysiology, 170–172
     phases of response, 170t
     recurrence of kidney disease in
          transplant, 174–176
     surgical complications, 171
     terminology, 170b
     tissue typing, 174
Triamterene, 44
Triple phosphate, 123
TS. *See* Tuberous sclerosis
TTP. *See* Thrombotic thrombocytopenic
     purpura
Tuberous sclerosis (TS), 116–117
Tubular transport processes, 6–11
     collecting duct, 9–11
     distal convoluted tubule, 9
     loop of Henle, 8–9
     proximal tubule, 7–8
Tubuloglomerular feedback, 6, 44.
     See also Autoregulation
Type I RTA, 82, 83t
Type II RTA, 82, 83t
Type IV RTA, 82, 83t

U

Ultrafiltration, 161
Ultrasonography, 200
Urea reduction ratio (URR), 163
Uremia, 19, 132, 148
Urinalysis, 121–129
     dipstick urine testing, 121–122
     microscopic analysis, 122–123
     microalbuminuria, 124–126
     nephritic syndrome, 126–127
     nephrotic syndrome, 126
     quantification of urinary protein,
          123–124
     syndromes, 126–127
     urine sediment, 122–123
Urinary glucose, 122
Urine crystals, 123, 125f, 125t
Urine osmolality, 32–33
Urine sediment, 122–123
     casts, 123, 124t, 124f
     crystals, 123, 125f, 125t
     fat globules, 123
     malignant cells, 123
     RBCs, 122

Urine sediment *(Continued)*
 renal tubular epithelial cells, 123
 WBCs, 123
URR. *See* Urea reduction ratio

V
Vasa recta, 2
Vascular system, 2
Vasopressin, 10

VHL. *See* von Hippel-Lindau syndrome
Visceral epithelial cells, 3
von Hippel-Lindau (VHL) syndrome, 117

W
Water balance, 29–31
Water deprivation test, 33
Water input, 29

Water metabolism. *See* Disorders of
 water metabolism
Water output, 29
Wegener's granulomatosis,
 103–104

X
Xenogeneic graft, 170b
Xenograft, 170b